Nutrition and Growth of Preterm Neonates during Hospitalization: Impact on Childhood Outcomes

Nutrition and Growth of Preterm Neonates during Hospitalization: Impact on Childhood Outcomes

Guest Editors

Antonios K. Gounaris
Rozeta Sokou

MDPI

Basel • Beijing • Wuhan • Barcelona • Belgrade • Novi Sad • Cluj • Manchester

Guest Editors
Antonios K. Gounaris
Department of Medicine
University of Thessaly
Larissa
Greece

Rozeta Sokou
Department of Neonatology
National and Kapodistrian
University of Athens
Athens
Greece

Editorial Office
MDPI AG
Grosspeteranlage 5
4052 Basel, Switzerland

This is a reprint of the Special Issue, published open access by the journal *Nutrients* (ISSN 2072-6643), freely accessible at: https://www.mdpi.com/journal/nutrients/special_issues/Nutrition_Preterm_Neonates.

For citation purposes, cite each article independently as indicated on the article page online and as indicated below:

Lastname, A.A.; Lastname, B.B. Article Title. *Journal Name* **Year**, *Volume Number*, Page Range.

ISBN 978-3-7258-5455-4 (Hbk)
ISBN 978-3-7258-5456-1 (PDF)
https://doi.org/10.3390/books978-3-7258-5456-1

Contents

About the Editors

Antonios K. Gounaris

Antonios K. Gounaris MD, PhD, Professor of Neonatology. Head of the neonatal clinic and NICU of the Regional General Hospital "Agios Panteleimon" Piraeus for 7 years. Professor and Head of the neonatal clinic and NICU, of the Regional General University Hospital, Medical School, University of Thessaly, Larissa Greece for 8 years.

Today, Emeritus Professor of Neonatology with contribution to research in the Medical School and participation in postgraduate courses of University of Thessaly. Scientific Associate of the Neonatal clinic and NICU, "REA" Maternity Hospital SA, Athens. Recent research activity: feeding and growth of VLBW newborns, effect of hospitalization on the late outcome of preterm neonates.

Rozeta Sokou

Rozeta Sokou, MD, MSc, PhD, PostDoctorate, Assistant Professor of Pediatrics Neonatology, National and Kapodistrian University of Athens, Medical School. Rozeta Sokou works in the Neonatal Department at the National and Kapodistrian University of Athens, Aretaieio Hospital, Greece. She has authored over 125 publications in international peer-reviewed journals and contributed chapters to Greek scientific books. Her research focuses on neonatal hematology, neonatal hemostasis and transfusion medicine, nutrition, growth, and the comprehensive care of preterm neonates, with particular emphasis on their long-term health and well-being. She has received 12 awards for her research from both Greek and international scientific congresses.

nutrients

MDPI

Editorial

Nutrition and Growth of Preterm Neonates during Hospitalization: Impact on Childhood Outcomes

Antonios K. Gounaris [1] and Rozeta Sokou [2,*]

[1] Neonatal Intensive Care Unit, University Hospital of Larissa, 413 34 Larissa, Greece; angounaris@med.uth.gr
[2] Neonatal Intensive Care Unit, Nikea General Hospital "Agios Panteleimon", 184 54 Piraeus, Greece
* Correspondence: sokourozeta@yahoo.gr

1. Introduction

The Special Issue has been completed with the publication of 13 review and research articles. Throughout the content of the articles and their relevant literature, two major themes emerged in our opinion.

Firstly, it is evident that the change in feeding protocols after the year 2000, especially for very premature neonates (VPNs), and despite some ongoing discussions that these changes generated, contributed significantly to improvements in survival and long-term morbidity even of neonates on the "grey zone" of viability (22–24^{+6} weeks) [1–3]. This is a monumental positive change in the treatment of premature neonates post 2000 that constitutes in our opinion a separate third era in Neonatology, rather than being a part of the second era. The adoption of this definition by Perinatal Societies would help to focus perinatal care on the growth and development of VPNs during hospitalization.

The second issue emerging in our opinion is that the time has come for the implementation of universal neonatal feeding protocols, based on the 2021 and 2022 ESPGHAN guidelines [4,5]. Despite some valid criticisms from eminent colleagues regarding the paucity of large-scale studies confirming the long-term outcomes of those policies, in our opinion, the wealth of studies showcasing the integral role of improved nutrition for long-term VPN prognosis should not be ignored by the scientific community. The choice to wait for large-scale studies is not a neutral one, as it will further entrench the huge inequalities in neonatal nutritional care currently observed between countries or even within neonatal units of the same country, with the associated disparity of outcomes.

Two studies explored growth patterns with the monitoring of head circumference (HC) and weight trajectory of VPNs. Lin et al. (contribution 1) showed an association between feeding progress in the first 56 days of life and HC at term and corrected ages of 6, 12 and 24 months, as well as neurodevelopment at 24 months corrected age. Infants showing slow feeding progress had a high risk of stunted HC growth or even microcephaly with associated neurodevelopmental disorders in early childhood. In the study of Peter et al. (contribution 2), there was an evaluation of a group of very-low-birth-weight (VLBW) infants that required surgical intervention and colostomy formation because of either necrotizing enterocolitis (NEC), spontaneous intestinal perforation (SIP) or meconium-related ileus (MI). It was found that the duration of inflammation and their growth velocity during hospitalization, as evidenced by their HC and weight, had a significant impact on the risk of cholestasis and adverse neurodevelopmental outcomes at 24 months irrespective of the etiology of the enteral surgery. These two studies further confirm the prevailing consensus that the delay of appropriate nutrition and growth in the neonatal period and up to 40 weeks corrected gestational age is detrimental to neurodevelopment at 24 months of age [6–9]. In the cases requiring surgical intervention, aiming to reduce ongoing inflammation, the early reintroduction of feeding and nutritional supplementation to aid in catch-up growth will help minimize those observed adverse effects.

Along the same vein, in a review article, Kosmeri et al. (contribution 3) collate and present the current knowledge around the nutritional needs of fetal growth-restricted (FGR)/small for gestational age (SGA) premature neonates of singleton and multiple pregnancies. They note from the reviewed literature that premature FGR/SGA babies experience cumulative nutritional deficiencies because of a multitude of factors: malnutrition at the fetal stage, comorbidities in the first few weeks of life, delayed initiation and slow advancement of enteral nutrition [10,11]. This finding is more common in neonates born <29 weeks and is confirmed by the latest study of Sériès et al. [6].

From those findings, the writers conclude that FGR/SGA VPNs require more aggressive feeding in the neonatal period in order to make up for these nutritional deficits.

Two studies focus on the methods of monitoring and evaluating VPN growth during their NICU stay. Kakatsaki et al. (contribution 4) compared the prevalence of SGA and extrauterine growth restriction (EUGR) among extremely and very preterm neonates (GA < 32 weeks) using the Fenton13 and Intergrowth-21 growth charts. They showed a significant difference in the prevalence of neonates meeting the SGA and EUGR definitions using these two different charts, something that has been confirmed by separate studies [12–16] and that, in practice, hinders the implementation of more universal clinical and feeding practices for VPNs. It is necessary, according to the authors, to determine a growth chart that enables the appropriate optimal monitoring of these neonates.

In an opinion piece, Gounaris et al. (contribution 5) argue that the variable definitions of the terms intrauterine growth restriction (IUGR), extrauterine growth restriction (EGR) and postnatal growth failure (PGF) in the international literature directly contribute to the absence of a universally accepted feeding and growth strategy for this infant population. In their opinion, the term EGR is more appropriate compared to PGF, as it focuses on a defined period of growth, up to 40 weeks corrected gestational, age that usually corresponds with the duration of hospital stay and during which nutritional interventions have maximum impact. In contrast, PGF refers to growth during an ill-defined period that can be extended up to the first year of life. Considering which growth paradigm should be considered safe, they argue that based on studies [17] showing that VPN growth > 10th centile at 36 weeks corrected gestational age (CGA) or at discharge did not increase neurodevelopmental risks, and that aiming for growth above the traditional definition of growth restriction (<10th centile for CGA) is both a safe and feasible target until a more precise one is determined through large scale studies. In terms of the adoption of a universal feeding policy, in the authors opinion the latest ESPGHAN guidelines from 2021 and 2022 can be used as a blueprint and a stepping stone to that direction [4,5].

Over the last few years, multiple studies have highlighted the benefits of breast milk for premature neonates, something reflected in the five studies focusing on breast feeding and breast milk. Seliga-Siwecka et al. (contribution 6) did not find a significant difference between targeted and standard breast milk fortification in terms of growth velocity during NICU stay, as reflected in HC, length and weight gain. This goes on to show that even if targeted breast milk fortification is not technically feasible, standard fortification has similar effects on VPN growth.

In the study by Gialeli et al. (contribution 7), it was found that donor breast milk (DBM) from mothers of premature neonates resulted in a significantly improved intake of protein ($p = 0.006$) and improved weight gain ($p = 0.019$) compared to term DBM, a finding that strengthens the argument that term DBM should be fortified in a targeted way when administered to VPNs. The study of Sokou et al. (contribution 8) confirmed the low levels of breast feeding among neonates hospitalized in NICUs, which are far lower than the targets set out by the WHO and CDC [18,19], and defined the causative factors behind them.

In a systematic review by Dimitroglou et al. (contribution 9), it was noted that SARS-CoV-2 infection promotes an IgA immune response in breast milk, whereas COVID vaccinations mainly caused an IgG response. In both cases, the levels of IgG immunoglobulins in maternal blood are closely correlated with immunoglobulin levels in breast milk.

The authors conclude that breast milk from mothers who have been infected or received a vaccination against the virus could help protect their babies during the pandemic.

A review by Sokou et al. (contribution 10) explored the ability of women affected by long-term conditions to breast feed. Cumulative evidence shows that women with long term health conditions achieve lower levels of breast feeding compared to healthy controls as a result of a multitude of contributing factors. This study examines in detail how each of the main long-term health morbidities affects exclusive breast-feeding levels. Interventions that support both maternal health and caregiving abilities will help reverse this trend.

Two reviews focus on the short- and long-term effects of BPD, one of the major morbidities of prematurity. In a literature review by Karatza et al. (contribution 11), the authors conclude that this population should receive sufficient calories and nutrients, both during and after their NICU stay, in order to achieve an adequate level of growth that will support lung alveolarization. The precise monitoring of growth both during and after discharge from hospital is necessary according to the authors as minimizing growth restriction will help improve lung function.

Likewise in their review, Briana and Malamitsi (contribution 12) examined the relationship between the parameters of hospital stay of extremely/very premature neonates and their long-term respiratory prognosis. Long-term observational studies have concluded that extremely/very premature birth is significantly associated with Chronic Obstructive Pulmonary Disease (COPD), something that respiratory physicians should be aware of. The authors here infer that the recent data underscore the significance of beneficial nutritional interventions in the neonatal period, for the long-term development of the lungs and their capacity to recover from damage [20,21]. The above findings could positively contribute to the long-term prognosis of extremely/very premature neonates.

The effects of prematurity on later life were explored in the study of Wood et al. (contribution 13) by examining the correlation between gestational age (GA) and the metabolic and muscle function during adolescence using 3IP-MRS. It was found that GA at birth was predictive of oxidative skeletal muscle function (T1/2 PCr) in adolescence. This finding demonstrates, according to the authors, the persistence of the metabolic impact of prematurity on later life.

In conclusion, these 13 studies along with their literature provide enough support to the argument for the more 'intense' nutrition of VPNs in the neonatal period, including breast milk fortification and closely following ESPHGHAN guidelines. Especially in the cases of neonates that are IUGR, SGA, born <29 weeks GA or affected by major morbidities such as BPD, strict adherence to guidelines with nutritional deficit replacement is necessary as it can make a positive difference in the lives of these neonates in years to come.

Author Contributions: Writing—original draft preparation, A.K.G. and R.S. All authors have read and agreed to the published version of the manuscript.

Conflicts of Interest: The authors declare no conflict of interest.

List of Contributions:

1. Lin: Y.-C.; Chu, C.-H.; Chen, Y.-J.; Chen, R.-B.; Huang, C.-C. Early Life Slow Enteral Feeding Progression Pattern Is Associated with Longitudinal Head-Size Growth Faltering and Neurodevelopmental Impairment Outcomes in Extremely Preterm Infants. *Nutrients* **2023**, *15*, 1277.
2. Peter, C.; Abukhris, A.; Brendel, J.; Böhne, C.; Bohnhorst, B.; Pirr, S. Growth and Duration of Inflammation Determine Short- and Long-Term Outcome in Very-Low-Birth-Weight Infants Requiring Abdominal Surgery. *Nutrients* **2023**, *15*, 1668.
3. Kosmeri, C.; Giapros, V.; Rallis, D.; Balomenou, F.; Serbis, A.; Baltogianni, M. Classification and Special Nutritional Needs of SGA Infants and Neonates of Multiple Pregnancies. *Nutrients* **2023**, *15*, 2736.
4. Kakatsaki, I.; Papanikolaou, S.; Roumeliotaki, T.; Anagnostatou, N.H.; Lygerou, I.; Hatzidaki, E. The Prevalence of Small for Gestational Age and Extrauterine Growth Restriction among

Extremely and Very Preterm Neonates, Using Different Growth Curves, and Its Association with Clinical and Nutritional Factors. *Nutrients* **2023**, *15*, 3290.

5. Gounaris, A.K.; Sokou, R.; Gounari, E.A.; Panagiotounakou, P.; Grivea, I.N. Extrauterine Growth Restriction and Optimal Growth of Very Preterm Neonates: State of the Art. *Nutrients* **2023**, *15*, 3231.
6. Seliga-Siwecka, J.; Fiałkowska, J.; Chmielewska, A. Effect of Targeted vs. Standard Fortification of Breast Milk on Growth and Development of Preterm Infants ($\leq$32 Weeks): Results from an Interrupted Randomized Controlled Trial. *Nutrients* **2023**, *15*, 619.
7. Gialeli, G.; Kapetanaki, A.; Panagopoulou, O.; Vourna, P.; Michos, A.; Kanaka-Gantenbein, C.; Liosis, G.; Siahanidou, T. Supplementation of Mother's Own Milk with Preterm Donor Human Milk: Impact on Protein Intake and Growth in Very Low Birth Weight Infants—A Randomized Controlled Study. *Nutrients* **2023**, *15*, 566.
8. Sokou, R.; Parastatidou, S.; Ioakeimidis, G.; Tavoulari, E.-F.; Makrogianni, A.; Isaakidou, E.; Iaou, N.; Konstantinidi, A. Breastfeeding in Neonates Admitted to an NICU: 18-Month Follow-Up. *Nutrients* **2022**, *14*, 3841.
9. Dimitroglou, M.; Sokou, R.; Iaou, N.; Pouliakis, A.; Kafalidis, G.; Boutsikou, T.; Iliodromiti, Z. Anti-SARS-CoV-2 Immunoglobulins in Human Milk after Coronavirus Disease or Vaccination—Time Frame and Duration of Detection in Human Milk and Factors That Affect Their Titers: A Systematic Review. *Nutrients* **2023**, *15*, 1905.
10. Sokou, R.; Parastatidou, S.; Iliodromiti, Z.; Lampropoulou, K.; Vrachnis, D.; Boutsikou, T.; Konstantinidi, A.; Iaou, N. Knowledge Gaps and Current Evidence Regarding Breastfeeding Issues in Mothers with Chronic Diseases. *Nutrients* **2023**, *15*, 2822.
11. Karatza, A.A.; Gkentzi, D.; Varvarigou, A. Nutrition of Infants with Bronchopulmonary Dysplasia before and after Discharge from the Neonatal Intensive Care Unit. *Nutrients* **2022**, *14*, 3311.
12. Briana, D.D.; Malamitsi-Puchner, A. An Update on Lung Function of Extremely and Very Preterm Infants in Later Life: The Role of Early Nutritional Interventions. *Nutrients* **2023**, *15*, 3353.
13. Wood, C.L.; Tinnion, R.; Hollingsworth, K.G.; Trenell, M.I.; Pearce, M.S.; Cheetham, T.D.; Embleton, N.D. Muscle Function, Body Composition, Insulin Sensitivity and Physical Activity in Adolescents Born Preterm: Impact of Gestation and Vitamin D Status. *Nutrients* **2022**, *14*, 5045.

References

1. Schuler, R.; Bedei, I.; Oehmke, F.; Zimmer, K.P.; Ehrhardt, H. Neonatal Outcome and Treatment Perspectives of Preterm Infants at the Border of Viability. *Children* **2022**, *9*, 313. [CrossRef] [PubMed]
2. Mustapha, M.; Wilson, K.A.; Barr, S. Optimising nutrition of preterm and term infants in the neonatal intensive care unit. *Paediatr. Child Health* **2021**, *31*, 38–45. [CrossRef]
3. Ehrenkranz, R.A. Early nutritional support and outcomes in ELBW infants. *Early Hum. Dev.* **2010**, *86* (Suppl. S1), 21–25. [CrossRef] [PubMed]
4. Moltu, S.J.; Bronsky, J.; Embleton, N.; Gerasimidis, K.; Indrio, F.; Köglmeier, J.; de Koning, B.; Lapillonne, A.; Norsa, L.; Verduci, E.; et al. Nutritional Management of the Critically Ill Neonate: A Position Paper of the ESPGHAN Committee on Nutrition. *J. Pediatr. Gastroenterol. Nutr.* **2021**, *73*, 274–289. [CrossRef] [PubMed]
5. Embleton, N.D.; Moltu, S.J.; Lapillonne, A.; van den Akker, C.H.P.; Carnielli, V.; Fusch, C.; Gerasimidis, K.; van Goudoever, J.B.; Haiden, N.; Iacobelli, S.; et al. Enteral Nutrition in Preterm Infants (2022): A Position Paper From the ESPGHAN Committee on Nutrition and Invited Experts. *J. Pediatr. Gastroenterol. Nutr.* **2023**, *76*, 248–268. [CrossRef] [PubMed]
6. Sériès, T.; Guillot, M.; Angoa, G.; Pronovost, E.; Ndiaye, A.; Mohamed, I.; Simonyan, D.; Lavoie, P.M.; Synnes, A.; Marc, I. Does Growth Velocity Affect Associations between Birth Weight and Neurodevelopment for Infants Born Very Preterm? *J. Pediatr.* **2023**, *260*, 113531. [CrossRef] [PubMed]
7. Coviello, C.; Keunen, K.; Kersbergen, K.J.; Groenendaal, F.; Leemans, A.; Peels, B.; Isgum, I.; Viergever, M.A.; de Vries, L.S.; Buonocore, G.; et al. Effects of early nutrition and growth on brain volumes, white matter microstructure, and neurodevelopmental outcome in preterm newborns. *Pediatr. Res.* **2018**, *83*, 102–110. [CrossRef] [PubMed]
8. Embleton, N.D.; Korada, M.; Wood, C.L.; Pearce, M.S.; Swamy, R.; Cheetham, T.D. Catch-up growth and metabolic outcomes in adolescents born preterm. *Arch. Dis. Child.* **2016**, *101*, 1026–1031. [CrossRef] [PubMed]
9. Lapillonne, A.; Griffin, I.J. Feeding preterm infants today for later metabolic and cardiovascular outcomes. *J. Pediatr.* **2013**, *162*, S7–S16. [CrossRef] [PubMed]
10. Shah, M.D.; Shah, S.R. Nutrient deficiencies in the premature infant. *Pediatr. Clin. N. Am.* **2009**, *56*, 1069–1083. [CrossRef] [PubMed]
11. Fleig, L.; Hagan, J.; Lee, M.L.; Abrams, S.A.; Hawthorne, K.M.; Hair, A.B. Growth outcomes of small for gestational age preterm infants before and after implementation of an exclusive human milk-based diet. *J. Perinatol.* **2021**, *41*, 1859–1864. [CrossRef] [PubMed]

12. Murray, Y.L.; Paul, I.M.; Miller, J.R.; Thrash, S.Z.; Kaiser, J.R. Variability in the use of growth curves between preterm and term infants in NICUs and newborn nurseries. *Pediatr. Res.* **2021**, *89*, 711–713. [CrossRef] [PubMed]
13. Ribas, S.A.; Paravidino, V.B.; Soares, F.V.M. Comparison of growth curves in very low birth weight preterm infants after hospital discharge. *Eur. J. Pediatr.* **2022**, *181*, 149–157. [CrossRef] [PubMed]
14. El Rafei, R.; Jarreau, P.H.; Norman, M.; Maier, R.F.; Barros, H.; Reempts, P.V.; Pedersen, P.; Cuttini, M.; Zeitlin, J. Variation in very preterm extrauterine growth in a European multicountry cohort. *Arch. Dis. Child. Fetal Neonatal Ed.* **2021**, *106*, 316–323. [CrossRef] [PubMed]
15. Silveira, R.C.; Procianoy, R.S. Preterm newborn's postnatal growth patterns: How to evaluate them. *J. Pediatr.* **2019**, *95*, S42–S48. [CrossRef] [PubMed]
16. Hokken-Koelega, A.C.; van der Steen, M.; Boguszewski, M.C.; Cianfarani, S.; Dahlgren, J.; Horikawa, R.; Mericq, V.; Rapaport, R.; Alherbish, A.; Braslavsky, D. International consensus guideline on small for gestational age: Etiology and management from infancy to early adulthood. *Endocr. Rev.* **2023**, *44*, 539–565. [CrossRef] [PubMed]
17. Shah, P.S.; Wong, K.Y.; Merko, S.; Bishara, R.; Dunn, M.; Asztalos, E.; Darling, P.B. Postnatal growth failure in preterm infants: Ascertainment and relation to long-term outcome. *J. Perinat. Med.* **2006**, *34*, 484–489. [CrossRef] [PubMed]
18. WHO. Breastfeeding. Available online: https://www.who.int/health-topics/breastfeeding#tab=tab_1 (accessed on 20 July 2022).
19. CDC. Breastfeeding Report Card. Available online: https://www.cdc.gov/breastfeeding/data/reportcard.htm (accessed on 24 July 2022).
20. Panagiotounakou, P.; Sokou, R.; Gounari, E.; Konstantinidi, A.; Antonogeorgos, G.; Grivea, I.N.; Daniil, Z.; Gourgouliannis, K.I.; Gounaris, A. Very preterm neonates receiving "aggressive" nutrition and early nCPAP had similar long-term respiratory outcomes as term neonates. *Pediatr. Res.* **2019**, *86*, 742–748. [CrossRef] [PubMed]
21. Groene, S.G.; Spekman, J.A.; Te Pas, A.B.; Heijmans, B.T.; Haak, M.C.; van Klink, J.M.M.; Roest, A.A.W.; Lopriore, E. Respiratory distress syndrome and bronchopulmonary dysplasia after fetal growth restriction: Lessons from a natural experiment in identical twins. *EClinicalMedicine* **2021**, *32*, 100725. [CrossRef] [PubMed]

nutrients MDPI

Systematic Review

Anti-SARS-CoV-2 Immunoglobulins in Human Milk after Coronavirus Disease or Vaccination—Time Frame and Duration of Detection in Human Milk and Factors That Affect Their Titers: A Systematic Review

Margarita Dimitroglou †, Rozeta Sokou *,†, Nicoletta Iacovidou *, Abraham Pouliakis, Georgios Kafalidis, Theodora Boutsikou and Zoi Iliodromiti

Neonatal Department, Medical School, National and Kapodistrian University of Athens, Aretaieio Hospital, 11528 Athens, Greece
* Correspondence: sokourozeta@yahoo.gr (R.S.); niciac58@gmail.com (N.I.)
† These authors contributed equally to this work.

Abstract: Human milk (HM) of mothers infected with or vaccinated against SARS-CoV-2 contains specific immunoglobulins, which may protect their offspring against infection or severe disease. The time frame and duration after infection or vaccination, during which these immunoglobulins are detected in HM, as well as the major factors that influence their levels, have not been fully elucidated. This systematic review aimed to collect the existing literature and describe the immune response, specifically regarding the immunoglobulins in HM after COVID-19 disease or vaccination in non-immune women. We conducted a systematic search of PubMed and Scopus databases to identify studies published up until 19 March 2023. In total, 975 articles were screened, and out of which 75 were identified as being relevant and were finally included in this review. Infection by SARS-CoV-2 virus primarily induces an IgA immune response in HM, while vaccination predominantly elevates IgG levels. These immunoglobulins give HM a neutralizing capacity against SARS-CoV-2, highlighting the importance of breastfeeding during the pandemic. The mode of immune acquisition (infection or vaccination) and immunoglobulin levels in maternal serum are factors that seem to influence immunoglobulin levels in HM. Further studies are required to determine the impact of other factors, such as infection severity, lactation period, parity, maternal age and BMI on immunoglobulin level in HM.

Keywords: human milk; COVID-19; SARS-CoV-2 virus; immunoglobulin levels; milk-transferred antibody; breastfeeding; immunology

1. Introduction

The global COVID-19 pandemic has resulted in more than 6.85 million deaths worldwide with about 0.1% of incidents occurring in neonates and children under 5 years [1,2]. The widespread availability of vaccines has played a crucial role in controlling transmission rates and reducing morbidity and mortality. The Center for Disease Control and Prevention (CDC) recommends vaccination for individuals aged 6 months and older, including neonates and non-vaccinated infants [3].

Younger or unvaccinated infants are defenseless against SARS-CoV-2 virus. Breastfeeding could be a protective factor against severe infection for these infants. Human milk (HM) contains various bioactive nutrients, such as immunoglobulins that block the penetration of microorganisms into the endothelium [4]. Initial concerns regarding the safety of breastfeeding during maternal infection led to previous recommendations for infected women to avoid breastfeeding. However, since June 23, 2020, the World Health Organization (WHO) strongly recommends breastfeeding, as the benefits outweigh the potential risks [5]. Recent studies indicate that maternal vaccination against SARS-CoV-2 virus reduces the risk of hospitalization in infants by approximately 60% [6].

SARS-CoV-2 virus is a single-stranded RNA virus, and its RNA is enveloped to a nucleocapsid. Its genome encodes four structural proteins: N(Nucleocapsid), M(Membrane), S(Spike) and E(Envelope) proteins [7]. The N protein is found in the virus core, and it forms complexes with viral RNA. It is also found in infected cells, so it is a common target for antigen tests [8,9]. The other three proteins are found in the viral envelope. The S protein interacts with the Angiotensin-converting enzyme 2(ACE2) receptor and mediates SARS-CoV-2 to be inserted into the host's cells. The S protein consists of two subunits: the S1 subunit which contains an exposed receptor-binding domain (RBD), the part of the S protein that binds to the ACE2 receptor, and the S2 subunit for membrane fusion [10]. Tests that are used to evaluate the immune response after the vaccination target S protein or a subunit of it. Serology tests that are used in cases of COVID-19 disease, can target the N protein as well.

Nicolaidou V. et al., in a recent systematic review, reported that the HM of vaccinated lactating women contains neutralizing immunoglobulins against SARS-CoV-2 [11]. The presence of specific antibodies against the virus in the HM of vaccinated women has also been confirmed by another recent meta-analysis by Whited and Cervantes [12]. COVID-19 disease leads to an immune response in maternal organisms as well, and neutralizing antibodies are detected in their HM [13]. However, the duration that these antibodies remain in detectable levels, the time frame in which the immune response begins to wane, the factors that influence their levels in HM and the differences in the immune response between infected women and those who are vaccinated still remain unclear. We conducted a systematic review of the current literature from the beginning of the pandemic until March 19, 2023, in order to synthesize the current knowledge regarding the presence of antibodies against SARS-CoV-2 in HM after COVID-19 disease or vaccination, among non-previously immune pregnant or lactating women.

2. Materials and Methods

In order to perform this systematic review, we followed the Preferred Reporting Items for Systematic Reviews and Meta-Analyses guidelines' (PRISMA) recommendation (presented as Supplementary Material) [14]. The systematic review was not registered in Prospero. We searched the Pubmed and Scopus databases from 1 December 2019 to 19 March 2023. We searched the existing literature only written in the English language.

The keywords used for the literature search were as follows: "SARS-CoV-2", "Covid 19", "novel coronavirus", "Immunoglobulin*", "antibody", "IgG", "IgA", "secretory IgA", "sIgA", "immunological", "immune system", "immunogenicity", "immunology", "milk transferred antibody", "breast milk", "maternal milk", "human milk", "breastmilk", "colostrum", "breastfeeding", "donor milk", "lactating women" and "lactation", combined with Boolean logical operators (AND, OR).

Additionally, we searched all of the references of the relevant studies and of previous corresponding systematic reviews in order to confirm the study saturation.

2.1. Study Eligibility Criteria

All selected studies examined the immunological response in the HM of pregnant or lactating women after COVID-19 disease or vaccination. After the duplicates were deleted, two investigators (M.D. and R.S.) independently checked the titles and abstracts of the retrieved papers, and consequently studied the full texts to decide which of them were eligible for the review. Any disagreements between the two researchers were analyzed and resolved by a third researcher (Z.I.).

Studies included in the present review met the following eligibility criteria: (1) women vaccinated against or infected by SARS-CoV-2 virus during pregnancy or lactating period were the study population, (2) there was no history of previously confirmed COVID-19 disease or vaccination, (3) current COVID-19 disease was confirmed via a PCR positive test, serology test or other laboratory method and (4) data on HM-specific immunoglobulins against SARS-CoV-2 were described in the studies that were included in the review as well. Irrelevant or non-original studies, case reports or studies with indecisive data were excluded from this review, as well as studies in any language other than English.

2.2. Data Extraction

The 2 researchers (M.D. and R.S.) separately studied the eligible studies and extracted useful data in an electronical database (Microsoft Excel). Complete information included the name of the first author, date of publication, country of origin, duration and population of the study, diagnosis method or vaccine type, time of HM collection, studied immunoglobulins and main outcomes or results of the study. Any disagreement between the two researchers was analyzed and resolved by a third researcher (Z.I.). Finally, the selected studies were examined again by another investigator (N.I) to check for eligibility and for duplication, and the extracted data were checked for their accuracy.

3. Results

A total of 975 articles were initially retrieved. After excluding duplicates and articles with titles and abstracts not related to our review object, 122 studies were selected for their full text to be studied. In these studies, the full text was comprehensively studied and 75 studies finally met the eligibility criteria. The searching and selection processes are depicted in a PRISMA graph (Figure 1).

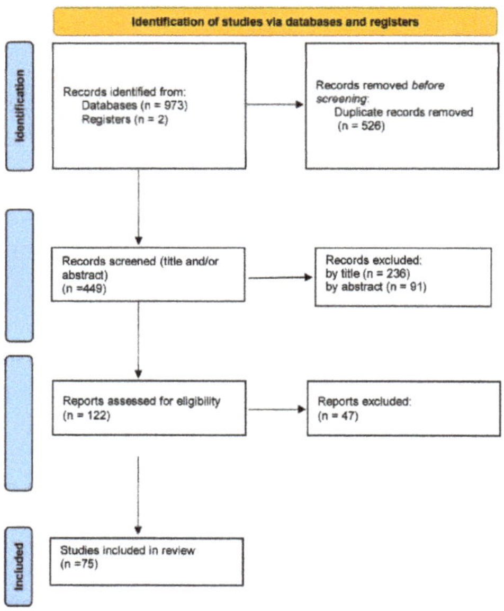

Figure 1. Flow chart of the study selection process.

Seventeen studies out of the total included women infected for the first time during pregnancy (Table 1) [9–26]. Another 17 studies examined women infected for the first time during lactation (Table 2) [27–43]. Six more studies included vaccinated pregnant women not previously immunized (Table 3) [22,25,27,29,44,45]. Finally, 40 studies examined vaccinated lactating women not previously immunized (Table 4) [22,25,32,38,42,46–80]. Ten studies included more than one participant group, and therefore they have been put into more than one table [22,25,27,29,32,38,42,44,46,47].

Table 1. Characteristics of included studies referring to first-time-infected pregnant women.

Author (Year, Country)	Duration of Study	Pregnant Women (N)	Diagnostic Test	Time of Sample HM Collection	Studied Immunoglobulins	Antibody Measurement Method	Outcome/Results
Gao X. et al. (2020, China) [18]	20 days	12	PCR or serology test	Within 7 days postpartum	Anti-SARS-CoV-2 antibodies (IgM and IgG)	CLIA commercial kit/NAL	Neutralizing antibodies present in 3 samples of HM. SARS-CoV-2 virus was not detected in any sample.
Narayanaswamy V. et al. (2021, USA) [15]	5 months	15	PCR test	Within 48 hours postpartum	Anti-RBD antibodies (IgA, IgM and IgG)	Homemade ELISA	Present antibodies in colostrum (IgA in 73%, IgG in 73% and IgM in 33% of the samples).
Larcade R. et al. (2022, Argentina) [16]	2.5 months	58	PCR test	Within 96 h postpartum	Anti-RBD antibodies (IgA)	Homemade ELISA	Antibodies present in the HM of 87% of participants. No significant correlation with time of infection. Positive correlation between serum IgG titers and IgA titers in HM.
Bobik T.V. et al. (2021, Switzerland) [19]	NA	41	PCR test	Postpartum	Anti-S and anti-N antibodies (sIgA)	Homemade ELISA	Anti-RBD antibodies detected even in the HM of women infected during the first trimester.
Peng S. et al. (2020, China) [20]	NA	19	PCR test	Days 3,7,14,21, 28,42,56,70 postpartum	Anti-SARS-CoV-2 antibodies (IgM and IgG)	ELISA commercial kit	IgM present in the HM of 47% of participants. IgG was not detected in any sample. SARS-CoV-2 virus was not detected in any sample.

Table 1. *Cont.*

Author (Year, Country)	Duration of Study	Pregnant Women (N)	Diagnostic Test	Time of Sample HM Collection	Studied Immunoglobulins	Antibody Measurement Method	Outcome/Results
Bäuerl C. et al. (2021, Spain) [21]	8 months	60	PCR or serology test	Postpartum	Anti-RBD antibodies (IgA, IgM and IgG)	Homemade ELISA	Antibodies present in about 85% of samples. IgA titers remained stable in high titers over time. IgG titers were rising over time. Positive correlation between total IgA titers and anti-RBD IgA titers in HM.
Collier-ARY. et al. (2021, USA) [22]	1 year	22	PCR test	Postpartum	Anti-RBD antibodies (IgA and IgG)	Homemade ELISA	Antibodies present in HM.
Conti MG. et al. (2021, Italy) [23]	6 months	28	PCR test	2 days and 2 months postpartum	Anti-S antibodies (IgA and IgG)	ELISA commercial kit	IgA present in all samples. Higher titers in 48 h compared to 2 months post delivery. IgG titers remain low and stable over time.
Luo QQ. et al. (2021, China) [24]	43 days	4	PCR test	1 week postpartum	Anti-SARS-CoV-2 antibodies (IgM and IgG)	Homemade ELISA	IgM present in all samples of confirmed disease. Positive correlation between IgM titers in HM and in serum. IgG was not detected in any sample. SARS-CoV-2 virus was not detected in any sample.
Conti, M. G. et al. (2022, USA) [25]	2 months	28	PCR test	5 days and 2 months after infection	Anti-S antibodies (IgA and IgG)	ELISA commercial kit	IgA present in higher titers than IgG in HM. No correlation between IgA titers in HM and in serum.

Table 1. *Cont.*

Author (Year, Country)	Duration of Study	Pregnant Women (N)	Diagnostic Test	Time of Sample HM Collection	Studied Immunoglobulins	Antibody Measurement Method	Outcome/Results
Decenti, E. C. et al. (2022, Italy) [26]	16 months	141	PCR test	Postpartum	Anti-SARS-CoV-2 antibodies (IgM and IgG)	CLIA, ELISA, ECLIA, CMIA commercial kits	IgG present in 3.0% and IgM in 7.5% of HM.
Gu, Y. et al. (2022, Singapore) [81].	NA	8	PCR test	1–3 months postpartum	Anti-S and anti-RBD antibodies (IgA and IgG)	Homemade ELISA	Antibodies present in minimal levels 0–3 months postpartum.
Leung, H. Y. H. et al. (2022, China) [44]	NA	18	Laboratory-confirmed	3–192 days post infection (median = 45 days)	Anti-RBD antibodies (IgA)	Homemade ELISA/BA-Nabs	Antibody titers wane over time. Neutralizing antibodies present in HM. Positive correlation between antibody titers and binding capacity.
Martin-Vicente, M. et al. (2022, Spain) [82]	NA	46	PCR or serology test	Postpartum	Anti-S antibodies (IgA, IgM and IgG)	Homemade ELISA/NAA	Antibodies' titers correlate positively with neutralizing capacity. IgA detected in higher titers than IgM and IgG.
Olearo, F. et al. (2022, Germany) [27]	6 months	9	PCR test	Monthly for 6 months postpartum	Anti-S antibodies (IgA) and anti-RBD antibodies (IgA, IgM and IgG)	Homemade ELISA/NAA	Presence of neutralizing antibodies in HM.
Szczygioł, P. et al. (2022, Poland) [28]	2.5 months	72	PCR test	1–229 days after infection (median 68)	Anti-RBD antibodies (IgA and IgG)	ELISA commercial kit	No correlation between antibody titers and severity of disease or time of infection.

Table 1. *Cont.*

Author (Year, Country)	Duration of Study	Pregnant Women (N)	Diagnostic Test	Time of Sample HM Collection	Studied Immunoglobulins	Antibody Measurement Method	Outcome/Results
Nir O. et al. (2022, Israel) [29]	2 months	11	PCR test	Postpartum	Anti-RBD antibodies (IgG)	Homemade ELISA	Positive correlation between IgG titers in HM and serum.
Fox, A. et al. (2022, USA) [43]	10 months	74	PCR test	4–6 weeks after infection and 4–10 months after infection	Anti-S antibodies (IgA and IgG)	Homemade ELISA/PNA	Detectable IgA in 89% of samples 4–6 weeks after infection. Detectable IgG in 75% of samples 4–6 weeks after infection. Detectable IgA even 4–10 months after infection. Increased neutralizing capacity of HM after infection.
Dutra LV. et al. (2023, Brazil) [83]	1 year	165	PCR test	1–2 days postpartum	Anti-S antibodies (IgA and IgG)	ELISA commercial kit	Detectable IgA in about 70% of participants. Negative correlation between IgA titers in colostrum and neonatal symptoms.
Wachman EM. et al. (2023, USA) [84]	1 year	31	PCR test	At delivery and 6 weeks postpartum	Anti-RBD and anti-N antibodies (IgA, IgM and IgG)	Homemade ELISA	Higher titers of anti-RBD IgA in the HM of women infected during first or second trimester. Positive correlation between IgG titer in maternal HM and serum.
Clabretto M. et al. (2023, Italy) [85]	8 months	12	PCR test	Postpartum	Anti-N antibodies (IgA) and anti-S antibodies (IgM and IgG)	CLIA and ELISA commercial kits	Presence of IgA in 66% of samples. Presence of IgM and IgG in no sample.

Anti-N antibodies = antibodies against nucleocapsid, anti-S antibodies = antibodies against Spike protein, anti-RBD = antibodies against receptor-binding domain, BA-Nabs = binding assay for screening neutralizing antibodies, CLIA = Chemiluminescent Immuno Assay, CMIA = Chemiluminescent Microparticle Immuno Assay, ECLIA = Electrochemiluminescent Immuno Assay, ELISA = enzyme-linked immunosorbent assay, IgA = Immunoglobulin A, IgG = Immunoglobulin G, IgM = Immunoglobulin M, NA = not acquired, NAAs = neutralizing antibody assays, PCR test = Polymerase chain reaction, PNA = Pseudovirus neutralization assay.

Table 2. Characteristics of included studies referring to first-time-infected lactating women.

Author (Year, Country)	Duration of Study	Lactating Women (N)	Diagnostic Test	Time of Sample HM Collection	Studied Immunoglobulins	Antibody Measurement Method	Outcome/Results
Pace R.M. et al. (2020, Moscow) [30]	NA	18	PCR test	12.0 ± 8.9 days after infection	Anti-SARS-CoV-2 antibodies (IgA and IgG)	Homemade ELISA/MNA	Antibodies present in HM samples. Positive correlation between anti-RBD antibodies' titers and neutralizing capacity. SARS-CoV-2 virus was not detected in any sample.
van Keulen, BJ. (2021, Switzerland) [31]	NA	19	PCR test	5.9 (SD = 2.6) weeks after infection	Anti-S antibodies (IgA and IgG), anti-RDB and anti-N antibodies (IgA, IgM, IgG)	Homemade ELISA/PNA	Antibodies present in the HM of 83% of participants. No correlation between antibody titers and neutralizing capacity.
Demers-Mathieu V. (2021, USA) [32]	NA	10	PCR test	63 ± 40 days after infection	Anti-RBD antibodies (sIgA/IgA, sIgM/IgM and IgG)	Homemade ELISA/PNA	Antibodies present in HM. Higher inhibiting capacity against binding RBD to its receptor in women with previous COVID-19 infection compared to controls.
Demers-Mathieu V. et al. (2021, USA) [33]	NA	8	PCR test	2 months after infection	Anti-RBD antibodies (sIgA/IgA, sIgM/IgM and IgG)	Homemade ELISA	Antibodies present in HM.
Junker H.G. et al. (2021, The Netherlands) [34]	3.5 months	165	PCR test	8 weeks (mean time) after infection	Anti-SARS-CoV-2 antibodies (IgA)	Homemade ELISA	Detectable antibodies in HM even 10 months after infection.

Table 2. *Cont.*

Author (Year, Country)	Duration of Study	Lactating Women (N)	Diagnostic Test	Time of Sample HM Collection	Studied Immunoglobulins	Antibody Measurement Method	Outcome/Results
Pullen K.M. (2021, USA) [35]	NA	20	PCR test	66 days (mean time) after infection	Anti-SARS-CoV-2 antibodies (IgA, IgM and IgG)	Systems serology	Antibodies present in HM. IgG detected in significantly lower titers. IgG functionally attenuated. Positive correlation between IgG titers in HM and serum. No correlation between IgA titers in HM and serum.
Pace, R.M. et al. (2021, USA) [36]	NA	18	PCR test	12 ± 8,9 days after infection	Anti-RBD, anti-S2, anti-N (IgA and IgG)	Homemade ELISA/MNA	IgA present in 76% of samples and IgG in 80% of samples. Total of 62% of samples had neutralization capacity. SARS-CoV-2 virus was not detected in any sample.
Demers-Mathieu V. et al. (2021, USA) [37]	NA	7	PCR test	3 ± 2 months after infection	Anti-RBD antibodies (sIgA/IgA, sIgM/IgM and IgG)	Homemade ELISA	Positive correlation between sIgA/IgA titers and time from infection. No correlation detected between antibody titers and maternal age, infant gender and severity of symptoms.
Young BE. et al. (2021, USA) [38]	5 months	47	PCR test	0, 3, 7, 10, 28 and 90 days after infection	Anti-RBD antibodies (IgA and IgG)	Homemade ELISA/MNA	IgA-dominant response. Detectable IgA in almost-stable titers even 3 months after infection. Increased neutralizing capacity of HM after infection. SARS-CoV-2 virus was not detected in any sample.

Table 2. *Cont.*

Author (Year, Country)	Duration of Study	Lactating Women (N)	Diagnostic Test	Time of Sample HM Collection	Studied Immunoglobulins	Antibody Measurement Method	Outcome/Results
Juncker HG. et al. (2021, The Netherlands) [39]	3 months	29	PCR test	1,2,3,4 and 5 months after infection	Anti-S antibodies (IgA)	Homemade ELISA	Antibodies present even 5 months after infection. Not significant decrease in antibody titers over time.
Pace RM. et al. (2021, The Netherlands) [40]	8 months	64	PCR test	1,2,3,4 and 8 weeks after infection	Anti-RBD antibodies (IgA)	Homemade ELISA	Maximum IgA concentration was higher in symptomatic women. SARS-CoV-2 virus was not detected in any sample.
Demers-Mathieu V. et al. (2021, USA) [41]	NA	7	PCR test	47 +/− 24 days after infection	Anti-S1 or S2 subunit antibodies (sIgA/IgA, sIgM/IgM and IgG)	ELISA	Present anti-S2 IgA antibodies.
Juncker HG. et al. (2021, Switzerland) [42]	70 days	18	PCR test	Every 2 weeks after infection for at least 70 days	Anti-SARS-CON-2 antibodies (IgA)	Homemade ELISA	Detectable IgA antibodies even 70 days after infection.
Longueira, Y. et al. (2022, Argentina) [46]	12 months	11	PCR test	After infection	Anti-S antibodies (IgA and IgG)	ELISA commercial kit	Antibodies present in HM.
Narayanaswamy, V. et al. (2022, USA) [86]	4 months	30	PCR test	Every 3 days (for the 1st month after infection) and 4 months after infection	Anti-RBD antibodies (IgA, IgM and IgG)	Homemade ELISA/NAA	Detectable neutralizing antibodies. Detectable IgA and IgG in the majority of participants even 4 months after infection.
Wang, J. et al. (2022, USA) [47]	28 days	45	PCR test	0, 3, 10, 19 and 28 days after enrolled day (within 14 days from infection)	Anti-S and anti-N antibodies (IgA and IgG)	LUMINEX assay	Antibodies present in HM. Positive correlation between IgG titers in HM and serum. No correlation between IgA titers in HM and serum.

Table 2. *Cont.*

Author (Year, Country)	Duration of Study	Lactating Women (N)	Diagnostic Test	Time of Sample HM Collection	Studied Immunoglobulins	Antibody Measurement Method	Outcome/Results
L. Bode. et al. (2022, USA) [87]	7 months	21	PCR test	Around infection	Anti-S, anti-RBD, anti-NTD and anti-N antibodies (IgA and IgG)	ECLIA	IgA was mainly against N protein and less against S protein. No difference was observed in IgG isotype. Heterogeneity in responses between participants.

Anti-N antibodies = antibodies against nucleocapsid, anti-NTD = antibodies against N-terminal domain, anti-S antibodies = antibodies against Spike protein, anti-RBD = antibodies against receptor-binding domain, CLIA = Chemiluminescent Immuno Assay, CMIA = Chemiluminescent Microparticle Immuno Assay, ECLIA = Electrochemiluminescent Immuno Assay, ELISA = enzyme-linked immunosorbent assay, IgA = Immunoglobulin A, IgG = Immunoglobulin G, IgM = Immunoglobulin M, MNA = microneutralizing assay, NA = not acquired, NAA, neutralizing antibody assay, PCR test = Polymerase chain reaction, PNA = Pseudovirus neutralization assay.

Table 3. Characteristics of included studies referring to vaccinated pregnant women not previously infected or vaccinated.

Author (Year, Country)	Duration of Study	Pregnant Women (N)	Vaccine Type	Time of Sample HM collection	Studied immunoglobulins	Antibody Measurement Method	Outcome/Results
Conti, M. G. et al. (2022, USA) [25]	NA	11	BNT162b2 2 doses	2 months after 2nd dose	Anti-S antibodies (IgA and IgG)	ELISA commercial kit	Higher IgG titers in vaccinated women compared to those who were infected. Positive correlation between IgG titers in HM and serum.

Table 3. *Cont.*

Author (Year, Country)	Duration of Study	Pregnant Women (N)	Vaccine Type	Time of Sample HM collection	Studied immunoglobulins	Antibody Measurement Method	Outcome/Results
Leung, H. Y. H. et al. (2022, China) [44]	NA	8	COVID-19 vaccination	0–334 days post 1st dose (median = 71 days)	Anti-RBD antibodies (IgA)	ELISA commercial kit/BA-Nabs	Neutralizing antibodies present in HM. Antibody titers wane over time. Higher binding capacity after infection than vaccination. Positive correlation between antibody titers and binding capacity.
Olearo, F. et al. (2022, Germany) [27]	6 months	5	BNT162b2 2 doses	Monthly for 6 months postpartum	Anti-S antibodies (IgA) Anti-RBD antibodies (IgA, IgM and IgG)	Homemade ELISA	Higher titers of antibodies compared to recovered women.
Nir O. et al. (2022, Israel) [29]	2 months	64	BNT162b2 2 doses	Postpartum, within a few days	Anti-RBD antibodies (IgG)	Homemade ELISA	Positive correlation between IgG titers in HM and serum.
Collier-ARY. et al. (2021, USA) [22]	4 months	30	mRNA-1273/BNT162b2 2 doses	Close after each dose and 2–8 weeks after 2nd dose	Anti-RBD antibodies (IgA and IgG)	Homemade ELISA	Neutralizing antibodies present in HM.
Marshall N.E. et al. (2022, USA) [45]	NA	78	mRNA-1273/BNT162b2 2 doses	Between 0–12 months postpartum	Anti-RBD antibodies (IgG)	Homemade ELISA	Half life of IgG in HM is about 2 months. Positive correlation between IgG titers in HM and serum. IgG1 and IgG3 are present in higher titers compared to IgG4.

Anti-S antibodies = antibodies against Spike protein, anti-RBD = antibodies against receptor-binding domain, BA-Nabs = binding assay for screening neutralizing antibodies, ELISA = enzyme-linked immunosorbent assay, IgA = Immunoglobulin A, IgG = Immunoglobulin G, IgM = Immunoglobulin M, NA = not acquired.

Table 4. Characteristics of included studies referring to vaccinated lactating women not previously infected or vaccinated.

Author (Year, Country)	Duration of Study	Lactating Women (N)	Vaccine Type	Time of Sample HM Collection	Studied Immunoglobulins	Antibody Measurement Method	Outcome/Results
Demers-Mathieu V. (2021, USA) [32]	NA	19	mRNA-1273/BNT162b2 2 doses	37 ± 20 days after vaccination	Anti-RBD antibodies (sIgA/IgA, sIgM/IgM and IgG)	Homemade ELISA/PNA	Antibodies present in HM. Higher IgG titers in vaccinated compared to infected women. Higher neutralizing capacity in vaccinated women compared to controls.
Young BE. et al. (2021, USA) [38]	5 months	30	mRNA-1273/BNT162b2 2 doses	Prevaccination, 18 days after 1st dose, 18 and 90 days after 2nd dose	Anti-RBD antibodies (IgA and IgG)	Homemade ELISA/MNT	IgG-dominant response. Increased IgG titers after each dose. Declined IgG titers by 3 months. Increased IgA titers only after the first dose. Increased neutralization capacity after vaccination.
Juncker HG. et al. (2021, Switzerland) [42]	70 days	26	BNT162b2 2 doses	Prevaccination 3, 5, 7, 9, 11, 13, 15–17 days after 1st dose and 2nd dose and 70 days after 1st dose	Anti-S antibodies (IgA)	Homemade ELISA	Biphasic response of IgA antibodies. Detectable antibodies in 96% of participants after 2 doses. Detectable antibodies in about 40% of participants 70 days post vaccination. No significant difference between IgA titers in the HM of lactating women either infected or vaccinated. No severe adverse effect after vaccination.

Table 4. *Cont.*

Author (Year, Country)	Duration of Study	Lactating Women (N)	Vaccine Type	Time of Sample HM Collection	Studied Immunoglobulins	Antibody Measurement Method	Outcome/Results
Conti, M. G. et al. (2022, USA) [25]	NA	12	BNT162b2 2 doses	10 days after 2nd dose	Anti-S antibodies (IgA and IgG)	ELISA commercial kit	Higher IgG titers in vaccinated women compared to the infected group. Positive correlation between IgG titers in HM and serum.
Esteve-Palau, E. et al. (2022, Spain) [48]	6 months	33	BNT162b2 2 doses	2 weeks after 1st dose and 2,4,12 and 24 weeks after 2nd dose	Anti-S1 and anti-N antibodies (IgG)	Serology test, commercial kit	Peak anti-S1-IgG titers 2 weeks after 2nd dose. Positive correlation between IgG titers in HM and serum. IgG titers wane over a 6 month period.
Longueira, Y. et al. (2022, Argentina) [46]	12 months	27	Sputnik V, ChAdOx1-S or BBIBP-CorV	21 and 65 days after first and 21, 65 and 120 days after second dose (mean time)	Anti-SARS-CoV-2 antibodies (IgA and IgG)	ELISA commercial kit	2.8-fold increase in IgG titer after the 2nd dose. IgA remained constant between 1st and 2nd dose. 1.6-fold decrease in IgG titers, but stable levels of IgA over a 3-month period. Higher titer of IgG in participants who received adenoviral-based vaccines compared to those who received inactivated SARS-CoV-2 Sinopharm. No difference in IgA titers.

Table 4. *Cont.*

Author (Year, Country)	Duration of Study	Lactating Women (N)	Vaccine Type	Time of Sample HM Collection	Studied Immunoglobulins	Antibody Measurement Method	Outcome/Results
Low, J. M. et al. (2022, Singapore) [49]	6 weeks	46	BNT162b2 2 doses	Prevaccination 3–7 days and 4–6 weeks after 2nd dose	Anti-RBD antibodies (IgA)	Homemade ELISA	Peak titers of IgA observed 3–5 days after 2nd dose. Total of 30% reduction in binding capacity of antibodies in Beta, Gamma and Delta variants compared to Wuhan-Hu-1 strain.
Narayanaswamy, V. et al. (2022, USA) [50]	NA	27	mRNA-1273/BNT162b2 2 doses	Prevaccination after 1st and 2nd dose	Anti-RBD antibodies (IgA IgM and IgG)	ELISA commercial kit/V-PLEX commercial kit	IgG-dominant immune response. No increase in IgA titers after 2nd dose. No correlation between lactation stage and antibody titers.
Bender, J. M. et al. (2022, USA) [51]	10 months	10	mRNA-1273/BNT162b2 2 doses	Prevaccination 1, 3, 6 months after 1st dose	Anti-RBD antibodies (IgA, IgM and IgG)	Homemade ELISA/sVNT	Peak antibody titers one month after the 1st dose. No significant increase in IgM titers. Positive correlation between IgG titers in serum, and IgG and IgA titers in HM. Increased neutralizing capacity after vaccination.
Collier-ARY et al. (2021, USA) [22]	4 months	16	mRNA-1273/BNT162b2 2 doses	Close to each dose and 2–8 weeks after 2nd dose	Anti-RBD antibodies (IgA and IgG)	Homemade ELISA]	Neutralizing antibodies present in HM.
Pieri, M. et al. (2022, Switzerland) [55]	7 months	43	mRNA-1273/BNT162b2 ChAdOx1-S 2 doses	Prevaccination 1 day before the 2nd dose, 3 weeks after the 2nd	Anti-SARS-CoV-2 antibodies (sIgA/IgA and IgG)	ELISA commercial kit	Higher titers of IgG and IgA after the 2nd dose. Stable high antibody titers 3 weeks after the 2nd dose.

Table 4. *Cont.*

Author (Year, Country)	Duration of Study	Lactating Women (N)	Vaccine Type	Time of Sample HM Collection	Studied Immunoglobulins	Antibody Measurement Method	Outcome/Results
Pietrasanta, C. et al. (2022, Italy) [53]	90 days	24	BNT162b2 2 doses	Prevaccination before 2nd dose and 30, 60 and 90 days after 2nd dose	Anti-S and anti-RBD antibodies (IgA, IgA1, IgA2 and IgG)	Homemade ELISA	Vaccination induced IgG and IgA (mainly IgA1) immune responses. Antibodies waned over time, but they were still in detectable titers 90 days after vaccination. No severe adverse effect after vaccination.
Ricciardi, A. et al. (2022, Italy) [54]	2,5 months	18	BNT162b2 2 doses	Prevaccination at the 2nd dose, 3 weeks after 2nd dose and 6 months after 1st dose	Anti-S antibodies (sIgA and sIgG)	ELISA commercial kit	Increased sIgA titers after the 1st dose. Peak sIgA titers 3 weeks after the 2nd dose. Significant decrease in sIgA titers 6 months post vaccination. Peak sIgG titers 6 months after the first dose.
Agostinis C. et al. (2023, Italy) [80]	6 months	22	BNT162b2/ ChAdOx1-S 2 doses	Post vaccination (max 75 days post vaccination)	Anti-S antibodies (IgA and IgG)	Homemade ELISA	Range of antibody titers among participants. Positive correlation between IgG titers in serum and HM. No correlation between time of sample collection and antibody titers. Presence of IgG antibodies that can activate the complement.

Table 4. *Cont.*

Author (Year, Country)	Duration of Study	Lactating Women (N)	Vaccine Type	Time of Sample HM Collection	Studied Immunoglobulins	Antibody Measurement Method	Outcome/Results
Selma-Royo, M. et al. (2022, Spain) [52]	NA	75	mRNA-1273/BNT162b2/ ChAdOx1-S 2 doses	Prevaccination 1,2,3–4 weeks after 1st and 2nd dose In ChAdOx1-S group, a sample collected before 2nd dose	Anti-RBD antibodies (IgA and IgG)	Homemade ELISA	Peaked IgG titers 2 weeks after 2nd dose. Peaked IgA titers 1 week after the 1st dose for mRNA vaccines. IgA titers did not increase further after the 2nd dose. Higher IgG and IgA titers after vaccination with mRNA vaccines compared to those vaccinated with adeno-vectored vaccine. No significant difference observed between 2 mRNA vaccines.
Guida M. et al. (2021, Italy) [59]	NA	10	BNT162b2 2 doses	20 days after 1st dose and 7 days after 2nd dose	Anti-S antibodies (total)	ECLIA commercial kit	Higher antibody titers after 2nd dose. No correlation between total anti-S antibodies in HM and serum.
Stafford, L. et al. (2022, USA) [56]	12 months	8	mRNA-1273/BNT162b2 2 doses Ad.26.COV2.S 1 dose	Prevaccination 15–30 after 1st dose (for mRNA-based vaccines) and 7–30 days, 60–75 days, 90–105 days and 6 months after last dose	Anti-SARS-CoV-2 antibodies (IgA and IgG)	ELISA commercial kit/PVA	Antibody titers wane over time. Detectable levels 6 months post vaccination. More significant decline in IgG titers compared to IgA titers. Positive correlation between IgG levels in serum and HM 6 months post vaccination. Increased neutralizing capacity of HM after vaccination, especially 6 months post vaccination.

Table 4. *Cont.*

Author (Year, Country)	Duration of Study	Lactating Women (N)	Vaccine Type	Time of Sample HM Collection	Studied Immunoglobulins	Antibody Measurement Method	Outcome/Results
Valcare V. et al. (2021, USA) [60]	4 months	22	mRNA-1273/BNT162b2 2 doses	Prevaccination, post 1st and 2nd dose	Anti-S antibodies (IgA and IgG)	ELISA	Detectable antibodies in HM after vaccination.
Trofin, F. et al. (2022, Romania) [57].	7 months	28	mRNA -1273/BNT162b2 2 doses	30 and 60 days post 2nd dose	Anti-RBD antibodies (IgA and IgG)	ELISA commercial kit	No significant decrease in antibody levels 60 days post vaccination. Positive correlation of antibodies with lactation period. Negative correlation with child parity. No correlation between antibody titers and maternal age or vaccine type.
Wang, J. et al. (2022, USA) [47]	40 days	30	mRNA-1273/BNT162b2 2 doses	Prevaccination, 18 days after 1st and 2nd dose	Anti-Spike antibodies (IgA and IgG)	Homemade ELISA	Peak IgG titers after the 2nd dose. Peak IgA after the 1st dose. Total of 10-fold and 100-fold increase in IgA and IgG post vaccination, respectively. Detectable IgG titers even 187 days after the 2nd dose. Positive correlation between IgG titers in HM and serum. No correlation between IgA titers in HM and serum.

Table 4. *Cont.*

Author (Year, Country)	Duration of Study	Lactating Women (N)	Vaccine Type	Time of Sample HM Collection	Studied Immunoglobulins	Antibody Measurement Method	Outcome/Results
Yang, X. et al. (2022, USA and UK) [58]	NA	54	mRNA-1273/BNT162b2 2 doses ChAdOx1-S/Ad.26.COV2.S 2 or 1 dose	Prevaccination and 14 days or 21–35 (J&J) days post last dose	Anti-Spike antibodies (IgA and IgG)	Homemade ELISA	mRNA vaccines induce higher IgA antibody titers compared to adenovirus-vectored vaccines. Detectable IgG titers in 86–100% of mRNA-vaccinated women and in 33–38% of adenovirus-vector-vaccinated women. Detectable IgA in 52–71% of mRNA-vaccinated women and in 17–23% of adenovirus-vector-vaccinated women. Vaccination does not lead to significant increase in secretory antibody titers. (<50% of samples had specific secretory antibodies.) Moderna vaccine induces 2-fold higher levels of secretory antibodies compared with other vaccines.
Ramirez DSR et al. (2021, Spain) [69]	2 months	93	mRNA-1273/BNT162b2 2 doses	14 days post 2nd dose	Anti-RBD antibodies (IgA, IgM and IgG)	ELISA commercial kit/NAA commercial kit	Detectable IgG and IgA but not IgM. Positive correlation between IgG titers in HM and serum, positive correlation between IgA and IgG titers in HM. No correlation between antibody levels and maternal age and BMI.

Table 4. *Cont.*

Author (Year, Country)	Duration of Study	Lactating Women (N)	Vaccine Type	Time of Sample HM Collection	Studied Immunoglobulins	Antibody Measurement Method	Outcome/Results
Lechosa-Muñiz C. et al. (2021, Spain) [61]	1 month	110	mRNA-1273/BNT162b2 2 doses ChAdOx1-S 1 dose	30 days after the last dose	Anti-SARS-CoV-2 antibodies (IgA and IgG)	Homemade ELISA, CLIA commercial kit	Higher titers of IgA and IgG in HM after mRNA vaccine compared to adenovirus-vectored vaccine (the latter received only 1 dose).
Gray KJ. et al. (2021, USA) [67]	NA	31	mRNA-1273/BNT162b2 2 doses	At time of 1st and 2nd dose, 2–5.5 weeks post 2nd dose	Anti-S and anti-RBD antibodies (IgA, IgM and IgG)	Homemade ELISA/LUMINEX	Robust IgG titers, but not IgA and IgM titers after the 2nd dose. Higher IgA titers detected to Moderna group after the 2nd dose.
Perez S.E. et al. (2021, USA) [62]	14 months	27	mRNA-1273/BNT162b2 2 doses	Prevaccination, 1, 3 and 6 months post vaccination	Anti-SARS-CoV-2 antibodies (IgA, IgM and IgG)	Homemade ELISA/sVNT commercial kit	Detectable IgG in all samples, IgA in about 1/2 of the samples and IgM in about 1/4 of samples. IgG reached their peak levels 1 month post vaccination. Detectable IgG titers even 6 months post vaccination. Detectable IgA and IgM titers even 3 months post vaccination. Positive correlation between IgG and IgA titers in HM and IgG titers in serum. Neutralizing capacity of HM even at 6 months post vaccination. Neutralizing capacity correlates positively with IgG titers.

Table 4. *Cont.*

Author (Year, Country)	Duration of Study	Lactating Women (N)	Vaccine Type	Time of Sample HM Collection	Studied Immunoglobulins	Antibody Measurement Method	Outcome/Results
Golan Y. et al. (2021, USA) [63]	NA	48	mRNA-1273/BNT162b2 2 doses	Prevaccination before 2nd dose and 4–10 weeks after 2nd dose	Anti-RBD antibodies (IgA and IgG)	Homemade ELISA	Higher IgA titers after the 1st dose. No further increase after the 2nd dose. Detectable IgA titers in 75% of participants. IgG titers increase after 1st dose, with further increase in their titers after 2nd dose. No significant difference in the immune response between mRNA-based vaccines. Positive correlation between IgG titers in HM and maternal serum. No severe adverse effect after vaccination.
Scaggs Huang F. et al. (2021, USA) [79]	3 months	98	mRNA-1273/BNT162b2 2 doses	14 days post 2nd dose	Anti-S1 (IgA, IgM and IgG) and anti-N antibodies (IgG)	Serology test/NAA	Anti-S1 IgG and IgA antibodies present in HM. IgM antibodies were not detectable in any sample. Positive correlation between IgG titers in serum and HM.
Jakuszko K. et al. (2021, Switzerland) [64]	3 months	28	BNT162b2 2 doses	8 ± 1, 22 ± 2, 29 ± 3 and 43 ± 4 after 1st dose	Anti-Spike antibodies (IgA, IgM and IgG)	ELISA commercial kit	Peak antibody titers 7 ± 3 days after 1st dose. Higher IgA titers in the HM of serum-positive IgA women compared to serum-negative ones. No IgM was detectable in any sample. Positive correlation between IgG titers in HM and serum.

Table 4. *Cont.*

Author (Year, Country)	Duration of Study	Lactating Women (N)	Vaccine Type	Time of Sample HM Collection	Studied Immunoglobulins	Antibody Measurement Method	Outcome/Results
Schwartz A. et al. (2021, Israel) [77]	5 months	61	BNT162b2 2 doses	Post vaccination	Anti-RBD antibodies (IgA and IgG)	ELISA	IgG antibodies were detectable in all samples. Positive correlation between IgG titers in serum and HM. Neutralizing antibodies were detected in about 40% of samples. Secretory IgA was detected in 15% of samples.
Perl SH. et al. (2021, Israel) [65]	8 weeks	84	BNT162b2 2 doses	Prevaccination 2, 3, 4, 5 and 6 weeks post 1st dose	Anti-SARS-CoV-2 antibodies (IgA and IgG)	CLIA commercial kit	Detectable IgA titers in 61.8% and 86.1% of participants at 2 and 4 weeks after the 1st dose, respectively. Increased IgA titers after the 1st and 2nd dose. Detectable IgA titers 6 weeks after the 1st dose. IgG titers increased 1 week after the 2nd dose. IgG was detectable in 97% of samples 5 and 6 weeks after the 1st dose. No severe adverse effects after vaccination.
Yeo KT. et al. (2021, Singapore) [76]	4,5 months	34	BNT162b2 2 doses	Prevaccination 1, 3, 7, 14 and 21 days after 1st and 2nd dose	Anti-RBD antibodies (IgA, IgM and IgG)	Homemade ELISA/s-VNA commercial kit	Neutralizing antibodies in HM increased after the 2nd dose. Neutralizing antibodies in HM were detectable even 3 weeks after 2nd dose. Dominance of IgG1 response post vaccination.

Table 4. *Cont.*

Author (Year, Country)	Duration of Study	Lactating Women (N)	Vaccine Type	Time of Sample HM Collection	Studied Immunoglobulins	Antibody Measurement Method	Outcome/Results
Low JM. et al. (2021, Singapore) [66]	NA	14	BNT162b2 2 doses	Prevaccination 1–3 and 7–10 days post 1st dose, 3–7 days and 4–6 weeks post 2nd dose	Anti-Spike and anti-RBD antibodies (IgA and IgG)	Homemade ELISA	Presence of IgA antibodies in 93% of participants. Higher IgA titers 3–7 days after the 2nd dose. IgA titers waned 4–6 weeks after the 2nd dose. IgG antibodies detected in all samples. IgG titers increased after the 2nd dose. Stable high IgG titers even 4–6 weeks after the 2nd dose. No severe adverse effects in participants.
Baird JK. et al. (2021, USA) [68]	NA	7	mRNA-1273/BNT162b2 2 doses	Prevaccination 1, 4, 7 and 14 days post 1st and 2nd dose and 1 day before 2nd dose	Anti-S and anti-RBD antibodies (IgA and IgG)	Homemade ELISA	Vaccination mainly induced IgG response. No significant difference between 2 vaccines. Antibodies present even 80 days after vaccination in 1 sample collected.
Juncker HG. et al. (2021, The Netherlands) [70]	1 month	20	BNT162b2 2 doses	Prevaccination 3, 5, 7, 9, 11, 13 and 15–17 days after 1st and 2nd doses and 1 day before 2nd dose	Anti-SARS-CoV-2 antibodies (IgA)	Homemade ELISA	Increased IgA titers 5–7 days after the 1st dose. IgA titers decreased by 50% between Day 15 and 21. IgA titers increased by 1.3 times after the 2nd dose compared to the 1st one.

Table 4. *Cont.*

Author (Year, Country)	Duration of Study	Lactating Women (N)	Vaccine Type	Time of Sample HM Collection	Studied Immunoglobulins	Antibody Measurement Method	Outcome/Results
Rosenberg-Friedman M. et al. (2021, Israel) [71]	NA	10	BNT162b2 2 doses	7 and 14 days post 1st and 2nd doses	Anti-S and anti-RBD antibodies (IgA and IgG)	Homemade ELISA	IgG titers peaked 7 days after the 2nd dose. IgG titers remained high on Day 14 after the 2nd dose. Increased IgA titers 7 days post the 2nd dose. Increased neutralizing capacity observed after vaccination.
Scrimin F. et al. (2022, Switzerland) [72]	6 months	40	mRNA-1273/BNT162b2 2 doses ChAdOx1-S 2 or 1 dose	20–30 days, 1–2 months or 3–4 months post 2nd dose	Anti-SARS-CoV-2 antibodies (IgA and IgG)	ELISA commercial kit/NAA	IgG antibodies detected in all samples. IgG present even 4 months after the 2nd dose. No severe adverse effects in participants.
Marshall N.E. et al. (2022, USA) [45]	NA	28	mRNA-1273/BNT162b2 2 doses	Between 0–12 months postpartum	Anti-RBD antibodies (IgG)	Homemade ELISA	Half life of IgG in HM is about 2 months. Positive correlation between IgG titers in HM and serum. IgG1 and IgG3 are present in higher titers compared to IgG4 antibodies.
Esteve-Palau E. et al. (2021, Spain) [75]	NA	33	mRNA -based BNT162b2 2 doses	2 weeks after 1st dose and 2 and 4 weeks after 2nd dose	Anti-S antibodies (IgG)	Serology test	Increased IgG titers after 2nd dose. Positive correlation between serum and HM IgG titers.

Table 4. *Cont.*

Author (Year, Country)	Duration of Study	Lactating Women (N)	Vaccine Type	Time of Sample HM Collection	Studied Immunoglobulins	Antibody Measurement Method	Outcome/Results
Gonçalves J. et al. (2021, Portugal) [74]	7 months	23	mRNA-1273/BNT162b2 2 doses	Prevaccination, a median of 10 days after 1st and 2nd dose	Anti-S antibodies (sIgA/IgA, IgM and IgG)	Homemade ELISA	Antibodies present in the HM of 96% of participants. Increased IgG titers after the 2nd dose. Increased IgA titers after the 1st dose. Poorly increased IgM antibodies after vaccination. Positive correlation between IgA and IgG titers in HM. Positive correlation between IgA titers in serum and HM. Antibody titers were not correlated with maternal age.
Lechosa-Muniz C. et al. (2023, Spain) [88]	6 months	62	mRNA-1273/BNT162b2 2 doses ChAdOx1-S 1 dose	6 months post vaccination	Anti-S antibodies (IgA and IgG)	Homemade ELISA/CLIA commercial kit	No significant difference in antibody levels according to vaccine type.
Charepe N. et al. (2021, Portugal) [73]	2 months	14	BNT162b2 2 doses	1–3 weeks post 1st and 2nd dose	Anti-S antibodies (IgA, IgM and IgG)	Homemade ELISA	Increased IgG titers after the 2nd dose. IgA peaked after the 1st dose. No IgM response was observed.
Kelly JC. et al. (2021, USA) [78]	NA	5	BNT162b2 2 doses	Prevaccination within 24 h after 1st dose and a week post vaccination	Anti-S antibodies (IgA and IgG)	ELISA	Anti-S antibodies were present in HM.

Anti-S antibodies = antibodies against Spike protein, anti-RBD = antibodies against receptor-binding domain, CLIA = Chemiluminescent Immuno Assay, ELISA = enzyme-linked immunosorbent assay, IgA = Immunoglobulin A, IgG = Immunoglobulin G, IgM = Immunoglobulin M, MNA = microneutralizing assay, NA = not acquired, NAA, neutralizing antibody assay, PCR test = Polymerase chain reaction, PNA = Pseudovirus neutralization assay, sVNT = surrogate virus neutralization assay.

In total, 874 infected pregnant women, 537 infected lactating women, 196 vaccinated pregnant women and 1450 vaccinated lactating women were included in this systematic review. In the case of pregnant women, all samples were collected postpartum and most of them were collected within the 1st week postpartum. In some cases, samples were collected later, even 6 months after delivery in one study [27]. HM samples from lactating women were collected in variable time-points, with the longest being 6–10 months post infection or vaccination [43,51,54,56,62]. All studies detected specific immunoglobulins against SARS-CoV-2. Infection mainly induces the production of specific IgA antibodies [17,30–43,46,47,83–86], while vaccination mostly elicits the IgG response [22,25,27,29,32,38,42,44,46,47]. From the included studies, it seems that maternal age and BMI do not influence antibody titers. Yet, the general immune response of the mother and consequently the titers of some immunoglobulins in HM and maternal serum seem to correlate with the levels of other immunoglobulins in HM [16,21].

SARS-CoV-2 virus was not detected in HM samples in any study [18,20,24,30,36,38,40], and no study reported severe side effects after vaccination [42,53,63,65,66,72].

4. Discussion

Breastfeeding is the best dietary choice for infants [4]. HM contains specific immunoglobulins that are produced in response to exposure of the mother to pathogens. These immunoglobulins maintain their structural integrity in the infant's stomach, bind to intestinal mucus and prevent pathogens from entering the bloodstream [89–91]. The presence of specific immunoglobulins against SARS-CoV-2 in the HM of infected or vaccinated mothers could potentially shield neonates and infants from future infections or even from severe disease.

4.1. Post Infection Immune Response

This systematic review affirms that specific immunoglobulins against SARS-CoV-2 virus were detected in the HM of women who were infected during pregnancy or lactation. These immunoglobulins were mainly IgA, and specifically secretory IgA antibodies, and less IgM and IgG were found [17,20,25,28,32,35,36,43,82], which is compatible with the known proportion of antibody isotypes in human milk [92]. They also primarily (80%) targeted the RBD domain of the S1 subunit [17].

4.1.1. Anti-SARS-CoV-2 IgA Immunoglobulins

IgA titers in HM increase one week after infection, and these titers are even higher 2 weeks post COVID-19 disease [40]. Many studies indicate that they remain high in HM and detectable even 2–3 months after infection [27,31,34,35,38–40,42,43,83,85,86]. Pace RM et al. reported that IgA remained positive in 77% of 64 lactating women 2 months after infection [40]. Junker HG et al. found that HM conversion was observed after a median of 15 days and IgA levels peaked after 35 days. After 70 days, however, IgA was detectable only in 33% of HM samples [42]. Conti MG et al. reported that IgA was detectable in all HM samples of 28 lactating women even 2 months after delivery [23]. These women had been infected during pregnancy, which indicates that IgA may persist for a longer period of time. Indeed, other studies confirm their persistence in HM even 5–10 months post COVID-19 disease [34,39,43]. Fox A. et al. reported that all of the 28 tested women in their study had detectable IgA in HM 4–10 months after infection and 43% of them had even higher titers than what they had at 1 month after the infection [43]. The presence of specific IgA against SARS-CoV-2 in HM is optimal for infants. According to a recent cross-sectional study in Brazil, the titers of IgA in the HM of women infected during pregnancy were negatively correlated with the presence of clinical symptoms in their neonates [83].

Various factors influence anti-SARS-CoV-2 IgA levels in HM. The concentration of specific IgA immunoglobulins in HM is positively correlated with the levels of total IgA, IgM and IgG titers in HM [21]. Additionally, levels of specific IgG in maternal serum are also significantly correlated with IgA levels in HM [16]. However, this is not the case for

IgA titers in serum. There is no reported association between IgA titers in HM and maternal serum [25,35,47]. This is logical as IgA in HM after natural infection is not of serum origin, but of muscular origin [93].

As for the time from infection, the data are conflicting. Some report a negative correlation with antibody titers [21,23], while others report a positive correlation [37]. Infection induces a humoral response and antibody titers begin to rise. After an unknown period of time, they reach a peak, and then they begin to wane over time [94]. Therefore, contradicting results in the studies may be due to different time-points of sample collection.

Additionally, not all types of antibodies have the same response over time. Bobik T.V. et al. tested sIgA against specific epitopes of SARS-CoV-2 virus (N protein, linear NTD, RBD-SD1 and RBD) and reported that the levels of sIgA against N-protein and against linear NTD and RBD-SD1 were higher in women that were infected during the third trimester compared to women infected during the first and second trimesters. Regarding sIgA against RBD, they found that their levels were similar, independent of the trimester of pregnancy when infection occurred [19]. No correlation between time of infection during pregnancy and anti-RBD antibodies was reported by Szczygioł, P. et al. either [28]. This indicates that this kind of antibody is more stable over time. Interestingly, Wachman EM et al. reported that anti-RBD IgA titers were not stable but significantly higher in women infected during the first or second trimester of pregnancy [84].

The severity of COVID-19 disease is another factor, but its impact on antibody titers has not yet been clarified. Pace, R.M et al. reported higher concentrations of antibodies in the HM of women with symptomatic COVID-19 disease than in the HM of asymptomatic women; yet, the difference was not significantly important [40]. In other relevant studies, no association between the two parameters has been found [28,83]. Probably, the severity of the disease has a positive impact on antibody levels. Many other studies on the general population have reported that antibody titers are higher in people with severe/moderate COVID-19 disease [94]. More studies are required to reach safe conclusions. From the existing data in the literature, no correlation has been found between IgA levels in HM and maternal age or infant gender [35,37].

4.1.2. Anti-SARS-CoV-2 IgM Immunoglobulins

IgM immunoglobulins are the second most abundant antibodies in HM, and yet their titers are significantly lower than IgA titers. In a prospective study, Decenti EC detected anti-SARS-CoV-2 antibodies in only 7.5% of milk samples [26]. Specific IgM against 2 SARS-CoV-2 was mainly detected in samples collected 10–40 days after infection, and after that, their levels declined [20,21]. In a relevant study by Luo QQ et al., a positive correlation between IgM levels in HM and maternal serum was found [24]. The presence of IgM antibodies against infectious diseases in HM can provide passive immunity to infants, while simultaneously hindering the entry and transportation of viruses, such as HIV, to the infant [95,96]. Given these findings, it is plausible that breastfeeding by SARS-CoV-2-infected mothers offers postpartum protection to the infant through antibodies, reducing the risk of viral transmission.

4.1.3. Anti-SARS-CoV-2 IgG Immunoglobulins

HM contains low titers of IgG immunoglobulins, and in some studies they were not even detectable [20,24]. Decenti, E. C. et al. studied HM samples from 141 women, and they detected IgG only in 3% of the study population [26]. Bauerl et al. reported low IgG titers in HM, with an increase in these titers from Day 40 to Day 205 after COVID-19 disease [21]. Pullen KM et al. detected IgG in a low concentration, but they did not observe any significant change in the titers over time (the mean time of sample collection was 66 days post infection). They also claimed that IgG was functionally attenuated compared to IgA and IgM [35]. In another 2 studies, low titers of IgG 0–3 months after delivery were reported [23,81]. Contrarily to the previous studies, Fox. A. et al. reported that they detected anti-S IgG antibodies in 75% of participants, with 13% of them being present in high titers [43]. The factors that influence their titers in HM are not all clear, but there is a positive correlation between IgG titers in HM and serum [29,35,47].

4.2. Post Vaccination Immune Response

The vaccination of pregnant or lactating women against SARS-CoV-2 also induces the secretion of specific anti-spike antibodies in HM. However, there are some differences in this immune response compared to the one after natural infection. First of all, vaccination mainly induces an IgG response and less of an IgA response [22,25,32,38,42,46–79]. After mRNA vaccination, a 10-fold and 100-fold increase in IgA and IgG titers was observed, respectively [47]. Vaccination induces no significant increase in secretory antibodies' titers. IgA seems to be almost exclusively of systemic and not mucosal origin [55]. Pietrasanta et al. measured two subtypes of specific anti-S IgA antibodies, IgA1, which has systemic origin, and IgA2, which is mainly detected in mucosal secretions, and they observed that the antibodies were mainly IgA1 [53]. These differences in immune response are probably due to the intramuscular route of vaccine administration [50,67].

4.2.1. Anti-SARS-CoV-2 IgG Immunoglobulins

IgG titers were detected in 87–100% of women post vaccination [50,62,65,66,72,77]. Only in one study was a moderate IgG immune response (43% of women) observed [73]. IgG titers in HM increase after each dose [38,47,50,52,55,63,67,71,74,75]. The peak of anti-S1-IgG titers occurs about 1–2 weeks after the 2nd dose and after that they wane [48,51–53,56,62,65,66,71]. A recent longitudinal study reported that IgG antibodies' half lives in HM are about 2 months [45]. In other relevant studies, no significant difference in IgG titers was observed between 30 and 60 days post vaccination [57,80]. Even IgG levels wane over time, but remain in detectable levels 2 [57], 3 [38,53,72] and 6 months post vaccination [49,73]. Contrarily with total IgG levels, secretory IgG antibodies continuously increase even 6 months after the first dose of mRNA vaccines [54]. The main IgG subclasses in HM after 2 doses of mRNA-based vaccines are IgG1 and IgG3, which are the main subclasses of IgG that emerge after viral infections [45,97]. Interestingly, Agostinis C. et al., in a recent study, demonstrated that the presence of anti-S IgG in the HM of vaccinated lactating women is capable of activating in vitro the complement [80]. All of these data indicate that vaccinated mothers are capable of providing protective antibodies to their offspring for a long time after their primary vaccination.

As for the factors influencing antibody levels in HM, numerous studies have confirmed a significant positive correlation between IgG titers in HM and maternal serum [25,29,45,47,48,51,56,62–64,69,75,77,79,80]. A positive correlation between the lactation period and the total antibody titers was also reported in a study by Trofin F. et al. (lactating period between 3 and 36 months) [57]. However, this was not confirmed in other studies during the lactation period between 1.5 and 23 months [50,73]. A negative correlation was reported with parity [57], while no correlation was confirmed between IgG levels and maternal age or BMI [57,69,74].

4.2.2. Anti-SARS-CoV-2 IgA Immunoglobulins

IgA immunoglobulins in detectable levels are present in 75–95% of vaccinated women at 2 weeks after the 2nd dose [42,63,65,66,74]. In a prospective study, though, detectable levels were present in just 36% of women post vaccination [73]. Yet, it is not clear if IgA rises mainly after the 1st dose, without any additional increase after the 2nd dose [38,47,63,67,73,74], or whether their titers present a biphasic model after vaccination [42,52,55,65,66,70,71]. Many studies indicate waning IgA titers about one month after the 1st vaccine dose [44,49,51,56]. Contrarily, Juncker HG et al. reported that IgA titers peaked 2 weeks after the 1st dose, and then they waned until the 2nd dose, when they finally reached a second peak 5 days after vaccination [70]. Ricciardi et al. studied secretory IgA and they observed peak titers at 3 weeks after the 2nd dose, while their concentration significantly decreased at 6 months post vaccination [54]. Perez SE et al. detected IgA antibodies in about 50% and 25% of samples at 1 and 3 months post vaccination, respectively [62]. Finally, Narayanaswamy et al. observed no difference in anti-RBD IgA median titers before and after vaccination [50].

A positive correlation was found between IgA titers in HM and IgG titers in maternal serum [51,62,69,74]. A positive correlation may also exist between the IgA titers in HM and the IgA titers in maternal serum [25,47,64]; however, this finding is not supported by all studies [74]. The lactation period is also another factor which has an impact on IgA titers, and is not clearly defined by the included studies. A positive impact (lactation period between 3 and 36 months) [57] was reported in one study, while in others, either a negative (lactation period <18 months) [63] or no impact (lactation period 1.5–23 months for infants) [50] was reported. A negative correlation was found between antibody concentration and parity [57], and there was no correlation with maternal age [57,74].

4.2.3. Anti-SARS-CoV-2 IgM immunoglobulins

Vaccination does not significantly influence IgM levels in HM. In the majority of studies, they are not even detectable [50,51,64,69,73,79], and in others they are just poorly detected [62,74].

4.3. Differences in Immune Response after Infection or Vaccination

Higher IgG titers were observed in the HM of vaccinated women compared to those who were previously infected with SARS-CoV-2 [22,25,32]. In the case of IgA, the data are ambiguous, with some studies reporting higher antibody titers after vaccination [27], some reporting lower [52] and some reporting no significant difference after vaccination or infection [42]. As has already been mentioned, infection mainly induces IgA and, to a lesser extent, the IgM immune response, while vaccination primarily stimulates the production of IgG antibodies. IgA and IgG are found mainly in secretory form and they are released by mammary tissue to HM. After a natural infection with SARS-CoV-2, B-cells stimulated in the lymphoid tissues of the respiratory tract migrate to the mammary gland and release secretory antibodies into HM [93]. Contrarily, post vaccination antiSARS-CoV-2 antibodies in HM are derived from maternal serum [11]. Secretory IgA antibodies are attached to the gastrointestinal tract of breastfeeding infants, where they bind with local microorganisms and block their penetration [4]. On the other hand, IgG antibodies produced post vaccination have been found to be capable of activating the complement. Therefore, infants can benefit from both types of antibodies in different ways [80].

As for the type of immunoglobulins, vaccination induces anti-spike protein antibodies. Infection, on the other hand, mainly induces the anti-N protein. A relative study by Bobik T.V. et al. reported significantly lower levels of the anti-RBD antibody compared to anti-N antibodies in the HM of lactating women infected during the third trimester [19]. L.Bode et al., in a recent study, reported that IgA antibodies in the HM of infected women are mainly directed against the N protein (about 43%) and less against the S protein (about 24%), and there was heterogeneity in the type and quantity of antibodies.

4.4. Differences in Immune Response According to Vaccine Type

No difference between detected antibody titers was described in women vaccinated with Moderna or Pfizer/BioNtech vaccines [32,52,57,63,68,88]. Only in one study of Gray KJ et al. were higher IgA titers detected in the Moderna group after the 2nd dose [67]. However, compared to the adenovirus-vectored vaccines, mRNA vaccines induce higher titers of antibodies [52,58,61]. Yang X. et al. reported that IgG and IgA levels were detectable in 86–100% and 52–71%, respectively, in mRNA-vaccinated women, and in 33–38% and 17–23%, respectively, in the adenovirus-vector-vaccinated women [58]. The Moderna vaccine also induces significantly higher titers of secretory antibodies compared with the rest of the vaccines [58]. Yet, six months post vaccination, no significant difference in antibody titers was observed among three types of vaccines [88].

4.5. Neutralizing Capacity

Although specific antibodies against SARS-CoV-2 are present in HM after COVID-19 disease or vaccination, it is essential to clarify whether these antibodies have neutralizing capacity. A neutralizing antibody binds with the viral surface and blocks its replication cycle, and so it protects the subject from subsequent infection [98]. Both infection [18,27,30, 32,36,43,44,82] and vaccination [22,27,32,44,50,51,53,56,62,71,76,77] induce the production of neutralizing antibodies in HM, more intense, though, post infection [38,44].

In a study of 38 infected lactating women, no correlation between specific anti-SARS-CoV-2 antibody levels and the neutralization capacity of the HM was observed [31]. However, this is not in line with what other studies support. The neutralizing capacity against SARS-CoV-2 seems to be greater in the HM of infected women compared to the pre-pandemic controls, and it also seems to be positively correlated with antibody titers [18,27,30,32,36,43,44,82]. In a relevant study, 62% of the samples had neutralizing antibodies in vitro. Contrarily, the samples collected from the pre-pandemic controls had no neutralizing capacity [36]. Pace RM et al. reported that the HM neutralizing capacity post infection is significantly correlated with anti-RBD antibody levels [30].

Antibody titers also seem to influence the neutralizing capacity of the HM of vaccinated women [44,62]. As for variants, vaccination seems to be more beneficial against the Wuhan-Hu-1 strain and less against the Beta, Gamma and Delta variants. The binding capacity of antibodies is reduced by 30% to these strains [49]. In another study, less of a neutralizing capacity was reported against the Beta variant compared to D614G, Alpha and Gamma [50].

Our systematic review has some limitations. SARS-CoV-2 is a new virus. In the early stages of the pandemic, many studies were conducted with small sample sizes and lacked inclusion criteria. Furthermore, most of the tests used were homemade ELISA assays, which lacked standardization in terms of measurement units. Due to the great heterogeneity of the studies included, not only regarding the type of laboratory test, but also the differences in the timing of sampling between studies and study subjects (pregnant or lactating women), a meta-analysis was not deemed appropriate and instead we focused on presenting a systematic review of the available literature.

5. Conclusions

Infection with SARS-CoV-2 and vaccination against the virus elicit a maternal immune response in breastfeeding mothers with a short period of 1–2 weeks. Consequently, these mothers can transmit specific immunoglobulins with neutralizing capacity to their infants via HM. Therefore, it is recommended that breastfeeding is encouraged in mothers infected or vaccinated, as their HM can provide infants with specific antibodies even months after infection or vaccination.

Infection primarily induces an IgA-mediated immune response, while vaccination mainly elevates IgG immunoglobulins. Our data suggest that both IgA and IgG immunoglobulins contribute to the neutralizing capacity of HM, indicating clinical benefits for infants who receive HM from vaccinated or infected women. However, further studies are required to determine whether factors such as infection severity, lactation period, parity, maternal age and BMI have an impact on the levels of immunoglobulins in HM.

Supplementary Materials: The following supporting information can be downloaded at: https://www.mdpi.com/article/10.3390/nu15081905/s1, Supplement: PRISMA 2020 check list.

Author Contributions: Conceptualization, M.D., R.S., Z.I. and N.I.; methodology, R.S. and M.D.; data curation, M.D., A.P., R.S., T.B., G.K., N.I. and Z.I.; investigation, R.S. and N.I.; writing—original draft preparation, M.D., R.S. and N.I.; writing—review and editing, M.D., T.B., R.S., N.I. and Z.I. All authors have read and agreed to the published version of the manuscript.

Funding: This research received no external funding.

Institutional Review Board Statement: Not applicable.

Informed Consent Statement: Not applicable.

Data Availability Statement: Data are contained within the article.

Conflicts of Interest: The authors declare no conflict of interest.

References

1. WHO Coronavirus (COVID-19) Dashboard | WHO Coronavirus (COVID-19) Dashboard with Vaccination Data. Available online: https://covid19.who.int/ (accessed on 7 February 2023).
2. Newborn Mortality. Available online: https://www.who.int/news-room/fact-sheets/detail/levels-and-trends-in-child-mortality-report-2021 (accessed on 7 February 2023).
3. COVID-19 Vaccination for Children | CDC. Available online: https://www.cdc.gov/vaccines/covid-19/planning/children.html (accessed on 7 February 2023).
4. Dimitroglou, M.; Iliodromiti, Z.; Christou, E.; Volaki, P.; Petropoulou, C.; Sokou, R.; Boutsikou, T.; Iacovidou, N. Human Breast Milk: The Key Role in the Maturation of Immune, Gastrointestinal and Central Nervous Systems: A Narrative Review. *Diagnostics* **2022**, *12*, 2208. [CrossRef] [PubMed]
5. Clinical Management of COVID-19: Interim Guidance, 27 May 2020. Available online: https://apps.who.int/iris/handle/10665/332196 (accessed on 14 November 2022).
6. Halasa, N.B.; Olson, S.M.; Staat, M.A.; Newhams, M.M.; Price, A.M.; Boom, J.A.; Sahni, L.C.; Cameron, M.A.; Pannaraj, P.S.; Bline, K.E.; et al. Effectiveness of Maternal Vaccination with MRNA COVID-19 Vaccine during Pregnancy against COVID-19-Associated Hospitalization in Infants Aged. *MMWR Morb. Mortal. Wkly. Rep.* **2022**, *71*, 264–270. [CrossRef] [PubMed]
7. Huang, Y.; Yang, C.; Xu, X.-F.; Xu, W.; Liu, S.-W. Structural and Functional Properties of SARS-CoV-2 Spike Protein: Potential Antivirus Drug Development for COVID-19. *Acta Pharmacol. Sin.* **2020**, *41*, 1141–1149. [CrossRef] [PubMed]
8. Ye, Q.; Lu, S.; Corbett, K.D. Structural Basis for SARS-CoV-2 Nucleocapsid Protein Recognition by Single-Domain Antibodies. *Front. Immunol.* **2021**, *12*, 719037. [CrossRef]
9. Batra, M.; Tian, R.; Zhang, C.; Clarence, E.; Sacher, C.S.; Miranda, J.N.; De La Fuente, J.R.O.; Mathew, M.; Green, D.; Patel, S.; et al. Role of IgG against N-Protein of SARS-COV2 in COVID-19 Clinical Outcomes. *Sci. Rep.* **2021**, *11*, 3455. [CrossRef]
10. Cafaro, A.; Sangster, M.; Yuan, M.; Shah, P.; Canziani, G.A.; Carter, E.P.; Chaiken, I. The Case for S2: The Potential Benefits of the S2 Subunit of the SARS-CoV-2 Spike Protein as an Immunogen in Fighting the COVID-19 Pandemic. *Front. Immunol.* **2021**, *1*, 637651. [CrossRef]
11. Nicolaidou, V.; Georgiou, R.; Christofidou, M.; Felekkis, K.; Pieri, M.; Papaneophytou, C. Detection of SARS-CoV-2-Specific Antibodies in Human Breast Milk and Their Neutralizing Capacity after COVID-19 Vaccination: A Systematic Review. *Int. J. Mol. Sci.* **2023**, *24*, 2957. [CrossRef]
12. Whited, N.; Cervantes, J. Antibodies against SARS-CoV-2 in Human Breast Milk after Vaccination: A Systematic Review and Meta-Analysis. *Breastfeed. Med.* **2022**, *17*, 475–483. [CrossRef]
13. Low, J.M.; Low, Y.W.; Zhong, Y.; Lee, C.Y.C.; Chan, M.; Ng, N.B.H.; Amin, Z.; Ng, Y.P.M. Titres and Neutralising Capacity of SARS-CoV-2-Specific Antibodies in Human Milk: A Systematic Review. *Arch. Dis. Child. Fetal Neonatal Ed.* **2022**, *107*, F1–F7. [CrossRef]
14. Page, M.J.; McKenzie, J.E.; Bossuyt, P.M.; Boutron, I.; Hoffmann, T.C.; Mulrow, C.D.; Shamseer, L.; Tetzlaff, J.M.; Akl, E.A.; Brennan, S.E.; et al. The PRISMA 2020 Statement: An Updated Guideline for Reporting Systematic Reviews. *BMJ* **2021**, *372*, n71. [CrossRef]
15. Narayanaswamy, V.; Pentecost, B.; Alfandari, D.; Chin, E.; Minor, K.; Kastrinakis, A.; Lieberman, T.; Arcaro, K.F.; Leftwich, H. Humoral and Cell-Mediated Immune Response in Colostrum from Women Diagnosed Positive for SARS-CoV-2. *Breastfeed. Med.* **2021**, *16*, 987–994. [CrossRef] [PubMed]
16. Larcade, R.; DeShea, L.; Lang, G.A.; Caballero, M.T.; Ferretti, A.; Beasley, W.H.; Tipple, T.E.; Vain, N.; Prudent, L.; Lang, M.L.; et al. Maternal-Fetal Immunologic Response to SARS-CoV-2 Infection in a Symptomatic Vulnerable Population: A Prospective Cohort. *J. Infect. Dis.* **2021**, *225*, 800–809. [CrossRef] [PubMed]
17. Fox, A.; Marino, J.; Amanat, F.; Krammer, F.; Hahn-Holbrook, J.; Zolla-Pazner, S.; Powell, R.L. Robust and Specific Secretory IgA against SARS-CoV-2 Detected in Human Milk. *iScience* **2020**, *23*, 101735. [CrossRef] [PubMed]
18. Gao, X.; Wang, S.; Zeng, W.; Chen, S.; Wu, J.; Lin, X.; Liu, Y.; Sun, Z.; Feng, L. Clinical and Immunologic Features among COVID-19-Affected Mother-Infant Pairs: Antibodies to SARS-CoV-2 Detected in Breast Milk. *New Microbes New Infect.* **2020**, *37*, 100752. [CrossRef] [PubMed]
19. Bobik, T.V.; Kostin, N.N.; Skryabin, G.A.; Tsabai, P.N.; Simonova, M.A.; Knorre, V.D.; Mokrushina, Y.A.; Smirnov, I.V.; Kosolapova, J.A.; Vtorushina, V.V.; et al. Epitope-Specific Response of Human Milk Immunoglobulins in COVID-19 Recovered Women. *Pathogens* **2021**, *10*, 705. [CrossRef]
20. Peng, S.; Zhu, H.; Yang, L.; Cao, L.; Huang, X.; Dynes, M.; Narayan, A.; Xia, J.; Chen, Y.; Zhang, P.; et al. A Study of Breastfeeding Practices, SARS-CoV-2 and Its Antibodies in the Breast Milk of Mothers Confirmed with COVID-19. *Lancet Reg. Health -West. Pacific* **2020**, *4*, 100045. [CrossRef]

21. Bäuerl, C.; Randazzo, W.; Sánchez, G.; Selma-Royo, M.; García Verdevio, E.; Martínez, L.; Parra-Llorca, A.; Lerin, C.; Fumadó, V.; Crovetto, F.; et al. SARS-CoV-2 RNA and Antibody Detection in Breast Milk from a Prospective Multicentre Study in Spain. *Arch. Dis. Child. Fetal Neonatal Ed.* **2021**, *107*, 216–221. [CrossRef]
22. Collier, A.R.Y.; McMahan, K.; Yu, J.; Tostanoski, L.H.; Aguayo, R.; Ansel, J.; Chandrashekar, A.; Patel, S.; Apraku Bondzie, E.; Sellers, D.; et al. Immunogenicity of COVID-19 MRNA Vaccines in Pregnant and Lactating Women. *JAMA* **2021**, *325*, 2370–2380. [CrossRef]
23. Conti, M.G.; Terreri, S.; Piano Mortari, E.; Albano, C.; Natale, F.; Boscarino, G.; Zacco, G.; Palomba, P.; Cascioli, S.; Corrente, F.; et al. Immune Response of Neonates Born to Mothers Infected with SARS-CoV-2. *JAMA Netw. Open* **2021**, *4*, e2132563. [CrossRef]
24. Luo, Q.Q.; Xia, L.; Yao, D.J.; Wu, M.; Wang, H.B.; Luo, M.H.; Jiang, X.; Chen, H. Breastfeeding in Mothers with COVID-19: Insights from Laboratory Tests and Follow-up from Early Outbreak of the Pandemic in China. *J. Women's Health* **2021**, *30*, 1546–1555. [CrossRef]
25. Conti, M.G.; Terreri, S.; Terrin, G.; Natale, F.; Pietrasanta, C.; Salvatori, G.; Brunelli, R.; Midulla, F.; Papaevangelou, V.; Carsetti, R.; et al. Severe Acute Respiratory Syndrome Coronavirus 2 Infection versus Vaccination in Pregnancy: Implications for Maternal and Infant Immunity. *Clin. Infect. Dis.* **2022**, *75*, S37–S45. [CrossRef] [PubMed]
26. Decenti, E.C.; Salvatore, M.A.; Mancon, A.; Portella, G.; Rocca, A.; Vocale, C.; Donati, S. A Large Series of Molecular and Serological Specimens to Evaluate Mother-to-Child SARS-CoV-2 Transmission: A Prospective Study from the Italian Obstetric Surveillance System. *Int. J. Infect. Dis.* **2022**, *126*, 1–9. [CrossRef] [PubMed]
27. Olearo, F.; Radmanesh, L.S.; Felber, N.; von Possel, R.; Emmerich, P.; Pekarek, N.; Pfefferle, S.; Nörz, D.; Hansen, G.; Diemert, A.; et al. Anti-SARS-CoV-2 Antibodies in Breast Milk during Lactation after Infection or Vaccination: A Cohort Study. *J. Reprod. Immunol.* **2022**, *153*, 103685. [CrossRef]
28. Szczygioł, P.; Łukianowski, B.; Kościelska-Kasprzak, K.; Jakuszko, K.; Bartoszek, D.; Krajewska, M.; Królak-Olejnik, B. Antibodies in the Breastmilk of COVID-19 Recovered Women. *BMC Pregnancy Childbirth* **2022**, *22*, 635. [CrossRef] [PubMed]
29. Nir, O.; Schwartz, A.; Toussia-Cohen, S.; Leibovitch, L.; Strauss, T.; Asraf, K.; Doolman, R.; Sharabi, S.; Cohen, C.; Lustig, Y.; et al. Maternal-Neonatal Transfer of SARS-CoV-2 Immunoglobulin G Antibodies among Parturient Women Treated with BNT162b2 Messenger RNA Vaccine during Pregnancy. *Am. J. Obstet. Gynecol. MFM* **2022**, *4*, 100492. [CrossRef]
30. Pace, R.M.; Williams, J.E.; Järvinen, K.M.; Belfort, M.B.; Pace, C.D.; Lackey, K.A.; Gogel, A.C.; Nguyen-Contant, P.; Kanagaiah, P.; Fitzgerald, T.; et al. COVID-19 and Human Milk: SARS-CoV-2, Antibodies, and Neutralizing Capacity. *medRxiv Prepr. Serv. Health Sci.* **2020**, *12*. [CrossRef]
31. van Keulen, B.J.; Romijn, M.; Bondt, A.; Dingess, K.A.; Kontopodi, E.; van der Straten, K.; Den Boer, M.A.; Burger, J.A.; Poniman, M.; Bosch, B.J.; et al. Human Milk from Previously COVID-19-Infected Mothers: The Effect of Pasteurization on Specific Antibodies and Neutralization Capacity. *Nutrients* **2021**, *13*, 1645. [CrossRef]
32. Demers-Mathieu, V.; Hakansson, A.P.; Hall, S.; Lavangnananda, S.; Fels, S.; Medo, E. Functional Antibodies against SARS-CoV-2 Receptor Binding Domain Variants with Mutations N501Y or E484K in Human Milk from COVID-19-Vaccinated, -Recovered, and -Unvaccinated Women. *Breastfeed. Med.* **2022**, *17*, 163–172. [CrossRef]
33. Demers-Mathieu, V.; DaPra, C.; Fels, S.; Medo, E. Receptor-Binding Domain Severe Acute Respiratory Syndrome Coronavirus 2-Specific Antibodies in Human Milk from Mothers with Coronavirus Disease 2019 Polymerase Chain Reaction or with Symptoms Suggestive of Coronavirus Disease 2019. *J. Pediatr. Gastroenterol. Nutr.* **2021**, *73*, 125–128. [CrossRef]
34. Juncker, H.G.; Romijn, M.; Loth, V.N.; Ruhé, E.J.M.; Bakker, S.; Kleinendorst, S.; de Groot, C.J.M.; Pajkrt, D.; Korosi, A.; van Goudoever, J.B.; et al. Antibodies against SARS-CoV-2 in Human Milk: Milk Conversion Rates in The Netherlands. *J. Hum. Lact.* **2021**, *37*, 469–476. [CrossRef]
35. Pullen, K.M.; Atyeo, C.; Collier, A.R.Y.; Gray, K.J.; Belfort, M.B.; Lauffenburger, D.A.; Edlow, A.G.; Alter, G. Selective Functional Antibody Transfer into the Breastmilk after SARS-CoV-2 Infection. *Cell Rep.* **2021**, *37*, 109959. [CrossRef]
36. Pace, R.M.; Williams, J.E.; Järvinen, K.M.; Belfort, M.B.; Pace, C.D.W.; Lackey, K.A.; Gogel, A.C.; Nguyen-Contant, P.; Kanagaiah, P.; Fitzgerald, T.; et al. Characterization of SARS-CoV-2 RNA, Antibodies, and Neutralizing Capacity in Milk Produced by Women with COVID-19. *MBio* **2021**, *12*, e03192-20. [CrossRef] [PubMed]
37. Demers-Mathieu, V.; Dapra, C.; Medo, E. Comparison of Severe Acute Respiratory Syndrome Coronavirus 2-Specific Antibodies' Binding Capacity between Human Milk and Serum from Coronavirus Disease 2019-Recovered Women. *Breastfeed. Med.* **2021**, *16*, 393–401. [CrossRef] [PubMed]
38. Young, B.E.; Seppo, A.E.; Diaz, N.; Rosen-Carole, C.; Nowak-Wegrzyn, A.; Cruz Vasquez, J.M.; Ferri-Huerta, R.; Nguyen-Contant, P.; Fitzgerald, T.; Sangster, M.Y.; et al. Association of Human Milk Antibody Induction, Persistence, and Neutralizing Capacity with SARS-CoV-2 Infection vs. MRNA Vaccination. *JAMA Pediatr.* **2021**, *176*, 159. [CrossRef] [PubMed]
39. Juncker, H.G.; Romijn, M.; Loth, V.N.; Caniels, T.G.; de Groot, C.J.M.; Pajkrt, D.; van Gils, M.J.; van Goudoever, J.B.; van Keulen, B.J. Human Milk Antibodies against SARS-CoV-2: A Longitudinal Follow-up Study. *J. Hum. Lact.* **2021**, *37*, 485–491. [CrossRef]
40. Pace, R.M.; Williams, J.E.; Järvinen, K.M.; Meehan, C.L.; Martin, M.A.; Ley, S.H.; Barbosa-Leiker, C.; Andres, A.; Yeruva, L.; Belfort, M.B.; et al. Milk from Women Diagnosed with COVID-19 Does Not Contain SARS-CoV-2 RNA but Has Persistent Levels of SARS-CoV-2-Specific IgA Antibodies. *Front. Immunol.* **2021**, *12*, 801797. [CrossRef]
41. Demers-Mathieu, V.; Dapra, C.; Mathijssen, G.; Sela, D.A.; Järvinen, K.M.; Seppo, A.; Fels, S.; Medo, E. Human Milk Antibodies against S1 and S2 Subunits from SARS-CoV-2, HCoV-OC43, and HCoV-229E in Mothers with a Confirmed COVID-19 PCR, Viral SYMPTOMS, and Unexposed Mothers. *Int. J. Mol. Sci.* **2021**, *22*, 1749. [CrossRef]

42. Juncker, H.G.; Mulleners, S.J.; van Gils, M.J.; Bijl, T.P.L.; de Groot, C.J.M.; Pajkrt, D.; Korosi, A.; van Goudoever, J.B.; van Keulen, B.J. Comparison of SARS-CoV-2-Specific Antibodies in Human Milk after MRNA-Based COVID-19 Vaccination and Infection. *Vaccines* **2021**, *9*, 1475. [CrossRef]
43. Fox, A.; Marino, J.; Amanat, F.; Oguntuyo, K.Y.; Hahn-Holbrook, J.; Lee, B.; Zolla-Pazner, S.; Powell, R.L. The IgA in Milk Induced by SARS-CoV-2 Infection Is Comprised of Mainly Secretory Antibody That Is Neutralizing and Highly Durable over Time. *PLoS ONE* **2022**, *17*, e0249723. [CrossRef]
44. Leung, H.Y.H.; Leung, B.W.; Gil, M.M.; Rolle, V.; Moungmaithong, S.; Wang, C.C.; Poon, L.C. SARS-CoV-2-specific Antibodies and Neutralization Capacity in Breast Milk Following Infection vs. Vaccination. *Ultrasound Obstet. Gynecol.* **2022**, *60*, 425. [CrossRef]
45. Marshall, N.E.; Blanton, M.B.; Doratt, B.M.; Malherbe, D.C.; Rincon, M.; True, H.; Mcdonald, T.; Beauregard, C.; Adatorwovor, R.; Messaoudi, I. SARS-CoV-2 Vaccine Booster Elicits Robust Prolonged Maternal Antibody Responses and Passive Transfer via the Placenta and Breastmilk. *bioRxiv* **2022**, *11*, 518385. [CrossRef] [PubMed]
46. Longueira, Y.; Ojeda, D.S.; Battistelli, R.B.A.; Sanchez, L.; Oviedo Rouco, S.; Albano, D.; Guevara, E.; Valls, V.; Pando, M.A.; Gamarnik, A.V. SARS-CoV-2-Specific IgG and IgA Response in Maternal Blood and Breastmilk of Vaccinated Naïve and Convalescent Lactating Participants. *Front. Immunol.* **2022**, *13*, 5514. [CrossRef] [PubMed]
47. Wang, J.; Young, B.E.; Li, D.; Seppo, A.E.; Zhou, Q.; Wiltse, A.; Nowak-Wegrzyn, A.; Murphy, K.; Widrick, K.; Diaz, N.; et al. Broad cross-Reactive IgA and IgG against Human Coronaviruses in Milk Induced by COVID-19 Vaccination and Infection. *medRxiv Prepr. Serv. Health Sci.* **2022**, *10*, 980. [CrossRef] [PubMed]
48. Esteve-Palau, E.; Gonzalez-Cuevas, A.; Guerrero, M.E.; Garcia-Terol, C.; Alvarez, M.C.; Garcia, G.; Moreno, E.; Medina, F.; Casadevall, D.; Diaz-Brito, V. Quantification and Progress over Time of Specific Antibodies against Severe Acute Respiratory Syndrome Coronavirus 2 in Breast Milk of Lactating Women Vaccinated with BNT162b2 Pfizer-BioNTech Coronavirus Disease 2019 Vaccine (LacCOVID). *Open Forum Infect. Dis.* **2022**, *9*, ofac239. [CrossRef]
49. Low, J.M.; Gu, Y.; Ng, M.S.F.; Wang, L.W.; Amin, Z.; Zhong, Y.; Macary, P.A. Human Milk Antibodies after BNT162b2 Vaccination Exhibit Reduced Binding against SARS-CoV-2 Variants of Concern. *Vaccines* **2022**, *10*, 225. [CrossRef]
50. Narayanaswamy, V.; Pentecost, B.T.; Schoen, C.N.; Alfandari, D.; Schneider, S.S.; Baker, R.; Arcaro, K.F. Neutralizing Antibodies and Cytokines in Breast Milk after Coronavirus Disease 2019 (COVID-19) MRNA Vaccination. *Obstet. Gynecol.* **2022**, *139*, 181–191. [CrossRef]
51. Bender, J.M.; Lee, Y.; Cheng, W.A.; Marentes Ruiz, C.J.; Pannaraj, P.S. Coronavirus Disease 2019 Vaccine Booster Effects Are Seen in Human Milk Antibody Response. *Front. Nutr.* **2022**, *9*, 898849. [CrossRef]
52. Selma-Royo, M.; Bäuerl, C.; Mena-Tudela, D.; Aguilar-Camprubí, L.; Pérez-Cano, F.J.; Parra-Llorca, A.; Lerin, C.; Martínez-Costa, C.; Collado, M.C. Anti-SARS-CoV-2 IgA and IgG in Human Milk after Vaccination Is Dependent on Vaccine Type and Previous SARS-CoV-2 Exposure: A Longitudinal Study. *Genome Med.* **2022**, *14*, 42. [CrossRef]
53. Pietrasanta, C.; Darwich, A.; Ronchi, A.; Crippa, B.; Spada, E.; Mosca, F.; Pugni, L.; Rescigno, M. Humoral Response to Anti-SARS-CoV-2 Vaccine in Breastfeeding Mothers and Mother-to-Infant Antibody Transfer through Breast Milk. *NPJ Vaccines* **2022**, *7*, 63. [CrossRef]
54. Ricciardi, A.; Zelini, P.; Cassaniti, I.; Avanzini, M.A.; Colaneri, M.; De Silvestri, A.; Baldanti, F.; Bruno, R. Serum and Breastmilk SARS-CoV-2 Specific Antibodies Following BNT162b2 Vaccine: Prolonged Protection from SARS-CoV-2 in Newborns and Older Children. *Int. J. Infect. Dis.* **2022**, *122*, 905. [CrossRef]
55. Pieri, M.; Maniori, M.A.; Shahabian, L.; Kanaan, E.; Paphiti-Demetriou, I.; Pipis, S.; Felekkis, K.; Nicolaidou, V.; Papaneophytou, C. Survival of Vaccine-Induced Human Milk SARS-CoV-2 IgG, IgA and SIgA Immunoglobulins across Simulated Human Infant Gastrointestinal Digestion. *Nutrients* **2022**, *14*, 3368. [CrossRef] [PubMed]
56. Stafford, L.; Valcarce, V.; Henry, M.; Neu, J.; Parker, L.; Martina, M.; Vicuna, V.; Gowen, T.; Cato, E.; Kosik, I.; et al. Detection of SARS-CoV-2 IgA and IgG in Human Milk and Breastfeeding Infant Stool 6 Months after Maternal COVID-19 Vaccination. *J. Perinatol.* **2023**, 1–7. [CrossRef] [PubMed]
57. Trofin, F.; Nastase, E.V.; Iancu, L.S.; Constantinescu, D.; Cianga, C.M.; Lunca, C.; Ursu, R.G.; Cianga, P.; Dorneanu, O.S. Anti-RBD IgA and IgG Response and Transmission in Breast Milk of Anti-SARS-CoV-2 Vaccinated Mothers. *Pathogens* **2022**, *11*, 286. [CrossRef] [PubMed]
58. Yang, X.; Fox, A.; Decarlo, C.; Norris, C.; Griffin, S.; Wedekind, S.; Flanagan, J.M.; Shenker, N.; Powell, R.L. Comparative Profiles of SARS-CoV-2 Spike-Specific Human Milk Antibodies Elicited by MRNA-and Adenovirus-Based COVID-19 Vaccines. In *Breastfeeding Medicine*; Mary Ann Liebert, Inc.: New York, NY, USA, 2022; Volume 17, pp. 638–646. [CrossRef]
59. Guida, M.; Terracciano, D.; Cennamo, M.; Aiello, F.; La Civita, E.; Esposito, G.; Gargiulo, V.; Maruotti, G.M.; Portella, G.; Sarno, L. COVID-19 Vaccine MRNABNT162b2 Elicits Human Antibody Response in Milk of Breastfeeding Women. *Vaccines* **2021**, *9*, 785. [CrossRef] [PubMed]
60. Valcarce, V.; Stafford, L.S.; Neu, J.; Cacho, N.; Parker, L.; Mueller, M.; Burchfield, D.J.; Li, N.; Larkin, J. Detection of SARS-CoV-2-Specific IgA in the Human Milk of COVID-19 Vaccinated Lactating Health Care Workers. *Breastfeed. Med.* **2021**, *16*, 1004–1009. [CrossRef] [PubMed]
61. Lechosa-Muñiz, C.; Paz-Zulueta, M.; Mendez-Legaza, J.M.; Irure-Ventura, J.; González, R.C.; Montes, J.C.; López-Hoyos, M.; Llorca, J.; Cabero-Pérez, M.J. Induction of SARS-CoV-2-Specific IgG and IgA in Serum and Milk with Different SARS-CoV-2 Vaccines in Breastfeeding Women: A cross-Sectional Study in Northern Spain. *Int. J. Environ. Res. Public Health* **2021**, *18*, 8831. [CrossRef] [PubMed]

62. Perez, S.E.; Luna Centeno, L.D.; Cheng, W.A.; Marentes Ruiz, C.J.; Lee, Y.; Congrave-Wilson, Z.; Powell, R.L.; Stellwagen, L.; Pannaraj, P.S. Human Milk SARS-CoV-2 Antibodies up to 6 Months after Vaccination. *Pediatrics* **2022**, *149*, e2021054260. [CrossRef]
63. Golan, Y.; Prahl, M.; Cassidy, A.G.; Gay, C.; Wu, A.H.B.; Jigmeddagva, U.; Lin, C.Y.; Gonzalez, V.J.; Basilio, E.; Warrier, L.; et al. COVID-19 MRNA Vaccination in Lactation: Assessment of Adverse Events and Vaccine Related Antibodies in Mother-Infant Dyads. *Front. Immunol.* **2021**, *12*, 4596. [CrossRef] [PubMed]
64. Jakuszko, K.; Kościelska-Kasprzak, K.; Żabińska, M.; Bartoszek, D.; Poznański, P.; Rukasz, D.; Kłak, R.; Królak-Olejnik, B.; Krajewska, M. Immune Response to Vaccination against COVID-19 in Breastfeeding Health Workers. *Vaccines* **2021**, *9*, 663. [CrossRef]
65. Perl, S.H.; Uzan-Yulzari, A.; Klainer, H.; Asiskovich, L.; Youngster, M.; Rinott, E.; Youngster, I. SARS-CoV-2-Specific Antibodies in Breast Milk after COVID-19 Vaccination of Breastfeeding Women. *JAMA* **2021**, *325*, 2013–2014. [CrossRef]
66. Low, J.M.; Gu, Y.; Ng, M.S.F.; Amin, Z.; Lee, L.Y.; Ng, Y.P.M.; Shunmuganathan, B.D.; Niu, Y.; Gupta, R.; Tambyah, P.A.; et al. Codominant IgG and IgA Expression with Minimal Vaccine MRNA in Milk of BNT162b2 Vaccinees. *NPJ Vaccines* **2021**, *6*, 105. [CrossRef] [PubMed]
67. Gray, K.J.; Bordt, E.A.; Atyeo, C.; Deriso, E.; Akinwunmi, B.; Young, N.; Baez, A.M.; Shook, L.L.; Cvrk, D.; James, K.; et al. COVID-19 Vaccine Response in Pregnant and Lactating Women: A Cohort Study. *medRxiv* **2021**, preprint. [CrossRef]
68. Baird, J.K.; Jensen, S.M.; Urba, W.J.; Fox, B.A.; Baird, J.R. SARS-CoV-2 Antibodies Detected in Mother's Milk Post-Vaccination. *J. Hum. Lact.* **2021**, *37*, 492–498. [CrossRef] [PubMed]
69. Ramirez, D.S.R.; Perez, M.M.L.; Perez, M.C.; Hernandez, M.I.S.; Pulido, S.M.; Villacampa, L.P.; Vilar, A.M.F.; Falero, M.R.; Carretero, P.G.; Millan, B.R.; et al. SARS-CoV-2 Antibodies in Breast Milk after Vaccination. *Pediatrics* **2021**, *148*, e2021052286. [CrossRef]
70. Juncker, H.G.; Mulleners, S.J.; van Gils, M.J.; de Groot, C.J.M.; Pajkrt, D.; Korosi, A.; van Goudoever, J.B.; van Keulen, B.J. The Levels of SARS-CoV-2 Specific Antibodies in Human Milk Following Vaccination. *J. Hum. Lact.* **2021**, *37*, 477–484. [CrossRef]
71. Rosenberg-Friedman, M.; Kigel, A.; Bahar, Y.; Werbner, M.; Alter, J.; Yogev, Y.; Dror, Y.; Lubetzky, R.; Dessau, M.; Gal-Tanamy, M.; et al. BNT162b2 MRNA Vaccine Elicited Antibody Response in Blood and Milk of Breastfeeding Women. *Nat. Commun.* **2021**, *12*, 6222. [CrossRef]
72. Scrimin, F.; Campisciano, G.; Comar, M.; Ragazzon, C.; Davanzo, R.; Quadrifoglio, M.; Giangreco, M.; Stabile, G.; Ricci, G. IgG and IgA Antibodies Post SARS-CoV-2 Vaccine in the Breast Milk and Sera of Breastfeeding Women. *Vaccines* **2022**, *10*, 125. [CrossRef]
73. Charepe, N.; Gonçalves, J.; Juliano, A.M.; Lopes, D.G.; Canhão, H.; Soares, H.; Serrano, E.F. COVID-19 MRNA Vaccine and Antibody Response in Lactating Women: A Prospective Cohort Study. *BMC Pregnancy Childbirth* **2021**, *21*, 632. [CrossRef]
74. Gonçalves, J.; Juliano, A.M.; Charepe, N.; Alenquer, M.; Athayde, D.; Ferreira, F.; Archer, M.; Amorim, M.J.; Serrano, F.; Soares, H. Secretory IgA and T Cells Targeting SARS-CoV-2 Spike Protein Are Transferred to the Breastmilk upon MRNA Vaccination. *Cell Rep. Med.* **2021**, *2*, 100468. [CrossRef]
75. Esteve-Palau, E.; Gonzalez-Cuevas, A.; Guerrero, M.E.; Garcia-Terol, C.; Alvarez, M.C.; Casadevall, D.; Diaz-Brito, V. Quantification of Specific Antibodies against SARS-CoV-2 in Breast Milk of Lactating Women Vaccinated with an MRNA Vaccine. *JAMA Netw. Open* **2021**, *4*, e2120575. [CrossRef]
76. Yeo, K.T.; Chia, W.N.; Tan, C.W.; Ong, C.; Yeo, J.G.; Zhang, J.; Poh, S.L.; Lim, A.J.M.; Sim, K.H.Z.; Sutamam, N.; et al. Neutralizing Activity and SARS-CoV-2 Vaccine MRNA Persistence in Serum and Breastmilk after BNT162b2 Vaccination in Lactating Women. *Front. Immunol.* **2022**, *12*, 5793. [CrossRef] [PubMed]
77. Schwartz, A.; Nir, O.; Toussia-Cohen, S.; Leibovich, L.; Strauss, T.; Asraf, K.; Doolman, R.; Sharabi, S.; Cohen, C.; Levin, E.G.; et al. Presence of SARS-CoV-2 Antibodies in Lactating Women and Their Infants Following BNT162b2 Messenger RNA Vaccine. *Am. J. Obstet. Gynecol.* **2021**, *225*, 577–579. [CrossRef] [PubMed]
78. Kelly, J.C.; Carter, E.B.; Raghuraman, N.; Nolan, L.S.; Gong, Q.; Lewis, A.N.; Good, M. Anti–Severe Acute Respiratory Syndrome Coronavirus 2 Antibodies Induced in Breast Milk after Pfizer-BioNTech/BNT162b2 Vaccination. *Am. J. Obstet. Gynecol.* **2021**, *225*, 101–103. [CrossRef] [PubMed]
79. Scaggs Huang, F. Are SARS-CoV-2 Antibodies Detectable in Human Milk after Vaccination against COVID-19? *J. Pediatric Infect. Dis. Soc.* **2022**, *11*, 126. [CrossRef]
80. Agostinis, C.; Toffoli, M.; Balduit, A.; Mangogna, A.; Yasmin, H.; Ragazzon, C.; Pegoraro, S.; Campisciano, G.; Stabile, G.; Zito, G.; et al. Anti-Spike Antibodies Present in the Milk of SARS-CoV-2 Vaccinated Mothers Are Complement-Activating. *Int. J. Mol. Sci.* **2023**, *24*, 4395. [CrossRef]
81. Gu, Y.; Low, J.M.; Tan, J.S.Y.; Ng, M.S.F.; Ng, L.F.P.; Shunmuganathan, B.; Gupta, R.; MacAry, P.A.; Amin, Z.; Lee, L.Y.; et al. Immune and Pathophysiologic Profiling of Antenatal Coronavirus Disease 2019 in the GIFT Cohort: A Singaporean Case-Control Study. *Front. Pediatr.* **2022**, *10*, 949756. [CrossRef]
82. Martin-Vicente, M.; Carrasco, I.; Muñoz-Gomez, M.J.; Lobo, A.H.; Mas, V.; Vigil-Vázquez, S.; Vázquez, M.; Manzanares, A.; Cano, O.; Alonso, R.; et al. Antibody Levels to SARS-CoV-2 Spike Protein in Mothers and Children from Delivery to Six Months Later. *Birth* **2022**. [CrossRef]
83. Dutra, L.V.; Silva, M.H.; Lebrão, C.W.; Affonso-Fonseca, F.L.; Suano-Souza, F.I. Impact of the Presence Anti-SARS-CoV-2 IgA in the Colostrum of Women Infected by COVID-19 During the Pregnancy in Neonatal Clinical Outcomes: A cross-Sectional Study. *Matern. Child Health J.* **2023**, *27*, 737. [CrossRef]

84. Wachman, E.M.; Snyder-Cappione, J.; Devera, J.; Boateng, J.; Dhole, Y.; Clarke, K.; Yuen, R.R.; Parker, S.E.; Hunnewell, J.; Ferraro, R.; et al. Maternal, Infant, and Breast Milk Antibody Response Following COVID-19 Infection in Early versus Late Gestation. *Pediatr. Infect. Dis. J.* **2023**, *42*, e70–e76. [CrossRef]
85. Calabretto, M.; D'Alisa, R.; Faraone, S.; Mazzuti, L.; Pecorini, F.; Turriziani, O. Detection of SARS-CoV-2 RNA and Antibodies in Breast Milk of Infected Mothers. *J. Med. Virol.* **2023**, *95*, e28142. [CrossRef]
86. Narayanaswamy, V.; Pentecost, B.T.; Telfer, J.C.; Burnside, A.S.; Schneider, S.S.; Alfandari, D.; Baker, R.L.; Saiju, A.; Nodiff, S.; Arcaro, K.F. Durable Antibody and Effector Memory T Cell Responses in Breastmilk from Women with SARS-CoV-2. *Front. Immunol.* **2022**, *13*, 985226. [CrossRef] [PubMed]
87. Bode, L.; Bertrand, K.; Najera, J.A.; Furst, A.; Honerkamp-Smith, G.; Shandling, A.D.; Chambers, C.D.; Camerini, D.; Campo, J.J. Characterization of SARS-CoV-2 Antibodies in Human Milk from 21 Women with Confirmed COVID-19 Infection. *Pediatr. Res.* **2022**, 1–8. [CrossRef] [PubMed]
88. Lechosa-Muñiz, C.; Paz-Zulueta, M.; Irure-Ventura, J.; Mendez-Legaza, J.M.; Cuesta González, R.; Gómez-Acebo, I.; López-Hoyos, M.; Llorca, J.; Cabero-Pérez, M.J. Development of SARS-CoV-2 Specific IgG and IgA Antibodies in Serum and Milk with Different SARS-CoV-2 Vaccines in Lactating Women. *Int. Breastfeed. J.* **2023**, *18*, 3. [CrossRef] [PubMed]
89. Demers-Mathieu, V.; Huston, R.K.; Markell, A.M.; McCulley, E.A.; Martin, R.L.; Dallas, D.C. Antenatal Influenza A-Specific IgA, IgM, and IgG Antibodies in Mother's Own Breast Milk and Donor Breast Milk, and Gastric Contents and Stools from Preterm Infants. *Nutrients* **2019**, *11*, 1567. [CrossRef]
90. Demers-Mathieu, V.; Underwood, M.A.; Beverly, R.L.; Dallas, D.C. Survival of Immunoglobulins from Human Milk to Preterm Infant Gastric Samples at 1, 2, and 3 Hours Postprandial. *Neonatology* **2018**, *114*, 242. [CrossRef]
91. Thai, J.D.; Gregory, K.E. Bioactive Factors in Human Breast Milk Attenuate Intestinal Inflammation during Early Life. *Nutrients* **2020**, *12*, 581. [CrossRef]
92. Hurley, W.L.; Theil, P.K. Perspectives on Immunoglobulins in Colostrum and Milk. *Nutrients* **2011**, *3*, 442–474. [CrossRef]
93. Goldman, A.S.; Chheda, S.; Keeney, S.E.; Schmalstieg, F.C. Immunology of Human Milk and Host Immunity. *Fetal Neonatal Physiol.* **2020**, *2011*, 1690–1701. [CrossRef]
94. Yaugel-Novoa, M.; Bourlet, T.; Paul, S. Role of the Humoral Immune Response during COVID-19: Guilty or Not Guilty? *Mucosal Immunol.* **2022**, *15*, 1170–1180. [CrossRef]
95. Michaud, E.; Mastrandrea, C.; Rochereau, N.; Paul, S. Human Secretory IgM: An Elusive Player in Mucosal Immunity. *Trends Immunol.* **2020**, *41*, 141–156. [CrossRef]
96. Van de Perre, P.; Simonon, A.; Karita, E.; Butera, J.B.; Hitimana, D.G.; Mukamabano, B.; Van Goethem, C.; Lepage, P.; Dabis, F.; Msellati, P. Infective and Anti-Infective Properties of Breastmilk from HIV-1-Infected Women. *Lancet* **1993**, *341*, 914–918. [CrossRef] [PubMed]
97. Vidarsson, G.; Dekkers, G.; Rispens, T. IgG Subclasses and Allotypes: From Structure to Effector Functions. *Front. Immunol.* **2014**, *5*, 520. [CrossRef] [PubMed]
98. Morales-Núñez, J.J.; Muñoz-Valle, J.F.; Torres-Hernández, P.C.; Hernández-Bello, J. Overview of Neutralizing Antibodies and Their Potential in COVID-19. *Vaccines* **2021**, *9*, 1376. [CrossRef] [PubMed]

nutrients

MDPI

Opinion

Extrauterine Growth Restriction and Optimal Growth of Very Preterm Neonates: State of the Art

Antonios K. Gounaris [1,*], Rozeta Sokou [2], Eleni A. Gounari [3], Polytimi Panagiotounakou [2] and Ioanna N. Grivea [1]

1 Neonatal Clinic-NICU, University Hospital of Larissa, 413 34 Larissa, Greece; ioanna.grivea@gmail.com
2 Neonatal Clinic-NICU, Nikea General Hospital "Agios Panteleimon", 184 54 Piraeus, Greece; sokourozeta@yahoo.gr (R.S.); ppppolytimi04@gmail.com (P.P.)
3 East Sussex Hospitals NHS Trust, Hastings TN37 7PT, UK; elenigounari@gmail.com
* Correspondence: angounaris@med.uth.gr; Tel.: +30-694-488-7522

Abstract: Over the last few decades, there has been an ongoing debate over both the optimal feeding mode for very premature neonates (VPN) as well as what their optimal growth should be. Despite the American Academy of Pediatric declaring since 1997 that the growth of VPN should follow the trajectory of intrauterine fetal growth, differences of opinion persist, feeding policies keep changing, and the growth and development of VPN remains extremely variable not only between countries, but even between neighboring neonatal units. Even the appropriate terminology to express poor postnatal growth (extrauterine growth restriction (EGR) and postnatal growth failure (PGF)) remains a subject of ongoing discussion. A number of recent publications have shown that by implementing breast milk fortification and closely following growth and adjusting nutrition accordingly, as per the consensus guidelines of the major Neonatal Societies, we could achieve growth that closely follows birth centiles. A recent position paper from EPSGAN recommending targeted nutritional support to cover the energy and protein deficits sustained by VPN during periods of critical illness further strengthens the above findings. Conclusion: We can promote better growth of VPN by ensuring a stable administration of sufficient calories and protein, especially in the first 2 weeks of life, implementing breast milk fortification, covering energy and protein deficits due to critical illness, and increasing feeding volumes as per the latest guidelines. The adoption of universal protocol for nutrition and growth of VPN is essential and will enable better monitoring of long-term outcomes for this population.

Keywords: very premature neonates; extrauterine growth restriction; postnatal growth failure; optimal growth; nutrition; feeding policies

1. Introduction

The third pregnancy trimester is a period of rapid fetal growth and development. The normal development of the fetus is disrupted during premature birth, and both intrauterine and extrauterine growth affect the long-term health of very premature neonates (VPN). In the last three decades, there has been ongoing discussion on what constitutes optimal growth for VPN. There are different opinions expressed and even different definitions/interpretations of the terms intrauterine growth restriction (IUGR), extrauterine growth restriction (EGR), and postnatal growth failure (PGF), resulting in the absence of a universally approved pathway for the nutrition and growth of this population.

Two recent major publications have put the issue of those definitions in the forefront, declaring the terms EGR and PGF as misnomers that need to be replaced [1] and suggesting new centile charts for VPN [2]. The esteemed authors of both articles cite multiple important reasons for their approach and particularly the risks that may arise from providing "excessive" nutrition in an effort for VPN to grow close to their birth centile at all costs.

Despite that, other recent publications [3,4] shed a different light on the issue as they achieved a significant reduction in VPN less than 10th centile at 36 weeks corrected age, without administering calories or protein in excess of what is recommended in the neonatal guidelines. It is evident from the above that it is important for the discussion on feeding policy and VPN growth to include the utility or not of the term EGR. It is noteworthy that although both the terms EGR and PGF are used to describe growth restriction, EGR, which implies a cut-off value at a determined point in life, refers to growth restriction until 40 weeks and is preferable to PGF, which implies a difference in growth velocity during an unspecified period that may extend to 1 year of life. Looking through the literature, it appears that the term EGR, defining neonates that are below the 10th percentile of intrauterine growth expectation, is too broad and can include neonates for whom the difference between birth and 36 weeks corrected gestational age (CGA) can range from −0.5 SD or −1 SD up to −2 SD. Clearly, neonates in the extremes of the EGR spectrum have vastly different risks of adverse outcomes. In this review, we will attempt to examine the validity, usefulness, and adequacy of the term EGR, and what would be considered optimal growth for VPN.

2. Feeding Policies Pre-2000 and Effect on VPN Growth and Prognosis

We need to remember that the term EGR was not commonly used prior to the year 2000. During that period, the initial enthusiasm from the widespread use of antenatal steroids and postnatal surfactant started to wane on the realization that the huge increase in survival, even at the extremes of viability, was not followed by an equivalent reduction in VPN with neurodisability. On the contrary, it resulted in an increase of the percentage of VPN surviving with significant neurodevelopmental abnormalities [5].

There were two further notable developments at that time. Firstly, it was established that the feeding policies, especially in terms of the amount of protein given, resulted in widespread growth restriction of VPN as demonstrated in the large NICHD/NNR study [6] where 97% of VP neonates were below 10th centile at 36 weeks CGA. Secondly, in the late 1990s, large prospective and retrospective studies showed that IUGR increased the risk of metabolic syndrome in later life [7]. Following those developments, the term EGR started coming into widespread use.

Many articles looking at the effects of different feeding strategies in the first and second era of neonatology found that prematurity and growth restriction before 40 weeks CGA increased the risk of adverse neurodevelopmental and metabolic outcomes (Figure 1) [8–13]. The understanding that the main reason for EGR in VPN was that nutrients and especially protein was less compared to the nutrients received through the placenta at different gestational ages led to a reconfiguration of feeding policies.

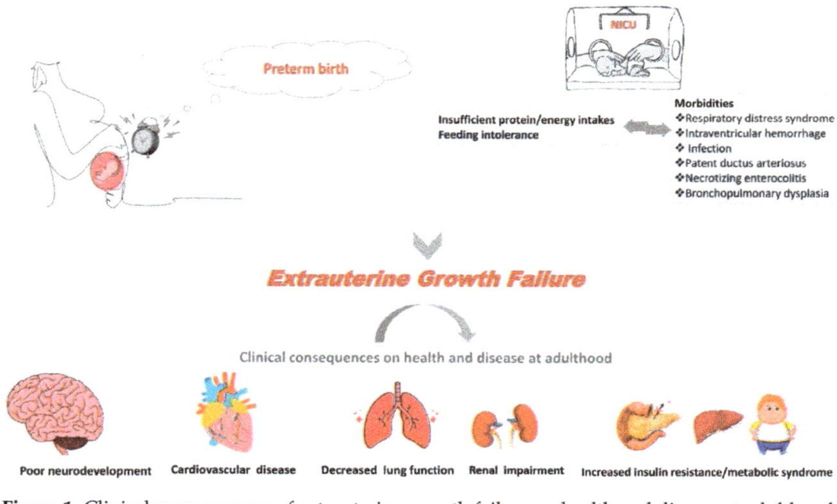

Figure 1. Clinical consequences of extrauterine growth failure on health and disease at adulthood.

3. The Effect of Early "Aggressive" Feeding Strategies Post-2000

In 2002, Ziegler et al. first used the term "aggressive" feeding to describe a feeding protocol that was in his opinion closer to the nutrition received by the mother through the placenta [14]. In the following decade, more authors and pediatric societies adopted a similar approach, suggesting feeding policies with more nutrients and focusing on protein content. The outcome of these policies was the marked reduction in the percentage of VPN with EGR, although it still remained high at around 50% [15]. In a more recent study, the percentage of VPN with EGR at 36 weeks CGA in 11 European countries showed a wide variation from 24% in Sweden to 60% in Portugal [16].

A large study of >90,000 VPN born between 2007 and 2018 showed that the mean value for weight and head circumference (HC) at 36 weeks CGA was >-1 SD for all gestational ages <32 weeks, and for neonates less than 28 weeks GA it reached -2 SD. It is clear that there are big variations in practice between different countries and between NICUs within the same country [2]. Embleton [17] asked in 2001 whether EGR is unavoidable, and this question still remains relevant today: is EGR unavoidable and, if so, to what degree?

A meta-analysis [18] and studies looking at associations between EGR and long-term prognosis of VPN born after 2000 have found a negative effect [19–22]. A recent study (LEMON study) compared monochorionic diamniotic twins from uncomplicated pregnancies that had differences in their intrauterine growth. Infants that had significant growth restriction compared to their twins had statistically significant risk of having lower IQ and exhibit moderate neurodevelopmental disorders [23].

In a very recent study, higher neonatal growth velocity in children born less than 29w GA was associated with modestly higher cognition and language score at 18–22 months CA [24]. These results were more profound among those born with the lower weight for gestational age, emphasizing the importance of postnatal growth in this population. It is clear that growth restriction of VPN either intrauterine or extrauterine can adversely affect their outcome, and the question posed by Embleton requires an urgent answer.

4. Factors Influencing Nutritional Supply and Growth of Preterm Infants

It is evident that prior to 2000, EGR of VPN was due to feeding policies with inadequate calorie and protein intake. The question remains, though, why the subsequent increases in nutrients provision did not solve the problem. In an effort to define the issue, some recent studies and meta-analyses have looked in more detail into the energy and nutrients provision of VPN. They found that infants with EGR were receiving fewer calories and less protein than the recommended from the Neonatal Societies' guidelines for variable periods of time and for a variety of reasons, mainly during the transition phase from the parenteral to enteral feeding [25–27]. Another possible cause is the lack of breast milk fortification.

4.1. Breast Milk Fortification

Is breast milk fortification necessary throughout admission? This remains controversial. A large study of over 45,000 VPN showed that of the VPN receiving breast milk, only 45.3% received fortification of some degree [28].

The results of some recent studies may aid decision making. Breast milk of mothers of premature neonates contains extra protein compared to that of term neonates only for the first month. The peak protein content is at 2 weeks (approx. 1.9 g/100 mL mean value) with subsequent gradual decrease in the following 2 weeks and without birth gestational age further affecting it [29,30]. In 2019, Li et al. [31], comparing VPN that received preterm breast milk with ones that received preterm breast milk with preterm formula, showed that the latter had better growth at 40 weeks CGA (mean difference 283 g; (95% CI: 121.6–445.6) without difference in body fat content on whole body MRI at 37–44 weeks. These results mean that the difference was down to the better growth of other vital tissues (lean tissue). The fortification rate of preterm breast milk was almost similar in all groups. In a recent paper, Perrin et al. [32] found that individualized fortification of human milk prevented postnatal weight loss in most infants and supported HC growth.

A 2023 study from Embleton et al. [33] showed that cow's milk-based fortifier did not adversely affect the gut microbiome when compared to human milk-based fortifier. Reservations on the use of breast milk fortifier focusing on intolerance to cow's milk and the risk of NEC do not appear to be substantiated on a meta-analysis of the data, which actually showed moderately better growth on VPN receiving fortifier [34], and a further recent study considers breast milk fortification necessary for adequate growth of VPN [35].

In our opinion and in view of those results, fortification of breast milk is necessary, as unfortified breast milk is not sufficient in the majority of cases, even in the first 4 weeks, to cover the nutritional needs of VPN.

4.2. VPN with Major Morbidities and Growth

Major morbidities (BPD, IVH, NEC, ROP, etc.) are complications that increase the risk of EGR. In the large study by Greenbury et al. [2], VPN with major morbidities had significantly restricted growth compared to the ones without. A likely contributing factor is the difficulty in administration of nutrients in this population. In a study by Milanesi et al. [36], VPN that eventually developed BPD did not receive the correct ratio of calories to protein for periods spanning from birth up to 4 weeks of age.

Ehrenkranz et al. [37] showed a correlation between major morbidities such as BPD and the development of VPN, considering EGR as a major factor underlying both. In another study, VPN with BPD that received an intense and targeted feeding regime and had similar growth to VPN without BPD did not show significant difference in their respiratory function at 8 years compared to VPN without BPD and term controls [38]. Groene et al. [39] showed that monochorionic twins with selective fetal growth restriction had significant increase in the prevalence of BPD despite the lowest incidence of respiratory distress syndrome compared to the larger co-twin, in spite of their identical genetic makeup and maternal risk factors, essentially in a form of a "natural experiment" that showcases the link between growth restriction and lung function. The above observations pose a question. Is a different feeding protocol needed for VPN with major morbidity in order to prevent further growth restriction and, if so, from what point in their disease?

Our opinion is that VPN with major morbidities should receive intense nutrition, to minimize their postnatal growth difference to those without major morbidities [40].

5. Feeding Policies and Reducing the Percentage of VPN with EGR

Several neonatologists from different countries have implemented feeding policies that have succeeded in reducing the percentage of VPN with EGR [3,4,41–43]. Some have achieved that by monitoring growth and correlating it with number and duration of interruptions in enteral feeding [41], others by providing higher protein content in the first 2 weeks of life [3,4], or by providing larger quantities of milk [42], with some giving more than 200 mL/kg/day of milk [43–45]. A common thread in most of those publications is breast milk fortification, close monitoring of growth at least on a weekly basis, and adjusting nutrition, according to the guidelines of Neonatal Societies, in order to achieve growth close to birth centiles.

In a 2022 publication from Rossholt et al. [46], close monitoring of growth resulted in only 3% of VPN having >-1 SD deviation from their birth centile at 36 weeks CGA. None of the above studies have recorded any instances of neonates receiving calories or protein in excess of the recommended guidelines.

6. And Now What: Current and Future Demands

Despite many different feeding protocols that promote growth and reduce EGR, it remains difficult to achieve that goal more broadly due to the absence of universally accepted policies and the variability between different countries and different NICUs. A characteristic example is a cluster of 10 different enteral feeding policies in one country reported by Greenbury et al. [28].

There are two distinct themes arising from the data above. Firstly, there is clear evidence that growth restriction of VPN up to 40 weeks CGA, despite the changes in feeding policies post 2000, increases the risk of metabolic syndrome and neurodevelopmental disorders. Whilst correlation does not equal causation, this evidence should not be ignored. Secondly there are NICUs that, by closely following the recommendations from the neonatal societies, have achieved reducing the percentage of VPN with EGR to less than 10%.

Two recent position papers form ESPGHAN can help in providing some answers to the questions we have posed above (Table 1) [47,48]. According to the 2021 EPSGHAN position, premature neonates with critical illness should have the energy and protein deficit sustained during that period replaced during the recovery phase in order to achieve catch-up growth. This, according to the authors, can be achieved by increasing calories during the recovery phase up to 160 kcal/kg/day, protein up to 4.5 g/kg/day, glucose up to 12.5 g/kg/day, and fat up to 8 g/kg/day for as long as required in order to replace nutrient/energy deficits sustained during the acute illness phase [47].

Table 1. ESPGHAN recommendations regarding energy and macronutrient requirements in preterm neonates.

Energy/Macronutrient	ESPGHAN 2022 Recommendations for Enteral Nutrient Intake; Embleton [48]	Energy/Nutrient Requirements in Critically Ill Neonates; Moltu [47]			
			Early Acute	Late Acute	Recovery
Energy (kcal/kg /day)	115–140 (160)	Enteral	40–55	70–95	110–160
		Parenteral	40–55	60–80	90–120
Fluid, mL/kg/d	135–200 (>200)	–	–	–	–
Glucose (g/kg/d)	11–15	Enteral	5–8	7–11	11–15 (18)
		Parenteral	5–8 (10)	7–10 (12)	11–14 (17)
Protein (g/kg/ day) *	3.5–4.0 (4.5)	Enteral	1.0–2.0	2.0–3.0	3.5–4.5
		Parenteral	1.0–2.0	2.0–3.0	2.5–3.5
Lipids (g/kg/ day)	4.8–8.1	Enteral	2.0–3.0	3.0–6.0	5.0–8.0
		Parenteral	1.0–2.0	2.0–3.0	3.0–4.0

Data in brackets represent upper intake; * to facilitate protein utilization, a non-protein energy to protein ratio of >25 kcal/g protein or a protein to energy ratio of 2.8–3.6 g/100 kcal is recommended.

The ESPGHAN position paper published in 2022 [48] alters previous guidelines published in 2010 [49] and for the first time recommends increasing calories up to 160 kcal/kg/day, protein up to 4.5 g/kg/day and milk up to 200 mL/kg/day or higher in some case of enterally fed VPN, in order to achieve improved growth. Those two ESPGHAN positions acknowledge that the period of up to 40 weeks CGA is critical for neonatal development and promote catch up growth following periods of growth restriction due to VPN complications.

Coming back to the initial question regarding EGR, the issue is not whether the term itself is correct. In our opinion, the issue is that this one term is too broad and can encompass a very wide range of neonates (from Z score > −0.70 up to >−1.70) that are likely to have vastly different risk profiles and sustain very different outcomes. We feel that a more nuanced approach that takes into account the vastly different risks at different points of the EGR spectrum is required.

What could be the target today? What level of VPN growth is both safe and realistic to achieve?

Based on the recent ESPGHAN recommendations and other recent publications, and using the traditional definition of EGR (<10th centile), it is achievable today for neonatologists to aim to limit the percentage of VPN with weight < 10th centile at 36 weeks or at discharge to around 10% of total [3,4]. In a 2006 study, it was shown that growth on the 10th centile for weight and HC at 36 weeks CGA did not increase the risk of neurodevelopmental disorders [50]. On that basis, a growth for VPN to achieve weight and HC > 10th centile at 36 weeks CGA is considered safe. Expressing EGR as a z score, this target would be a difference from birth weight centile of up to −0.70 or up −0.80 at 36 weeks CA [3,51]. For neonates born at less than 26 weeks GA, this difference could be a little bit higher but less than −1 z score.

Regarding the question of a universal feeding policy, in our view, the close monitoring of VPN growth and strict adherence to the latest ESPGHAN guidelines, especially the ones concerning catch-up growth following acute illness (Table 1), will significantly contribute to reducing neonates with growth restriction.

After all, in the era of constantly rising rates of extremely premature survivors, a universal definition EGR and relevant robust guidelines on neonatal feeding are both highly desirable.

In conclusion, we feel that the term EGR is useful, but it needs to be better defined in order to express its real effect in the early and late neonatal prognosis. From the reported data, it is obvious that very premature neonates require close monitoring of their growth and adequate and reliable administration of nutrients based on the latest guidelines, both via the parenteral and enteral route, including breast milk fortification and especially in the first 2 weeks of life. Any energy or nutrient deficits sustained during periods of acute illness or significant co-morbidities should be replaced within the 40 weeks GCA. Studies with nutritional practices that succeeded growth of VPN close to the birth centiles could today be the guide for the implementation of universal common feeding protocols and growth for the VPN.

Author Contributions: Conceptualization, A.K.G.; methodology, A.K.G. and R.S.; data curation, R.S., A.K.G., P.P., E.A.G. and I.N.G.; investigation, A.K.G.; writing—original draft preparation, A.K.G., R.S. and E.A.G. writing—review and editing, A.K.G., R.S., P.P., E.A.G. and I.N.G. All authors have read and agreed to the published version of the manuscript.

Funding: This research received no external funding.

Institutional Review Board Statement: Not applicable.

Informed Consent Statement: Not applicable.

Data Availability Statement: Data are contained within the article.

Conflicts of Interest: The authors declare no conflict of interest.

References

1. Fenton, T.R.; Cormack, B.; Goldberg, D.; Nasser, R.; Alshaikh, B.; Eliasziw, M.; Hay, W.W.; Hoyos, A.; Anderson, D.; Bloomfield, F.; et al. "Extrauterine growth restriction" and "postnatal growth failure" are misnomers for preterm infants. *J. Perinatol. Off. J. Calif. Perinat. Assoc.* **2020**, *40*, 704–714. [CrossRef] [PubMed]
2. Greenbury, S.F.; Angelini, E.D.; Ougham, K.; Battersby, C.; Gale, C.; Uthaya, S.; Modi, N. Birthweight and patterns of postnatal weight gain in very and extremely preterm babies in England and Wales, 2008–2019: A cohort study. *Lancet Child Adolesc. Health* **2021**, *5*, 719–728. [CrossRef] [PubMed]
3. Andrews, E.T.; Ashton, J.J.; Pearson, F.; Beattie, R.M.; Johnson, M.J. Early postnatal growth failure in preterm infants is not inevitable. *Arch. Dis. Child. Fetal Neonatal* **2019**, *104*, F235–F241. [CrossRef] [PubMed]
4. McKinley, L.T.; Przystac, L.; Tucker, R.; Trail-Burns, E.; Vohr, B.R.; Laptook, A.R.; Bliss, J.M. Implementation of a Nutrition Care Bundle and Improved Weight Gain of Extremely Preterm Infants to 36 Weeks Postmenstrual Age. *J. Pediatr.* **2022**, *241*, 42–47.e2. [CrossRef]
5. Wilson-Costello, D.; Friedman, H.; Minich, N.; Fanaroff, A.A.; Hack, M. Improved survival rates with increased neurodevelopmental disability for extremely low birth weight infants in the 1990s. *Pediatrics* **2005**, *115*, 997–1003. [CrossRef]
6. Lemons, J.A.; Bauer, C.R.; Oh, W.; Korones, S.B.; Papile, L.A.; Stoll, B.J.; Verter, J.; Temprosa, M.; Wright, L.L.; Ehrenkranz, R.A.; et al. Very low birth weight outcomes of the National Institute of Child health and human development neonatal research network, January 1995 through December 1996. NICHD Neonatal Research Network. *Pediatrics* **2001**, *107*, E1. [CrossRef] [PubMed]
7. Barker, D.J.; Eriksson, J.G.; Forsén, T.; Osmond, C. Fetal origins of adult disease: Strength of effects and biological basis. *Int. J. Epidemiol.* **2002**, *31*, 1235–1239. [CrossRef]
8. Sipola-Leppänen, M.; Vääräsmäki, M.; Tikanmäki, M.; Matinolli, H.M.; Miettola, S.; Hovi, P.; Wehkalampi, K.; Ruokonen, A.; Sundvall, J.; Pouta, A.; et al. Cardiometabolic risk factors in young adults who were born preterm. *Am. J. Epidemiol.* **2015**, *181*, 861–873. [CrossRef]

9. Franz, A.R.; Pohlandt, F.; Bode, H.; Mihatsch, W.A.; Sander, S.; Kron, M.; Steinmacher, J. Intrauterine, early neonatal, and postdischarge growth and neurodevelopmental outcome at 5.4 years in extremely preterm infants after intensive neonatal nutritional support. *Pediatrics* **2009**, *123*, e101–e109. [CrossRef]
10. Vohr, B.R.; Wright, L.L.; Dusick, A.M.; Mele, L.; Verter, J.; Steichen, J.J.; Simon, N.P.; Wilson, D.C.; Broyles, S.; Bauer, C.R.; et al. Neurodevelopmental and functional outcomes of extremely low birth weight infants in the National Institute of Child Health and Human Development Neonatal Research Network, 1993–1994. *Pediatrics* **2000**, *105*, 1216–1226. [CrossRef]
11. Zozaya, C.; Díaz, C.; Saenz de Pipaón, M. How Should We Define Postnatal Growth Restriction in Preterm Infants? *Neonatology* **2018**, *114*, 177–180. [CrossRef]
12. Sammallahti, S.; Pyhälä, R.; Lahti, M.; Lahti, J.; Pesonen, A.K.; Heinonen, K.; Hovi, P.; Eriksson, J.G.; Strang-Karlsson, S.; Andersson, S.; et al. Infant growth after preterm birth and neurocognitive abilities in young adulthood. *J. Pediatr.* **2014**, *165*, 1109–1115.e3. [CrossRef] [PubMed]
13. Crump, C.; Groves, A.; Sundquist, J.; Sundquist, K. Association of Preterm Birth with Long-term Risk of Heart Failure into Adulthood. *JAMA Pediatr.* **2021**, *175*, 689–697. [CrossRef] [PubMed]
14. Ziegler, E.E.; Thureen, P.J.; Carlson, S.J. Aggressive nutrition of the very low birthweight infant. *Clin. Perinatol.* **2002**, *29*, 225–244. [CrossRef] [PubMed]
15. Horbar, J.D.; Ehrenkranz, R.A.; Badger, G.J.; Edwards, E.M.; Morrow, K.A.; Soll, R.F.; Buzas, J.S.; Bertino, E.; Gagliardi, L.; Bellù, R. Weight Growth Velocity and Postnatal Growth Failure in Infants 501 to 1500 Grams: 2000–2013. *Pediatrics* **2015**, *136*, e84–e92. [CrossRef] [PubMed]
16. El Rafei, R.; Jarreau, P.-H.; Norman, M.; Maier, R.F.; Barros, H.; Van Reempts, P.; Pedersen, P.; Cuttini, M.; Zeitlin, J. Variation in very preterm extrauterine growth in a European multicountry cohort. *Arch. Dis. Child. Fetal Neonatal* **2021**, *106*, 316. [CrossRef]
17. Embleton, N.E.; Pang, N.; Cooke, R.J. Postnatal malnutrition and growth retardation: An inevitable consequence of current recommendations in preterm infants? *Pediatrics* **2001**, *107*, 270–273. [CrossRef]
18. Martínez-Jiménez, M.D.; Gómez-García, F.J.; Gil-Campos, M.; Pérez-Navero, J.L. Comorbidities in childhood associated with extrauterine growth restriction in preterm infants: A scoping review. *Eur. J. Pediatr.* **2020**, *179*, 1255–1265. [CrossRef]
19. Ehrenkranz, R.A.; Dusick, A.M.; Vohr, B.R.; Wright, L.L.; Wrage, L.A.; Poole, W.K. Growth in the neonatal intensive care unit influences neurodevelopmental and growth outcomes of extremely low birth weight infants. *Pediatrics* **2006**, *117*, 1253–1261. [CrossRef]
20. Belfort, M.B.; Rifas-Shiman, S.L.; Sullivan, T.; Collins, C.T.; McPhee, A.J.; Ryan, P.; Kleinman, K.P.; Gillman, M.W.; Gibson, R.A.; Makrides, M. Infant growth before and after term: Effects on neurodevelopment in preterm infants. *Pediatrics* **2011**, *128*, e899–e906. [CrossRef]
21. Ordóñez-Díaz, M.D.; Pérez-Navero, J.L.; Flores-Rojas, K.; Olza-Meneses, J.; Muñoz-Villanueva, M.C.; Aguilera-García, C.M.; Gil-Campos, M. Prematurity with Extrauterine Growth Restriction Increases the Risk of Higher Levels of Glucose, Low-Grade of Inflammation and Hypertension in Prepubertal Children. *Front. Pediatr.* **2020**, *8*, 180. [CrossRef] [PubMed]
22. Schneider, J.; Fischer Fumeaux, C.J.; Duerden, E.G.; Guo, T.; Foong, J.; Graz, M.B.; Hagmann, P.; Chakravarty, M.M.; Hüppi, P.S.; Beauport, L.; et al. Nutrient Intake in the First Two Weeks of Life and Brain Growth in Preterm Neonates. *Pediatrics* **2018**, *141*, e20172169. [CrossRef] [PubMed]
23. Groene, S.G.; Stegmeijer, K.J.J.; Tan, R.; Steggerda, S.J.; Haak, M.C.; Slaghekke, F.; Roest, A.A.W.; Heijmans, B.T.; Lopriore, E.; van Klink, J.M.M. Long-term effects of selective fetal growth restriction (LEMON): A cohort study of neurodevelopmental outcome in growth discordant identical twins in the Netherlands. *Lancet. Child Adolesc. Health* **2022**, *6*, 624–632. [CrossRef]
24. Sériès, T.; Guillot, M.; Angoa, G.; Pronovost, E.; Ndiaye, A.; Mohamed, I.; Simonyan, D.; Lavoie, P.M.; Synnes, A.; Marc, I. Does Growth Velocity Affect Associations Between Birth Weight and Neurodevelopment for Infants Born Very Preterm? *J. Pediatr.* **2023**, *260*, 113531. [CrossRef] [PubMed]
25. Hu, F.; Tang, Q.; Wang, Y.; Wu, J.; Ruan, H.; Lu, L.; Tao, Y.; Cai, W. Analysis of Nutrition Support in Very Low-Birth-Weight Infants with Extrauterine Growth Restriction. *Nutr. Clin. Pract. Off. Publ. Am. Soc. Parenter. Enter. Nutr.* **2019**, *34*, 436–443. [CrossRef]
26. Brennan, A.M.; Fenton, S.; Murphy, B.P.; Kiely, M.E. Transition Phase Nutrition Recommendations: A Missing Link in the Nutrition Management of Preterm Infants. *JPEN J. Parenter. Enter. Nutr.* **2018**, *42*, 343–351. [CrossRef]
27. Wang, N.; Zhang, J.; Wang, B.; Yu, Z.; Zhang, J.; Qu, L.; Tang, B. Relationship between nutrient intakes in the transition phase and postnatal growth of preterm infants: A systematic review. *Ital. J. Pediatr.* **2023**, *49*, 13. [CrossRef]
28. Greenbury, S.F.; Ougham, K.; Wu, J.; Battersby, C.; Gale, C.; Modi, N.; Angelini, E.D. Identification of variation in nutritional practice in neonatal units in England and association with clinical outcomes using agnostic machine learning. *Sci. Rep.* **2021**, *11*, 7178. [CrossRef]
29. Mills, L.; Coulter, L.; Savage, E.; Modi, N. Macronutrient content of donor milk from a regional human milk bank: Variation with donor mother-infant characteristics. *Br. J. Nutr.* **2019**, *122*, 1155–1167. [CrossRef]
30. Brown, J.V.; Embleton, N.D.; Harding, J.E.; McGuire, W. Multi-nutrient fortification of human milk for preterm infants. *Cochrane Database Syst. Rev.* **2016**, *5*, CD000343. [CrossRef]
31. Li, Y.; Liu, X.; Modi, N.; Uthaya, S. Impact of breast milk intake on body composition at term in very preterm babies: Secondary analysis of the Nutritional Evaluation and Optimisation in Neonates randomised controlled trial. *Arch. Dis. Child. Fetal Neonatal Ed.* **2019**, *104*, F306–F312. [CrossRef]

32. Perrin, T.; Pradat, P.; Larcade, J.; Masclef-Imbert, M.; Pastor-Diez, B.; Picaud, J.C. Postnatal growth and body composition in extremely low birth weight infants fed with individually adjusted fortified human milk: A cohort study. *Eur. J. Pediatr.* **2023**, *182*, 1143–1154. [CrossRef]
33. Embleton, N.D.; Sproat, T.; Uthaya, S.; Young, G.R.; Garg, S.; Vasu, V.; Masi, A.C.; Beck, L.; Modi, N.; Stewart, C.J.; et al. Effect of an Exclusive Human Milk Diet on the Gut Microbiome in Preterm Infants: A Randomized Clinical Trial. *JAMA Netw. Open* **2023**, *6*, e231165. [CrossRef] [PubMed]
34. Brown, J.V.; Lin, L.; Embleton, N.D.; Harding, J.E.; McGuire, W. Multi-nutrient fortification of human milk for preterm infants. *Cochrane Database Syst. Rev.* **2020**, *6*, CD000343. [CrossRef] [PubMed]
35. Arslanoglu, S.; Boquien, C.Y.; King, C.; Lamireau, D.; Tonetto, P.; Barnett, D.; Bertino, E.; Gaya, A.; Gebauer, C.; Grovslien, A.; et al. Fortification of Human Milk for Preterm Infants: Update and Recommendations of the European Milk Bank Association (EMBA) Working Group on Human Milk Fortification. *Front. Pediatr.* **2019**, *7*, 76. [CrossRef] [PubMed]
36. Milanesi, B.G.; Lima, P.A.; Villela, L.D.; Martins, A.S.; Gomes-Junior, S.C.S.; Moreira, M.E.L.; Méio, M. Assessment of early nutritional intake in preterm infants with bronchopulmonary dysplasia: A cohort study. *Eur. J. Pediatr.* **2021**, *180*, 1423–1430. [CrossRef]
37. Ehrenkranz, R.A.; Das, A.; Wrage, L.A.; Poindexter, B.B.; Higgins, R.D.; Stoll, B.J.; Oh, W.; Eunice Kennedy Shriver National Institute of Child Health and Human Development Neonatal Research Network. Early Nutrition Mediates the Influence of Severity of Illness on Extremely LBW Infants. *Pediatr. Res.* **2011**, *69*, 522–529. [CrossRef]
38. Panagiotounakou, P.; Sokou, R.; Gounari, E.; Konstantinidi, A.; Antonogeorgos, G.; Grivea, I.N.; Daniil, Z.; Gourgouliannis, K.I.; Gounaris, A. Very preterm neonates receiving "aggressive" nutrition and early nCPAP had similar long-term respiratory outcomes as term neonates. *Pediatr. Res.* **2019**, *86*, 742–748. [CrossRef]
39. Groene, S.G.; Spekman, J.A.; Te Pas, A.B.; Heijmans, B.T.; Haak, M.C.; van Klink, J.M.M.; Roest, A.A.W.; Lopriore, E. Respiratory distress syndrome and bronchopulmonary dysplasia after fetal growth restriction: Lessons from a natural experiment in identical twins. *EClinicalMedicine* **2021**, *32*, 100725. [CrossRef]
40. Gounaris, A.K.; Sokou, R.; Gounari, E.; Panagiotounakou, P.; Grivea, I.N. Post-natal growth of very preterm neonates. *Lancet. Child Adolesc. Health* **2022**, *6*, e9–e10. [CrossRef] [PubMed]
41. Stevens, T.P.; Shields, E.; Campbell, D.; Combs, A.; Horgan, M.; La Gamma, E.F.; Xiong, K.; Kacica, M. Statewide Initiative to Reduce Postnatal Growth Restriction among Infants <31 Weeks of Gestation. *J. Pediatr.* **2018**, *197*, 82–89.e2. [CrossRef] [PubMed]
42. Travers, C.P.; Wang, T.; Salas, A.A.; Schofield, E.; Dills, M.; Laney, D.; Yee, A.; Bhatia, A.; Winter, L.; Ambalavanan, N.; et al. Higher- or Usual-Volume Feedings in Infants Born Very Preterm: A Randomized Clinical Trial. *J. Pediatr.* **2020**, *224*, 66–71.e1. [CrossRef] [PubMed]
43. Gounaris, A.; Sokou, R.; Theodoraki, M.; Gounari, E.; Panagiotounakou, P.; Antonogeorgos, G.; Ioakeimidis, G.; Parastatidou, S.; Konstantinidi, A.; Grivea, I.N. "Aggressive" Feeding of Very Preterm Neonates and Body Mass Index at School Age. *Nutrients* **2021**, *13*, 1901. [CrossRef] [PubMed]
44. Klingenberg, C.; Muraas, F.K.; Isaksen, C.E.; Nilsen, T.; Torgersen, M.; Melum-Hansen, C. Growth and neurodevelopment in very preterm infants receiving a high enteral volume-feeding regimen–A population-based cohort study. *J. Matern. Neonatal Med.* **2019**, *32*, 1664–1672. [CrossRef]
45. Kosmeri, C.; Giapros, V.; Gounaris, A.; Sokou, R.; Siomou, E.; Rallis, D.; Makis, A.; Baltogianni, M. Are the current feeding volumes adequate for the growth of very preterm neonates? *Br. J. Nutr.* **2023**, 1–5. [CrossRef]
46. Rossholt, M.E.; Bratlie, M.; Wendel, K.; Aas, M.F.; Gunnarsdottir, G.; Fugelseth, D.; Stiris, T.; Domellöf, M.; Størdal, K.; Moltu, S.J. A standardized feeding protocol ensured recommended nutrient intakes and prevented growth faltering in preterm infants <29 weeks gestation. *Clin. Nutr. ESPEN* **2023**, *53*, 251–259. [CrossRef]
47. Moltu, S.J.; Bronsky, J.; Embleton, N.; Gerasimidis, K.; Indrio, F.; Köglmeier, J.; de Koning, B.; Lapillonne, A.; Norsa, L.; Verduci, E.; et al. Nutritional Management of the Critically Ill Neonate: A Position Paper of the ESPGHAN Committee on Nutrition. *J. Pediatr. Gastroenterol. Nutr.* **2021**, *73*, 274–289. [CrossRef]
48. Embleton, N.D.; Moltu, S.J.; Lapillonne, A.; van den Akker, C.H.P.; Carnielli, V.; Fusch, C.; Gerasimidis, K.; van Goudoever, J.B.; Haiden, N.; Iacobelli, S.; et al. Enteral Nutrition in Preterm Infants (2022): A Position Paper from the ESPGHAN Committee on Nutrition and Invited Experts. *J. Pediatr. Gastroenterol. Nutr.* **2023**, *76*, 248–268. [CrossRef]
49. Agostoni, C.; Buonocore, G.; Carnielli, V.P.; De Curtis, M.; Darmaun, D.; Decsi, T.; Domellöf, M.; Embleton, N.D.; Fusch, C.; Genzel-Boroviczeny, O.; et al. Enteral nutrient supply for preterm infants: Commentary from the European Society of Paediatric Gastroenterology, Hepatology and Nutrition Committee on Nutrition. *J. Pediatr. Gastroenterol. Nutr.* **2010**, *50*, 85–91. [CrossRef]
50. Shah, P.S.; Wong, K.Y.; Merko, S.; Bishara, R.; Dunn, M.; Asztalos, E.; Darling, P.B. Postnatal growth failure in preterm infants: Ascertainment and relation to long-term outcome. *J. Perinat. Med.* **2006**, *34*, 484–489. [CrossRef]
51. Rochow, N.; Raja, P.; Liu, K.; Fenton, T.; Landau-Crangle, E.; Göttler, S.; Jahn, A.; Lee, S.; Seigel, S.; Campbell, D.; et al. Physiological adjustment to postnatal growth trajectories in healthy preterm infants. *Pediatr. Res.* **2016**, *79*, 870–879. [CrossRef] [PubMed]

nutrients

MDPI

Review

Nutrition of Infants with Bronchopulmonary Dysplasia before and after Discharge from the Neonatal Intensive Care Unit

Ageliki A. Karatza, Despoina Gkentzi and Anastasia Varvarigou *

Department of Paediatrics, Neonatal Intensive Care Unit, University of Patras Medical School, 26504 Patras, Greece
* Correspondence: anastasiavarvarigou@upatras.gr; Tel.: +30-6932-544001; Fax: +30-2610-994533

Abstract: Bronchopulmonary dysplasia (BPD) represents a severe sequela in neonates born very prematurely. The provision of adequate nutritional support in this high-risk population is challenging. The development of the lungs and physical growth are closely linked together in infants with BPD. Growth deficiency has been associated with pulmonary dysfunction, whereas improvement in respiratory status results in growth acceleration. Currently, there is not enough data regarding optimal nutritional strategies in this population. Nutrition in these infants should provide sufficient calories and nutrients to establish growth, avoid growth retardation and assist alveolarization of the lungs. Meticulous follow-up is mandatory during and after discharge from the Neonatal Intensive care Unit (NICU) to minimize growth retardation and improve lung function. Despite the significant literature supporting the contribution of growth and nutrition in the avoidance of BPD, there is limited research regarding interventions and management of infants with established BPD. Our aim was to review clinical strategies applied in everyday clinical practice and identify debates on the nutritional approach of newborns with BPD. Well-organized interventions and clinical trials regarding the somatic development and nutrition of infants with BPD are warranted.

Keywords: extremely preterm neonate; extremely low birth weight infant; bronchopulmonary dysplasia; nutrition; feeding

1. Introduction

Bronchopulmonary dysplasia (BPD) represents a severe sequela in neonates born very prematurely [1]. Bronchopulmonary dysplasia was defined in 1967 by Northway as a disorder of the respiratory system in late preterm newborns who were supported for a long time with artificial ventilation and required increased administration of oxygen [2]. In the "Old BPD" cystic changes of the lungs and heterogeneous aeration have been documented, whereas the "New BPD" has a different phenotype and presents in extremely preterm neonates who have been exposed to antenatal steroids, have been given surfactant and have been supported with gentle modern ventilator techniques [3]. The main feature of new BPD is diffuse underdevelopment of the alveoli, which leads to a significantly diminished lung substrate for the elimination of CO_2 and the accretion of O_2, injury of the airways, inflammation, and pulmonary fibrosis. The alterations in the lungs are less profound than in old BPD [4]. BPD affects predominantly premature neonates born at a gestational age which is less than 28 weeks with 67% of them affected by a moderate or severe form of BPD resulting in a mortality of 19% [5]. The incidence of BPD remains stable despite the great progress in perinatal care leading to improved survival of very premature neonates [1].

BPD takes place in neonates born at the developmental stage of the lungs in which the transition from the canalicular to the saccular stage occurs. Its pathophysiology is multifactorial involving several antenatal and postnatal adverse events which derange lung development leading to severe disease with long-term consequences [6]. Chronic deprivation of nutrients and oxygen in pregnancy may result in alterations in the structure of the airways and the lung parenchyma affecting lung function, not only in neonates but also later in life. Deficient nutritional support in very premature infants deranges the development of the respiratory system and may contribute to the evolution of BPD [7]. Prematurity affects lower respiratory tract embryogenesis which has been attributed to unfavorable antenatal and postnatal events such as intrauterine growth retardation, inflammation, resuscitation, oxygen demand, ventilatory support and systemic infections, all of which can result in an arrest in pulmonary vascular development and alveolarization [3]. It is not known whether prematurity causes BPD or whether parameters that are associated with prematurity are its cause [6]. In children with severe BPD, the performance of the respiratory system does not ameliorate with chronological age. In a recent study, in two-thirds of the subjects enrolled, Forced expiratory volume at 1 s (FEV1) and the ratio to forced vital capacity (FEV_1/FVC) got worse over time. Lung function progress was better in adulthood in the subjects that were born after 1990 in comparison with children born before this period. This may be attributed to improved perinatal care in recent years [8]. Pulmonary hypertension has increased incidence in children with BPD. It is documented in 25% of children in the severe spectrum of BPD and represents a parameter that adversely affects morbidity and mortality in this population [9]. Survivors with neonatal BPD also have neurological sequelae, affecting motor and cognitive development and have lower academic progress compared to premature infants without BPD [10].

The real incidence of BPD is difficult to identify as different definitions have been used. This problem makes also difficult to identify variations in the incidence of BPD over time [11,12]. In a study performed in the USA during the last 20 years, improvements in pregnancy and neonatal management and minimization in overall morbidity have been documented; however, the incidence of BPD increased. Increased survival was documented for infants who were born at 23 to 24 weeks and survival without significant sequelae was shown for neonates that were born between 25 and 28 weeks [13]. BPD affects predominately neonates whose birth weight is less than 1500 g. There is an inverse relationship between the prevalence of BPD and gestational age as well as birth weight [13]. In Europe, 10–20% of infants with a gestational age of 23–31 weeks manifest BPD [14].

Increased fluid provision and inefficient loss of weight occurring in the first 10 days after birth have been linked to the augmented likelihood of BPD because of pulmonary congestion and edema [15]. Furthermore, it has been shown that in neonates born at less than 30 weeks, sodium provision should be deferred after 6% of birth weight is lost, an intervention that decreases oxygen requirements without affecting growth [16]. To avoid the development of BPD, extremely preterm and very preterm infants are often fluid-restricted to 120 mL/kg/day [12,15]. Commonly diuretics are prescribed; however, current information on the effectiveness of diuretics in the avoidance and therapy of BPD has been questionable [17]. Fluid restriction can lead to deficient caloric provision, compromised growth, and inadequate nutritional support, which are risk factors for BPD development [12,18]. It should be noted that premature neonates with established BPD have higher demands in calories because their work of breathing is higher and they require caloric support to assist in the alveolarization of the lungs and overcome pulmonary inflammation [19,20]. Preterm infants who develop BPD need medical support and supervision beyond neonatal intensive care unit hospitalization, including nutritional support and monitoring of growth status in the long term [6].

2. Growth of Neonates with Bronchopulmonary Dysplasia

The nutritional support of very preterm newborns was investigated in a cohort study that reported that 20.5% developed BPD. At term equivalent anthropometric measurements were smaller in the bronchopulmonary dysplasia group who initiated feeding by mouth and achieved full oral feeds at a more mature postnatal age, requiring prolonged intravenous nutritional support. The amount of protein given to both groups was the same, irrespective of whether they had bronchopulmonary dysplasia or not, but fluid volume and proteins given to those who developed BPD were lower after the fourteenth day. The ratio of calorie to protein (30 kcal/g protein) per day was achieved by almost 90% of the neonates that had no bronchopulmonary dysplasia on their 21st day of life. The bronchopulmonary dysplasia group received a lower amount until the fourteenth day and the deficiency persisted in 56.3% of them for one month. The authors conclude that an inadequate calorie/protein ratio was a fact in neonates who established bronchopulmonary dysplasia, and adequate nutritional support for this population is challenging. Somatic parameters were measured at birth and at term equivalent postnatal age apart from the weight which was measured every week for four weeks. Z-scores at birth were similar between the neonates who developed BPD and those who did not develop BPD. However, at term equivalent, head circumference and length Z-scores were significantly lower in infants with BPD. The decrease in the weight Z-scores in both groups was similar during the first month, but at term equivalent to postnatal age, the Z-scores of the weight of the premature neonates with BPD showed further decrease, while the preterm infants without BPD started to catch up [21].

Another study investigated the nutritional condition of neonates with BPD during the first month after birth and the probability of acquiring malnutrition. The infants in the BPD group received excessive fluids but fewer calories and proteins after the first 14 days of life, required mechanical ventilatory support for more days and needed more days to achieve oral feeding without the need for supplementation with parenteral nutrition, which was thus administered for more days. These disorders were more prevalent in the group of infants with malnutrition. Anthropometric measurements were significantly smaller in the BPD in comparison to the non-BPD infants and they were lower in infants with malnutrition than in those who were well nourished. The weight to length ratio, body mass index, triponderal mass index, and the velocity of weight gain in the population with BPD was significantly lower compared to the non-BPD group.

Days on artificial ventilatory support, provision of lipids at 4 weeks, time to achieve full feeding by mouth and parenteral nutrition days were independent risk factors for malnutrition [22].

Malikiwi et al. have investigated if there is a link between growth status, provision of nutrients and fluids in the first month after birth and the probability to acquire bronchopulmonary dysplasia. Infants with BPD received fewer calories and fluids during the first month of life. Z-scores of weight at birth and at one month were similar between the BPD and non-BPD neonates. The percentage of infants with weights below the 10th percentile and the mean weight velocity at one month also were similar between the groups. However, the adverse effect of BPD on somatic growth was preserved during infancy, so infants with BPD had significant growth retardation at 6 and 12 months of age.

The risk of establishing BPD was higher when infants were ventilator-dependent during the first month and were lower when a higher first-month provision of calories was achieved. The authors conclude that the BPD group received fewer calories and fewer fluids during the first month. Only two independent predictors for BPD establishment were identified and these were the dependency on an artificial ventilator and the provision of low caloric intake during the first month [23].

Another study investigated whether there is a relationship between the provision of nutrients during the first week of life and the severity of bronchopulmonary dysplasia in neonates born extremely preterm. Out of the 226 infants that were enrolled in the study 67% developed moderate–severe BPD. Participants with moderate–severe BPD were more immature, had a lower birth weight, and needed more prolonged ventilatory support compared to the infants that did not develop BPD. During the study period, the provision of nutrients was significantly less, whereas the provision of fluids was significantly more in the group who developed moderate–severe BPD compared to those who did not. Taking into consideration potential confounding factors, fluid provision, time on mechanical ventilation and low caloric provision were significant determinants of increased risk of moderate–severe BPD [24].

Another study aimed to investigate the role of nutritional support either by mouth or intravenously during the first 2 weeks of life to the risk of acquiring bronchopulmonary dysplasia. The neonates who acquired BPD received fewer calories compared to the controls. Carbohydrate and fat provision was also diminished in BPD patients. This study showed that neonates with BPD are provided with fewer calories and lipids during the first two weeks of life [25].

Preterm infants with BPD have growth retardation, with deficient total body fat and free fat mass identified at 6 weeks post-term; free fat mass and total body fat remain low compared with healthy term infants during the first year of life [26].

As already stated, premature neonates with BPD have an increased incidence of restriction in growth after birth. In a multicentered cohort study breastmilk feeding used exclusively was related to diminished growth but a reduction in the probability of developing bronchopulmonary dysplasia, Furthermore, the incidence of necrotizing enterocolitis and retinopathy of prematurity were decreased [27]. In a retrospective case–control study, neonates with bronchopulmonary dysplasia were provided with fewer calories and fluids in the first month of life. After adjustment for confounders, the requirement for mechanical ventilation and low one-month provision of calories were independently related to increased risk of BPD [23]. As previously mentioned energy requirements are increased in infants with BPD [19,20]. Another study evaluated whether providing more oral calories in preterm neonates with BPD can have a positive effect on growth. Growth was assessed in a cohort of premature neonates who were born before 32 weeks of gestation, their birth weight was less than 1500 g and needed oxygen support up to 28 days after birth who were fed individually tailored fortified breast milk and/or preterm formula, and was compared to a group of neonates with BPD who received fortified breast milk and/or pre-term formula [28]. Days of parenteral nutrition and oral protein intake did not differ between the two groups. However, the provision of oral calories was increased in the infants in the first group with mild or moderate BPD and in those with severe BPD. Rates of weight increase were higher in the neonates of the first group with mild or moderate BPD and in those with severe BPD. The percentage of neonates with growth restriction at 36 weeks was increased in the second group. The authors suggest that optimization of nutritional support improves growth rates after birth in premature neonates having bronchopulmonary dysplasia [25,28,29].

3. Nutritional Management in Infants with Established BPD, either in the Hospital or after Discharge

Currently, few data describe the ideal nutrition strategy in neonates with BPD before and after the exit from the NICU [30]. A recent meta-analysis with the use of PRISMA guidelines with thirty articles selected for inclusion concluded that although there is a lot of data supporting the significance of growth and nutritional support in the avoidance of BPD, there is limited research regarding policies and treatment of infants with BPD. Therefore, interventions and well-organized trials concerning growth and nutritional support in subjects with BPD are warranted. These ideally have to be multicenter as cases with BPD are few at each NICU [30].

Lung function and physical growth are interrelated in neonates developing bronchopulmonary dysplasia. Growth retardation is related to prolonged respiratory impairment and conversely, amelioration in lung function results in increased growth rates [31].

Energy demands in infants with BPD are 15–20% higher compared with infants without BPD [19,20]. This is probably due to laborious breathing, tachypnoea and oxygen demands. Patients born extremely preterm may have difficulties with oral feeding and experience gastroesophageal reflux, vomiting and other issues associated with discoordinated sucking, swallowing dysfunction, poor swallow breath coordination, and poor sucking endurance and performance [19,20]. Early recognition of feeding difficulties and gastroesophageal reflux is crucial for the nutritional management of these infants. Chronic stress and inflammation as well as the use of diuretics and corticosteroids may increase energy demands. Furthermore, necrotizing enterocolitis may require bowel resection and may result in short bowel syndrome with resultant malabsorption and limited energy intake orally or via intravenous nutritional support. Total parenteral nutrition is essential at the initial age of all very premature infants but may be warranted for the treatment of patients with short bowel syndrome in the long term [32].

Fluid restriction is essential for infants with BPD who should receive no more than 150 mL/kg/day and ideally 135 mL/kg/day [33–35]. The oral provision of energy should be optimized at 120–150 kcal/kg/day [30,34]. However, it is not always easy to establish satisfactory caloric provision by offering a restricted volume of fluids. A limited number of studies have investigated the needs of neonates with BPD in proteins, therefore it may be suggested that these are similar to the requirements of premature neonates that do not have BPD according to ESPGHAN [36]. These subjects have altered body composition, suggesting that the usual provision of protein may not be adequate [20]. Enteral protein intake should be at 4.0–4.5 g/kg/day in infants having a birth weight of less than 1000 g and at 3.5–4.0 g/kg/day in neonates with a birth weight of 1000–1800 g [36].

Lipids are an essential component for the growth of extremely premature neonates because they include essential fatty acids and assist to achieve energy requirements [36]. Moreover, lipids play an important role in the absorption of fat-soluble vitamins [20]. Total lipid intake should be 4.8–6.6 g/kg/day with 12–30 mg/kg/day of Arachidonic acid and 18–42 mg/kg/day of Docosahexaenoic acid [36]. Neonates should be provided with long-chain polyunsaturated fatty acids (LC-PUFAs) in adequate amounts to assist visual and cognitive development. For breastfeeding infants, LC-PUFA is provided by maternal milk; however, when breastfeeding is not the case, dietary LC-PUFAs should be supplemented during the first six months of life. Currently, there is not sufficient information for quantitative recommendations regarding LCPUFAs provision [37]. The results of a very recent meta-analysis were that provision with n-3 polyunsaturated fatty acids cannot prevent BPD. Therefore, the increased use of n-3 polyunsaturated fatty acids in premature infants to prevent BPD is not currently supported [37].

The recommended nutritional intakes for premature infants with bronchopulmonary dysplasia are presented in the table.

A bone disease of prematurity is an issue in neonates with BPD and has been associated with the use of postnatal steroids, diuretics and deficient intake of minerals [38].

Enteral feeding should provide a sufficient quantity of calcium and phosphorus; however, it is usually deficient due to its low amount in oral feeds, which has been attributed to the usage of breast milk without fortification, cholestatic liver disease or disorders of absorption [39]. Moreover, bone mineral deposition is reduced in infants with BPD who receive corticosteroids and diuretics usage increases the excretion of calcium. As expected osteopenia of prematurity, a disorder that is due to the insufficient nutritional provision of calcium and phosphorus is an important issue in neonates with bronchopulmonary dysplasia [34,35,37]. Enteral calcium and phosphorus intake should be optimized at 120–140 mg/kg/day of Ca or 150–220 mg/kg/day with 90 mg/kg/day or 75–140 mg/kg/day of phosphorus and Ca/P ratio of 2 [38,39]. In order to avoid volume overload diuretics are often prescribed causing hyponatremia as a complication that requires the provision of sodium which is necessary for optimal growth. Ideally serum Na levels should be >135 mEq/L [40]. Vitamin A and Vitamin E should be supplied at 400–1000 μg/kg/day or 1320–3300 IU/kg/day and 2.2–11 mg/kg/day, respectively [40]. The role of avoidance and therapy of anemia is also important and therefore iron supplementation is required at 4 mg/kg/day, starting at 1–2 months after birth and up to the age of 12 months [41].

Preterm infants have low selenium levels as its transfer through the placenta occurs mainly during the third trimester of pregnancy. The American Society for Clinical Nutrition (ASCN) recommends a parenteral Se intake of 2 μg/kg/day and the American Academy of Pediatrics Committee on Nutrition recommends enteral Se provision of 1.3–4.5 μg/kg/day in preterm neonates [42]. Darlow et al. found an association between low plasma selenium levels and increased risk of lung disease in very premature infants, defined as oxygen dependency on the 28th day of life [43]. A Cochrane review from 2003 showed that low plasma Se was associated with increased complications of prematurity including BPD, increased days of oxygen dependency, and increased risk of adverse respiratory outcomes [44].

Zinc promotes epithelial development, participates in the enzymatic reactions underlying the repair of tissue damage, protects against infection, and modulates the inflammatory response of the respiratory system [45]. Thus, it is reasonable to hypothesize a potential contribution of zinc in preventing bronchopulmonary dysplasia. However, clinical studies demonstrating a clear relationship between zinc and BPD are not yet available [46].

4. Human Breast Milk

A recent meta-analysis investigated the role of donor milk on the incidence of BPD in comparison with feeding with formula and found that the incidence of BPD was significantly lower in the donor milk-fed group [47]. Similar were the results of another study that compared feeding exclusively fresh maternal breast milk compared to maternal breast milk after pasteurization [48]. The participating infants were divided into two groups: one group received their mother's own fresh milk and another group was given their mother's milk post pasteurization. After controlling for confounding factors, the incidence of bronchopulmonary dysplasia was lower in the group who received their own mother's fresh milk. The provision of human milk exclusively, preferably using fresh maternal breast milk, is recommended in the treatment of neonates at the early stages of BPD [49]. The results of a large study involving premature neonates born before 32 weeks showed that maternal breastmilk used exclusively resulted in a decreased incidence of BPD, necrotizing enterocolitis and retinopathy of prematurity, although it was associated with decreased growth [50]. Furthermore, in infants with established BPD provision of breast milk for a longer period of time was related to reduced visits to the hospital emergency departments, less corticosteroid use, cough or chest congestion, and a lower incidence of admissions to the hospital [49].

Maternal milk is generally accepted as the ideal feeding for infants in the first 6 months after birth [51]. Breast milk has been proven to have short and long-term benefits and can be considered a public health issue. Hospitals should routinely support and encourage the initiation and continuation of breastfeeding exclusively during the first 6 months of life as suggested by the American Academy of Pediatrics and WHO/UNICEF [51].

In oxygen-dependent infants with BPD, a link has been documented between the time of oxygen support and gestational age, duration of ventilator support, hemoglobin concentration at the exit from the NICU, use of human milk exclusively and growth. An ambulatory Kangaroo Mother Care Program with established protocols and close follow-up showed that breastfeeding permits sufficient weight gain and assists stop of oxygen use in a safe way. Anemia, growth, and oxygen weaning in oxygen-dependent premature infants were significantly related to breastfeeding in this program [52].

Although breastfeeding should be supported and current evidence indicates its use as the ideal form of feeding for all neonates has positive consequences for human health both in infancy and childhood, human milk may not offer adequate nutritional support for very premature neonates. Using volumes of 120–150 mL/Kg may lead to impaired growth rates resulting in poor health outcomes including bronchopulmonary dysplasia. Fortification of maternal milk with a commercial product containing protein, calcium, and phosphate is suggested to achieve the higher nutritional needs of the very low birth weight neonates [53].

Although fortified maternal milk is the preferred type of feeding, nutrients provided by fortified breast milk often are insufficient to cover the nutritional requirements of neonates with bronchopulmonary dysplasia. This can be attributed to the low protein concentration of the fortifiers and changes in human milk's nutritional values over time.

Individualized human milk fortification has been suggested, such as adjusted fortification and target fortification to overcome this issue [20].

Adjustable fortification consisted of standard fortification and the addition of more quantity of fortifier and extra protein monitored by blood urea nitrogen measurements. Infants receiving the adjustable fortification regimen had increased provision of proteins during the first 3 weeks after birth and showed significantly greater anthropometric measurements compared to neonates in which the standard fortification formula was used. Anthropometric measurements were positively related to protein provision [54].

In another interventional cohort study, BPD infants were fed with specifically fortified breast milk and/or preterm formula with the addition of Duocal and MCT oil and were compared with a control group fed fortified breast milk and/or pre-term formula. The intervention group showed improved growth suggesting that optimization of nutritional support improves growth after birth in preterm infants with BPD [55]. Although the increased provision of calories may result in increased CO_2 release, the favorable growth outcome is more important in infants with BPD [20].

5. Premature Formulas and Caloric Supplementation

A study that enrolled 224 infants with BPD found that almost half started premature formula before exiting the NICU. Neonates who stopped human milk before exiting the NICU received human milk for a shorter period of time compared with those who continued to breastfeed after discharge [55]. Following the cessation of maternal milk based on the maturity of the infant and nutritional demands, feeding with a specific formula is suggested. The commercially available preterm formulas which are used in the NICU, contain increased amounts of energy, protein, calcium, and phosphorus, and the type of fat added in the formula is a blend of vegetable oils including long-chain triglycerides and MCT [56].

A nutrient-enriched formula containing high energy and micronutrients used on neonates with BPD up to 3 months after birth results in improved growth in comparison to neonates consuming an isoenergetic standard preterm formula. This implies that infants with BPD have increased growth rates when formulas richer in nutrients compared to standard ones are used [57].

Theile et al. have demonstrated that neonates with bronchopulmonary dysplasia born in the current period have better growth compared with infants born 10 years ago. The authors speculate that early parenteral nutrition including amino acids and caloric-dense feeding policies have contributed to this result. They speculated that growth acceleration depends on several factors; however, the administration of calorically dense (>24 kcal per oz) milk products that optimize the uptake of proteins in infants in which liberal provision of fluids is contraindicated plays an important role. Calorically dense milk contains about 3 g of protein/100 kcal compared to formulas given ten years ago, which provided about 2 g of protein/100 kcal. BPD patients in the current era BPD had improved growth and required ventilator support for a shorter period of time [58].

A pilot study compared the nutritional status of patients with BPD who were provided with either ready-to-feed formula having a caloric concentration of a 30 kcal/oz or a preterm formula including nutritional supplementation. The authors found that the nutritional supply of the two regimens was similar, whereas the 30 kcal/oz formula provided increased protein. Thus the 30 kcal/oz formula is a satisfactory choice for premature infants with BPD [59].

Following cessation of breast milk after discharge from the NICU post-discharge formulas improve growth rates. There is no sufficient information supporting the use of certain formulas in neonates with bronchopulmonary dysplasia. As respiratory function improves in parallel with growth velocity high caloric milk can be weaned and children can follow a normal diet [20]. However, a percentage of children with BPD which is severe will need high caloric supplementations in their childhood to maintain sufficient growth [20]. In addition, the introduction of solid foods may be different in term infants compared to those with BPD. The initiation of solid foods should not be based on chronological age as these children may be able to swallow solid foods at a later age as a result of prematurity and feeding difficulties. Thicker foods may easier to swallow [19].

6. Feeding Issues

Gastroesophageal reflux is a frequent problem in neonates that have bronchopulmonary dysplasia. A study of 131 infants with BPD assessed the occurrence of side effects with a follow-up time of 1.5 years. pH-multichannel intraluminal impedance and gastric sodium concentrations were assessed for 24 h in the study population when they reached 36 weeks and 18 months. The incidence of gastroesophageal reflux in BPD was about 40% and included both acid gastroesophageal reflux and duodenogastroesophageal reflux. Increased incidence of respiratory symptoms was documented in infants born before 30 weeks, having a birth weight less than 1500 g, those requiring mechanical ventilation > 7 days, and those who had had acid and duodenal gastroesophageal reflux. Infants with BPD and duodenal gastroesophageal reflux were at higher risk for late side effects compared to the rest of the infants studied [60].

Swallowing dysfunction is also a common problem in BPD patients that may affect respiratory function. Neonates that develop bronchopulmonary dysplasia have tachypnoea, experience more episodes of low saturations, have poor coordination between sucking and swallowing and have poor sucking endurance and performance. They also have recurrent episodes of cough, wheezing, vomiting, difficulties with feeding and choking [61].

7. Alternatives to Oral Feeding

As infants with BPD have a high incidence of difficulties with oral feeding very often alternative methods of feeding are applied, even after discharge home. Feeding by mouth has been shown to affect respiratory function in very premature neonates with severe BPD during NICU stay or even when they go home. This is a prolonged effect as these infants experience significantly lower saturations during feedings even at 2–6 months after birth. Another side effect documented in this population is that they also have growth restrictions at the same chronological age [61].

Studies concerning feeding strategies after discharge from the NICU have demonstrated that the use of nasogastric tube feeding is preferable to gastrostomy [62]. However, different institutions use different feeding protocols post-discharge. Nasogastric tube use in the population with established bronchopulmonary dysplasia seems to be a practical approach with lower numbers of babies needing the insertion of a gastrostomy tube. Brain magnetic resonance imaging abnormalities were more prevalent in infants in babies in which a gastrostomy tube was placed postdischarge [63].

Analysis of very premature infants from 25 centers found that among the infants requiring gastrostomy tube placement post-discharge, 77% had bronchopulmonary dysplasia. The gastrostomy tube was related to altered anthropometric parameters, neurodevelopmental delay, and feeding and prolonged lung issues at follow-up [64].

8. Monitoring of Growth and Nutritional Status

While being in hospital weight is monitored every day and length and head circumference once a week. Iron status should be monitored with complete blood count with reticulocyte count, serum ferritin levels, protein status with blood urea nitrogen and metabolic bone disease with phosphorus and alkaline phosphate concentrations. Regular electrolyte measurements should be measured in patients on diuretics and monitoring of vitamins and trace elements should be performed if there is suspicion of deficiency [20]. A similar plan should be employed after discharge with the general pediatrician and the aid of specialists in nutrition and feeding. The implementation of a multidisciplinary approach involving the consultation of specialists may be beneficial for these infants.

9. Conclusions

Nutrition of infants with BPD should focus on the supply of adequate caloric support and provision of nutrients to promote growth, prevent extrauterine growth retardation and assist in alveolarization of the lungs. Meticulous follow-up is warranted before and after discharge from the NICU to minimize growth deficiency and improve lung function. Currently, there is limited data regarding the optimal feeding strategies for this population of infants. Well-designed clinical studies are required to improve our practices regarding feeding and nutrition issues of infants with BPD.

Author Contributions: A.A.K. writing—original draft preparation; D.G. writing—review and editing; A.V. supervision. All authors have approved the submitted version and agree to be personally accountable for the author's own contributions and for ensuring that questions related to the accuracy or integrity of any part of the work, even ones in which the author was not personally involved, are appropriately investigated, resolved, and documented in the literature. All authors have read and agreed to the published version of the manuscript.

Funding: The study was funded by the research committee of the University of Patras Medical School, Greece.

Institutional Review Board Statement: N/A.

Informed Consent Statement: N/A.

Data Availability Statement: N/A.

Conflicts of Interest: The authors declare no conflict of interest.

References

1. Bonadies, L.; Zaramella, P.; Porzionato, A.; Perilongo, G.; Muraca, M.; Baraldi, E. Present and Future of Bronchopulmonary Dysplasia. *J. Clin. Med.* **2020**, *9*, 1539. [CrossRef] [PubMed]
2. Northway, W.H., Jr.; Rosan, R.C.; Porter, D.Y. Pulmonary disease following respirator therapy of hyaline-membrane disease: Bronchopulmonary dysplasia. *N. Engl. J. Med.* **1967**, *27*, 6357–6368. [CrossRef] [PubMed]
3. Hwang, J.S.; Rehan, V.K. Recent Advances in Bronchopulmonary Dysplasia: Pathophysiology, Prevention, and Treatment. *Lung* **2018**, *196*, 129–138. [CrossRef] [PubMed]
4. Baraldi, E.; Filippone, M. Chronic lung disease after premature birth. *N. Engl. J. Med.* **2007**, *357*, 1946–1955. [CrossRef]
5. Geetha, O.; Rajadurai, V.S.; Anand, A.J.; Dela Puerta, R.; Huey Quek, B.; Khoo, P.C.; Chua, M.C.; Agarwal, P. New BPD-prevalence and risk factors for bronchopulmonary dysplasia/mortality in extremely low gestational age infants 28 weeks. *J. Perinatol.* **2021**, *41*, 1943–1950. [CrossRef]
6. Cardoen, F.; Vermeulen, F.; Proesmans, M.; Moens, M.; De Boeck, K. Lung function evolution in children with old and new type bronchopulmonary dysplasia: A retrospective cohort analysis. *Eur. J. Pediatr.* **2019**, *178*, 1859–1866. [CrossRef]
7. Arigliani, M.; Spinelli, A.M.; Liguoro, I.; Cogo, P. Nutrition and Lung Growth. *Nutrients* **2018**, *10*, 919. [CrossRef]
8. Hansmann, G.; Sallmon, H.; Roehr, C.C.; Kourembanas, S.; Austin, E.D.; Koestenberger, M. European Pediatric Pulmonary Vascular Disease Network (EPPVDN). Pulmonary hypertension in bronchopulmonary dysplasia. *Pediatr. Res.* **2021**, *89*, 446–455. [CrossRef]
9. Cheong, J.L.Y.; Doyle, L.W. An update on pulmonary and neurodevelopmental outcomes of bronchopulmonary dysplasia. *Semin. Perinatol.* **2018**, *42*, 478–484. [CrossRef]
10. Jensen, E.A.; Schmidt, B. Epidemiology of bronchopulmonary dysplasia. *Birth Defects Res. A Clin. Mol. Teratol.* **2014**, *100*, 145–157. [CrossRef]
11. Van Marter, L.J. Epidemiology of bronchopulmonary dysplasia. *Semin. Fetal Neonatal Med.* **2009**, *14*, 358–366. [CrossRef]
12. Principi, N.; Di Pietro, M.G.; Esposito, S. Bronchopulmonary dysplasia: Clinical aspects and preventive and therapeutic strategies. *J. Transl. Med.* **2018**, *16*, 36. [CrossRef]
13. Stoll, B.J.; Hansen, N.I.; Bell, E.F.; Walsh, M.C.; Carlo, W.A.; Shankaran, S.; Laptook, A.R.; Sánchez, P.J.; Meurs, K.P.; Wyckoff, M.; et al. Trends in Care Practices, Morbidity, and Mortality of Extremely Preterm Neonates, 1993–2012. *JAMA* **2015**, *314*, 1039–1051. [CrossRef]
14. Gortner, L.; Misselwitz, B.; Milligan, D.; Zeitlin, J.; Kollee, L.; Boerch, K.; Agostino, R.; Van Reempts, P.; Chabernaud, J.L.; Bréart, G.; et al. Members of the MOSAIC Research Group. Rates of bronchopulmonary dysplasia in very preterm neonates in Europe: Results from the MOSAIC cohort. *Neonatology* **2011**, *99*, 112–117. [CrossRef]
15. Oh, W.; Poindexter, B.B.; Perritt, R.; Lemons, J.A.; Bauer, C.R.; Ehrenkranz, R.A.; Toll, B.J.; Poole, K.; Wright, L.L. Neonatal Research Network. Association between fluid intake and weight loss during the first ten days of life and risk of bronchopulmonary dysplasia in extremely low birth weight infants. *J. Pediatr.* **2005**, *147*, 786–790. [CrossRef]

16. Hartnoll, G.; Bétrémieux, P.; Modi, N. Randomised controlled trial of postnatal sodium supplementation on oxygen dependency and body weight in 25–30 week gestational age infants. *Arch. Dis. Child Fetal Neonatal Ed.* **2000**, *82*, F19–F23. [CrossRef]
17. Stewart, A.; Brion, L.P. Intravenous or enteral loop diuretics for preterm infants with (or developing) chronic lung disease. *Cochrane Database Syst. Rev.* **2011**, *2011*, CD001453. [CrossRef]
18. Uberos, J.; Jimenez-Montilla, S.; Molina-Oya, M.; García-Serrano, J.L. Early energy restriction in premature infants and bronchopulmonary dysplasia: A cohort study. *Br. J. Nutr.* **2020**, *123*, 1024–1031. [CrossRef]
19. Bauer, S.E.; Vanderpool, C.P.B.; Ren, C.; Cristea, A.I. Nutrition and growth in infants with established bronchopulmonary dysplasia. *Pediatr. Pulmonol.* **2021**, *56*, 3557–3562. [CrossRef]
20. Rocha, G.; Guimarães, H.; Pereira-da-Silva, L. The Role of Nutrition in the Prevention and Management of Bronchopulmonary Dysplasia: A Literature Review and Clinical Approach. *Int. J. Environ. Res. Public Health* **2021**, *18*, 6245. [CrossRef]
21. Milanesi, B.G.; Lima, P.A.T.; Villela, L.D.; Martins, A.S.; Gomes-Junior, S.C.S.; Moreira, M.E.L.; Baker Méio, M.D.B. Assessment of early nutritional intake in preterm infants with bronchopulmonary dysplasia: A cohort study. *Eur. J. Pediatr.* **2021**, *180*, 1423–1430. [CrossRef]
22. Jiang, H.; Lv, Y.; Hou, W.; Xu, X.; Zhu, L.L.; Zhang, H.; Shu, G. Association between neonatal malnutrition and bronchopulmonary dysplasia in very low-birth-weight infants: A propensity score-matched analysis. *Nutr. Clin. Pract.* 2022, *online ahead of print*. [CrossRef]
23. Malikiwi, A.I.; Lee, Y.M.; Davies-Tuck, M.; Wong, F.Y. Postnatal nutritional deficit is an independent predictor of bronchopulmonary dysplasia among extremely premature infants born at or less than 28 weeks gestation. *Early Hum. Dev.* **2019**, *131*, 29–35. [CrossRef]
24. Al-Jebawi, Y.; Agarwal, N.; Groh Wargo, S.; Shekhawat, P.; Mhanna, M.J. Low caloric intake and high fluid intake during the first week of life are associated with the severity of bronchopulmonary dysplasia in extremely low birth weight infants. *J. Neonatal Perinatal Med.* **2020**, *13*, 207–214. [CrossRef]
25. Uberos, J.; Lardón-Fernández, M.; Machado-Casas, I.; Molina-Oya, M.; Narbona-López, E. Nutrition in extremely low birth weight infants: Impact on bronchopulmonary dysplasia. *Minerva Pediatr.* **2016**, *68*, 419–426.
26. Huysman, W.A.; de Ridder, M.; de Bruin, N.C.; van Helmond, G.; Terpstra, N.; Van Goudoever, J.B.; Sauer, P.J. Growth and body composition in preterm infants with bronchopulmonary dysplasia. *Arch. Dis. Child. Fetal Neonatal Ed.* **2003**, *88*, F46–F51. [CrossRef]
27. Spiegler, J.; Preuss, M.; Gebauer, C.; Bendiks, M.; Herting, E.; Gopel, W. Does breastmilk influence the development of bronchopulmonary dysplasia? *J. Pediatr.* **2016**, *169*, 76–80. [CrossRef]
28. Gianni, M.L.; Roggero, P.; Colnaghi, M.R.; Piemontese, P.; Amato, O.; Orsi, A.; Morlacchi, L.; Mosca, F. The role of nutrition in promoting growth in pre-term infants with bronchopulmonary dysplasia: A prospective non-randomised interventional cohort study. *BMC Pediatr.* **2014**, *14*, 235. [CrossRef]
29. Yeh, T.F.; Mc Clenan, D.A.; Ajayi, O.A.; Pildes, R.S. Metabolic rate and energy balance in infants with bronchopulmonary dysplasia. *J. Pediatr.* **1989**, *114*, 448–451. [CrossRef]
30. Baner, S.E.; Huff, K.A.; Vanderpool, C.P.B.; Rose, R.S.; Cristea, A.I. Growth and nutrition in children with established bronchopulmonary dysplasia: A review of the literature. *Nutr. Clin. Pract.* **2022**, *37*, 282–298. [CrossRef]
31. De Meer, K.; Westerterp, K.R.; Houwen, R.H.J.; Brouwers, H.A.A.; Berger, R.; Okken, A. Total energy expenditure in infants with bronchopulmonary dysplasia is associated with respiratory status. *Eur. J. Pediatr.* **1997**, *156*, 299–304. [CrossRef]
32. Lauro, A.; Lacaille, F. Short bowel syndrome in children and adults: From rehabilitation to transplantation. *Expert Rev. Gastroenterol. Hepatol.* **2019**, *13*, 55–70. [CrossRef]
33. Bell, E.F.; Acarregui, M.J. Restricted versus liberal water intake for preventing morbidity and mortality in preterm infants. *Cochrane Database Syst. Rev.* **2014**, *2014*, CD000503. [CrossRef]
34. Barrington, K.J.; Fortin-Pellerin, E.; Pennaforte, T. Fluid restriction for treatment of preterm infants with chronic lung disease. *Cochrane Database Syst. Rev.* **2017**, *2*, CD005389. [CrossRef]
35. Zhang, R.; Lin, X.Z.; Chang, Y.M.; Liu, X.H.; Tong, X.M.; Ding, G.F. Nutritional Committee of Neonatology Branch of Chinese Medical Doctor Association. Editorial Committee of Chinese Journal of Contemporary Pediatrics Expert consensus on nutritional management of preterm infants with bronchopulmonary dysplasia. *Chin. J. Contemp. Paediatr.* **2020**, *22*, 805–814. [CrossRef]
36. Agostoni, C.; Buonocore, G.; Carnielli, V.P.; De Curtis, M.; Darmaun, D.; Decsi, T.; Domellöf, M.; Embleton, N.D.; Fusch, C.; Genzel-Boroviczeny, O.; et al. Enteral Nutrient Supply for Preterm Infants: Commentary FROM the European Society of Paediatric Gastroenterology, Hepatology and Nutrition Committee on Nutrition. *J. Pediatr. Gastroenterol. Nutr.* **2010**, *50*, 85–91. [CrossRef]
37. Wang, Q.; Zhou, B.; Cui, Q.; Chen, C. Omega-3 Long-chain Polyunsaturated Fatty Acids for Bronchopulmonary Dysplasia: A Meta-analysis. *J. Pediatr.* **2019**, *144*, e20190181. [CrossRef]
38. Chinoy, A.; Mughal, M.Z.; Padidela, R. Metabolic bone disease of prematurity: Causes, recognition, prevention, treatment and long-term consequences. *Arch. Dis. Child. Fetal Neonatal Ed.* **2019**, *104*, F560–F566. [CrossRef]
39. Abrams, S.A.; Bhatia, J.J.S.; Corkins, M.R.; De Ferranti, S.D.; Golden, N.H.; Silverstein, J. The Committee on Nutrition. Calcium and Vitamin D Requirements of Enterally Fed Preterm Infants. *Am. Acad. Pediatr.* **2013**, *131*, e1676–e1683. [CrossRef]
40. Poindexter, B.B.; Martin, C.R. Impact of Nutrition on Bronchopulmonary Dysplasia. *Clin. Perinatol.* **2015**, *42*, 797–806. [CrossRef]
41. Pereira-Da-Silva, L.; Virella, D.; Fusch, C. Nutritional Assessment in Preterm Infants: A Practical Approach in the NICU. *Nutrients* **2019**, *11*, 1999. [CrossRef]

42. Tindell, R.; Tipple, T. Selenium: Implications for outcomes in extremely preterm infants. *J. Perinatol.* **2018**, *38*, 197–202. [CrossRef]
43. Darlow, B.A.; Inder, T.E.; Graham, P.J.; Sluis, K.B.; Malpas, T.J.; Taylor, B.J.; Winterbourn, C.C. The relationship of selenium status to respiratory outcome in the very low birth weight infant. *Pediatrics* **1995**, *96*, 314–319. [CrossRef]
44. Darlow, B.A.; Austin, N.C. Selenium supplementation to prevent short-term morbidity in preterm neonates. *Cochrane Database Syst Rev.* **2003**, *4*, CD003312. [CrossRef]
45. Terrin, G.; Canani, R.B.; Di Chiara, M.; Pietravalle, A.; Aleandri, V.; Conte, F.; De Curtis, M. Zinc in Early Life: A Key Element in the Fetus and Preterm Neonate. *Nutrients* **2015**, *7*, 10427–11044. [CrossRef]
46. Wu, W.; Bromberg, P.A.; Samet, J.M. Zinc ions as effectors of environmental oxidative lung injury. *Free Radic. Biol. Med.* **2013**, *65*, 57–69. [CrossRef]
47. Villamor-Martínez, E.; Pierro, M.; Cavallaro, G.; Mosca, F.; Kramer, B.W.; Villamor, E. Donor Human Milk Protects against Bronchopulmonary Dysplasia: A Systematic Review and Meta-Analysis. *Nutrients* **2018**, *10*, 238. [CrossRef]
48. Dicky, O.; Ehlinger, V.; Montjaux, N.; Gremmo-Féger, G.; Sizun, J.; Rozé, J.C.; Arnaud, C.; Casper, C. EPIPAGE 2 Nutrition Study Group, EPINUTRI Study Group. Policy of feeding very preterm infants with their mother's own fresh expressed milk was associated with a reduced risk of bronchopulmonary dysplasia. *Acta Paediatr.* **2017**, *106*, 755–762. [CrossRef]
49. Johnston, M.; Landers, S.; Noble, L.; Szucs, K.; Viehmann, L. Breastfeeding and the use of human milk. *Pediatrics* **2012**, *129*, e827–e841. [CrossRef]
50. Kim, L.Y.; McGrath-Morrow, S.A.; Collaco, J.M. Impact of breast milk on respiratory outcomes in infants with bronchopulmonary dysplasia. *Pediatr. Pulmonol.* **2019**, *54*, 313–318. [CrossRef]
51. Gilfillan, M.; Bhandari, A.; Bhandari, V. Diagnosis and management of bronchopulmonary dysplasia. *BMJ* **2021**, *375*, n1974. [CrossRef] [PubMed]
52. Montealegre-Pomar, A.D.P.; Charpak, N. Anemia, nutrition, and ambulatory oxygen weaning in a cohort of oxygen-dependent premature infants. *Pediatr. Pulmonol.* **2021**, *56*, 1601–1608. [CrossRef] [PubMed]
53. Aslanoglu, S.; Boquien, C.Y.; King, K.; Lamireau, D.; Tonetto, P.; Barnett, D.; Bertino, E.; Gaya, A.; Gebauer, C.; Grovslien, A.; et al. Fortification of Human Milk for Preterm Infants: Update and Recommendations of the European Milk Bank Association (EMBA) Working Group on Human Milk Fortification. *Front. Pediatr.* **2019**, *7*, 76. [CrossRef] [PubMed]
54. Aslanoglu, S.; Moro, G.E.; Ziegler, E.E. Adjustable fortification of human milk fed to preterm infants: Does it make a difference? *J. Perinatol.* **2006**, *26*, 614–621. [CrossRef]
55. Seshadri, S.; Kim, L.Y.; McGrath-Morrow, S.A.; Collaco, J.M. Human Milk Cessation in the NICU in Infants with 55. Bronchopulmonary Dysplasia. *Am. J. Perinatol.* 2021, *Online ahead of print.* [CrossRef]
56. Hay, W.W.; Hendrickson, K.C. Preterm formula use in the preterm very low birth weight infant. *Semin. Fetal Neonatal Med.* **2017**, *22*, 15–22. [CrossRef]
57. Brunton, J.A.; Saigal, S.; Atkinson, S.A. Growth and body composition in infants with bronchopulmonary dysplasia up to 3 months corrected age: A randomized trial of a high-energy nutrient-enriched formula fed after hospital discharge. *J. Pediatr.* **1998**, *133*, 340–345. [CrossRef]
58. Theile, A.R.; Radmacher, P.G.; Anschutz, T.W.; Davis, D.W.; Adamkin, D.H. Nutritional strategies and growth in extremely low birth weight infants with bronchopulmonary dysplasia over the past 10 years. *J. Perinatol.* **2012**, *32*, 117–122. [CrossRef]
59. Puangco, M.A.; Schanler, R.J. Clinical experience in enteral nutrition support for premature infants with bronchopulmonary dysplasia. *J. Perinatol.* **2000**, *20*, 87–91. [CrossRef]
60. Wang, L.J.; Hu, Y.; Wang, W.; Zhang, C.Y.; Bai, Y.Z.; Zhang, S.C. Gastroesophageal Reflux Poses a Potential Risk for Late Complications of Bronchopulmonary Dysplasia: A Prospective Cohort Study. *Chest* **2020**, *158*, 1596–1605. [CrossRef]
61. Misuno, K.; Nishida, Y.; Taki, M.; Hibino, S.; Murase, M.; Sakurai, M.; Itabashi, K. Infants with bronchopulmonary dysplasia suckle with week pressures to maintain breathing during feeding. *Pediatrics* **2007**, *120*, e1035–e1042. [CrossRef] [PubMed]
62. Wang, L.Y.; Luo, H.J.; Hsieh, W.S.; Hsu, C.H.; Chen, P.S.; Chiu, N.C.; Lee, W.T.; Jeng, S.F. Severity of bronchopulmonary dysplasia and increased risk of feeding desaturation and growth delay in very low birth weight preterm infants. *Pediatr. Pulmonol.* **2010**, *45*, 165–173. [CrossRef] [PubMed]
63. Matharu, P.; Cristea, A.I.; Slaven, J.E.; Becker, S.; Niehaus, J.Z. Feeding Outcomes for Infants with Bronchopulmonary Dysplasia Discharged on Nasogastric Feeds. *Am. J. Perinatol.* **2021**, *38*, 897–900. [CrossRef] [PubMed]
64. Warren, M.G.; Do, B.; Das, A.; Smith, P.B.; Adams-Chapman, I.; Jadcherla, S.; Jensen, E.A.; Goldstein, R.F.; Goldberg, R.N.; Cotten, C.M.; et al. Gastrostomy Tube Feeding in Extremely Low Birthweight Infants: Frequency, Associated Comorbidities, and Long-term Outcomes. *J. Pediatr.* **2019**, *214*, 41–46. [CrossRef] [PubMed]

nutrients

MDPI

Review

Classification and Special Nutritional Needs of SGA Infants and Neonates of Multiple Pregnancies

Chrysoula Kosmeri [1], Vasileios Giapros [2,*], Dimitrios Rallis [2], Foteini Balomenou [2], Anastasios Serbis [1] and Maria Baltogianni [2]

[1] Department of Pediatrics, University Hospital of Ioannina, 455 00 Ioannina, Greece
[2] Neonatal Intensive Care Unit, School of Medicine, University of Ioannina, 455 00 Ioannina, Greece
* Correspondence: vgiapros@uoi.gr; Tel.: +0030-2651007546

Abstract: Data regarding the nutritional management of preterm small for gestational age (SGA) infants are scarce. In the recent report of ESPGHAN, the recommended energy for very preterm infants during hospitalization has been increased, yet this may not fit the needs of all preterm infants. It is important to distinguish fetal growth-restricted (FGR) infants from constitutional SGA infants, as well as preterm SGA from preterm AGA infants, since they may have different nutritional needs. Preterm FGR infants, and specifically infants < 29 weeks' gestation, accumulate nutrient deficits due to intrauterine malnutrition, prematurity, morbidities, delayed initiation of feeding, and feeding intolerance. Therefore, these infants may need more aggressive nutrition for optimal catch-up growth and neurologic development. However, a balance should be kept between optimal and excessive catch-up growth, since the combination of intrauterine malnutrition and excessive postnatal growth has been linked with later adverse metabolic consequences. Furthermore, multiple gestation is often complicated by FGR and prematurity. There is controversy in the definition of FGR in multiple gestations, and it should be noted that FGR in multiple gestation usually differs etiologically from FGR in singletons. The aim of this review is to summarize existing knowledge regarding the nutritional needs of preterm FGR and FGR infants of multiple gestation.

Keywords: nutrition; preterm; small for gestation age; fetal growth restriction; multiple pregnancy

1. Introduction

Although there is plenty of guidance for the nutritional management of preterm neonates, studies regarding the feeding of preterm small for gestational age (SGA) infants are scarce. Moreover, the special nutritional needs of preterm infants of multiple pregnancies, often SGA, are also practically missing. The ESPGHAN Committee on Nutrition of preterm infants has recently recommended to manage the nutrition of fetal growth restricted (FGR) or SGA infants in the same way as appropriate for gestational age (AGA) infants due to the paucity of data to propose specific recommendations. However, they also recommended an individualization of intakes [1].

However, preterm SGA infants may have different nutritional needs from preterm AGA infants, since preterm SGA infants often remain SGA at discharge, indicating accumulative nutrient deficits and failure to catch-up [2]. All preterm infants have deficits of important nutrients crossing the placenta mainly during the third trimester such as iron, calcium, vitamin A, and long-chain polyunsaturated fatty acids [3]. A preterm infant that is also FGR has experienced intrauterine malnutrition. Furthermore, comorbidities in the first days of life in preterm FGR infants, such as necrotizing enterocolitis (NEC) or feeding intolerance, often lead to delayed enteral feeding initiation [2,4]. Because of these factors, preterm FGR infants accumulate more nutrient deficits compared to preterm AGA infants. Furthermore, the combination of intrauterine malnutrition and excessive postnatal growth has been linked with metabolic changes and later adverse metabolic consequences in FGR infants [5,6]. All these factors render preterm FGR infants a special population with unique nutritional needs and a need for special nutritional management.

The two terms SGA and FGR should not be used as synonyms, since they refer to different conditions [7]. Various fetal, placental, maternal and genetic factors regulate intrauterine growth [8,9]. The definition of SGA includes infants with birth weight less than the 10th percentile, or at least two standard deviations below the mean for the infant's gestational age, based on data derived from a reference population [10,11]. This can be the consequence of a pathological process or can represent constitutionally small fetuses.

FGR defines a fetus that fails to reach his potential growth based on race and gender [9]. This term indicates that a neonate has undergone intrauterine malnutrition and growth compromise irrespective of their birth weight percentile [9]. This means that an AGA fetus can be also growth restricted if its intrinsic growth potential was higher [7]. These definitions are shown in Figure 1.

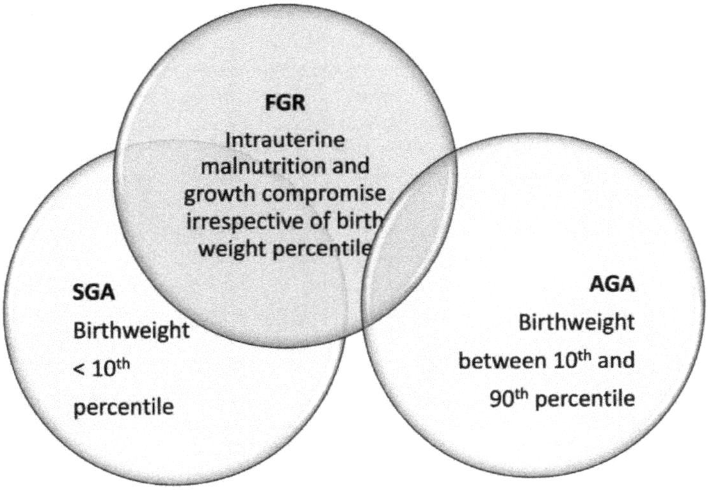

Figure 1. The definitions of small for gestational age (SGA), appropriate for gestational age (AGA) and fetal growth-restricted infants (FGR). Both SGA and AGA infants can be growth restricted.

It is challenging to assess the epidemiology of SGA and FGR infants, since some studies use the term SGA to refer to both FGR and constitutionally small infants. The incidence of SGA in well-resourced countries is 10% [12], while in low- and middle-income countries, almost 20% of term infants are SGA [13,14]. A recent study from cities in China found that the overall prevalence of SGA for 2014–2019 was 12.5% for term infants and 7.7% for preterm infants [15]. The prevalence of FGR is higher in resource-limited countries [14] and the incidence increases with decreasing gestational age [16,17]. Moreover, a significant part of all FGR occurs in AGA infants [7].

Even though FGR is a common condition, clear guidance for feeding these infants is lacking, and there is still debate on this subject. Studies addressing the optimal way of feeding FGR infants are scarce, and the terms SGA and FGR are often used as synonyms, despite referring to different conditions. Moreover, multiple pregnancies are often complicated with intrauterine restriction, especially when growth charts for singletons are used. This review will focus on existing knowledge and guidance regarding the different nutritional needs of preterm FGR infants and FGR infants of multiple gestation.

A thorough PubMed and Google Scholar search was conducted using the following terms: preterm infant, FGR, SGA, constitutionally small, multiple gestation, nutrition, and feeding. Relevant studies written in English up to April 2023 were included in this review, and specifically meta-analyses, systematic reviews, clinical trials and observational studies.

The reference lists of the articles were also reviewed in the search for other relevant articles that could have been missed in the initial search. The initial search retrieved 420 articles, and after title and abstract screening, a total of 71 articles were used in this narrative review.

2. The Distinction between Constitutional SGA and FGR Infants

It is important to distinguish FGR infants from constitutional SGA infants, since these two groups may have different nutritional needs. In the literature, SGA and FGR terms are often used as synonyms based on the idea that a small fetal size is associated with a higher possibility of growth restriction. However, the population is then diluted by healthy SGA fetuses and does not include AGA fetuses that are growth restricted [7]. On retrospective data, it is not possible to distinguish the two categories and exclude mature SGA infants. This is only possible in prospective studies that are designed to detect fetal growth deviations [18].

Ananth and Vitzileos hypothesized in their retrospective study that term SGA infants are mostly constitutionally small, while the group of preterm SGA may be comprised mainly by FGR fetuses, since biologic variability is not fully expressed at preterm gestations [19]. Large observational studies suggested that customized growth charts that adjust for the weight, height, ethnicity, and parity of the mother may be better compared to population-based charts in differentiating between constitutional SGA and FGR infants [20–23]. However, a Cochrane review in 2014 did not find randomized trials to assess the benefits and disadvantages of population-based growth charts compared with customized growth charts [24].

A 2016 consensus definition was established by experts in the field for the antenatal diagnosis of FGR through a Delphi procedure [25]. They concluded that an antenatal diagnosis of FGR includes an abnormal umbilical artery Doppler blood flow profile in addition to reduced growth velocity during fetal life. This means that both SGA and AGA fetuses can be diagnosed as FGR [25]. Furthermore, this consensus allowed for a distinction between early and late-onset FGR.

Therefore, constitutional SGA and FGR terms should not be used as synonyms, and studies in the literature have proposed effective ways to distinguish these two categories of infants.

3. Why Do FGR Infants Have Different Nutritional Needs?

It is still unclear what is the optimal nutritional management of FGR infants. On one hand, adequate catch-up growth is essential for the normal neurocognitive development of infants with intrauterine growth restriction [26]. However, excessive catch-up growth in the neonatal period and in infancy has been associated with later adverse cardiovascular and metabolic disorders [5,6,27,28]. A systematic review found an association between rapid infancy weight gain and higher absolute weight-for-length during the first 2 years of life with later obesity [29].

As already mentioned, premature infants have been found to have deficiencies of important nutrients acquired in the third trimester as well as deficiencies in zinc, copper, water- and fat-soluble vitamins and carnitine stores [3]. Infants with FGR have additional nutrient deficits, since they experience intrauterine malnutrition, resulting in chronic growth failure [9].

Because of intrauterine malnutrition, in order to survive, the fetus adapts by redistributing blood flow and nutrients to vital organs, mainly the brain, heart, and adrenal glands, at the expense of other organs. There is also an alteration in the production of placental and fetal hormones that affect fetal growth [9]. This developmental programming can cause epigenetic modifications that occur during a critical period of growth and maturation, resulting in long-term adverse effects. Retrospective studies comparing SGA with AGA infants linked SGA with increased visceral adiposity, increased risk of later hypertension, type 1 and 2 diabetes mellitus, and hyperlipidemia [5,27,28,30]. In multivariate analysis of a retrospective study, FGR was a significant risk factor for increased systolic blood pressure, while prematurity was not. FGR was also associated with reduced renal functional reserve, while prematurity alone was not [5]. A recent meta-analysis of 28 individual studies found that SGA children and adolescents had a 2.33-fold higher risk of type 2 diabetes [6].

In addition to these prenatal modifications, the excessive caloric intake after birth and a sedentary lifestyle later in life are associated with increased risk for metabolic syndrome, insulin resistance, and cardiovascular disease [31]. FGR infants can have increased appetite because they lack satiety due to an imbalance of their hypothalamic orexigenic/anorexigenic neuropeptides [9]. This may be beneficial leading to catch-up growth, but it may also contribute to later adverse metabolic effects.

Therefore, FGR infants may need special nutritional management, since neither iatrogenic malnutrition and insufficient catch-up growth nor excessive fat tissue gain are acceptable practices. Furthermore, FGR infants may accumulate nutrient deficits in the early postnatal life due to the higher risk of morbidities, the need for hospitalization, and the hesitation to start early feeding or the intolerance of feeding [4,32]. This is more prominent in preterm FGR infants.

One goal when feeding these infants is the administration of sufficient nutrients so postnatal growth would be similar to that of a normal fetus of the same gestational age or an infant with the same postmenstrual age. The intrauterine fetal growth is at least 15–20 g/kg/day. Tudehope et al. proposed in their review that a caloric intake of at least 110–135 kcal/kg/day with additional energy may be necessary for SGA infants for adequate catch-up growth to reach the rate of in utero growth [33].

On the other hand, constitutional SGA infants do not experience intrauterine malnutrition; therefore, they may have different metabolic needs. There are no studies focusing mainly on constitutional SGA infants except a prospective study of 58 constitutional SGA infants which found no increased risk for metabolic sequalae in the first 24 months of age [34]. Therefore, constitutional SGA infants should receive normal newborn care [33], although more prospective studies are needed.

4. The SGA Infant and Metabolic Consequences

The combination of poor fetal and accelerated postnatal growth rates in SGA infants appears to act in synergy in later metabolic adverse events [31]. In most SGA infants, catch-up growth occurs in the first 2 years of life and mostly in the first 6 months [35–37].

A systematic review of two randomized trials of term SGA infants concluded that enriched infant formulas that promoted early growth and contained 28–43% more protein and 6–12% more energy than the control formula increased fat mass, lean mass, and blood pressure at the age 5–8 years [38]. The authors of the two RCTs recommended that higher caloric intake and rapid weight gain are not optimal for these children, and therefore, breastfeeding should be preferred, since it was associated with slower weight and height gain [39,40]. However, a more recent systematic review of term SGA infants showed that children receiving exclusive breastfeeding had no body composition alteration or increased insulin resistance compared to children receiving a higher calorie formula [41]. Therefore, it seems that breastfeeding should be preferred over enriched infant formulas in term SGA infants.

Prospective and observational studies of term SGA infants showed that rapid weight gain and length catch-up growth during early postnatal life, specifically in the first 3 months of life, were associated with lower insulin sensitivity, lower HDL-cholesterol concentrations, higher triglyceride concentrations, obesity, and markers of atherosclerosis in early adulthood [42,43]. It is worth mentioning that these studies did not distinguish between constitutional SGA infants and FGR infants. Furthermore, it is important to note that these studies refer to term SGA infants, while similar data on preterm SGA infants are lacking. Therefore, it is unclear whether these findings apply to preterm SGA infants as well.

A recent systematic review and meta-analysis that included either preterm or SGA infants found that early macronutrient supplementation led to greater weight and length in toddlers without an increase in the risk for metabolic disease later in life. The data were mostly for toddlers and older children, while data for older ages were limited [44]. In a subgroup analysis, this study also found that supplementation decreased triglyceride concentrations but increased cholesterol concentrations at age older than 3 years and increased fasting insulin concentrations in adolescence only in SGA and not in AGA children. However, due to the small sample, since the three trials included only 25 SGA children, a safe conclusion about the effects of macronutrient supplementation on SGA infants could not be drawn [44].

Therefore, data indicate that term SGA infants may experience later adverse metabolic effects after excessive catch-up growth. However, available studies did not distinguish between FGR and constitutional small infants, and there is a paucity of data regarding the possible metabolic consequences in preterm FGR. Thus, future prospective and properly designed studies in SGA preterm are necessary to answer this question.

5. Fetal Growth Restriction in Multiple Gestation

There is controversy in the definition of FGR in multiple gestations. Twin pregnancies are often complicated with intrauterine growth restriction and prematurity. One or both fetuses can be restricted, and FGR infants have increased morbidity. In the cohort study LEMON of monochorionic diamniotic twins with selective FGR (sFGR), it was found that smaller twins had mild neurodevelopmental impairment compared to the larger twin, while no difference was found in children who had severe neurodevelopmental impairment between the two groups [45].

The FGR in singletons usually etiologically differs from FGR in twins, and the definition of FGR in multiple pregnancies is different in the literature. The National Institute for Health and Care Excellence (NICE, 2019) defines sFGR as the discordance of estimated fetal weight (EFW) 25% and above or EFW of one fetus below the 10th centile for gestational age [46]. The International Federation of Gynecology and Obstetrics (FIGO) recommends using twin-specific growth charts to avoid the overdiagnosis of sFGR [47].

A 2019 consensus definition was established by experts in the field for the sFGR through a Delphi procedure. The panel agreed that EFW of one twin < 3rd centile, irrespective of chorionicity, was adequate for a definition of sFGR. Moreover, at least two contributory parameters out of the following would define sFGR in monochorionic twin pregnancy: EFW of one twin < 10th centile, abdominal circumference of one twin < 10th centile, EFW discordance of $\geq$25%, umbilical artery pulsatility index of the smaller twin > 95th centile. In dichorionic twin pregnancy, EFW of one twin < 3rd centile and at least two out of three of the following contributory parameters was agreed to define sFGR: EFW of one twin < 10th centile, EFW discordance of $\geq$25%, umbilical artery pulsatility index of the smaller twin > 95th centile [48]. The Delphi definition recommends using singleton growth charts to assess fetal growth in twin pregnancies.

In a case-control study of 313 twin pregnancies, FGR was defined as one twin having a birth weight < 10th or <5th percentile for gestational age or a birth-weight discordance $\geq$ 20%. In this study, a twin with birth weight < 10th percentile was found in 47% of pregancies, at least one twin with a birth weight < 5th percentile was found in 27% of pregnancies, and in 16% of patients, there was a birth-weight discordance of $\geq$20% [49]. In these tables, the 10th percentile curve in singletons is similar to the 25th percentile curve in twins, demonstrating that almost 25% of twins are below the 10th percentile for birth weight based on singleton norms [49].

The incidence of FGR in twin pregnancies was reported 15 to 47% in the literature [49–51]. Selective FGR was found in 10–15% of all monochorionic pregnancies, and it was a cause of significant perinatal mortality and morbidity [52].

There are limited data to guide the management of twins affected by FGR, including optimal nutritional management, whereas the need for prospective nutritional studies seems to be imperative. The nutrition of FGR infants of multiple gestation will be discussed in this review together with the nutrition of preterm FGR infants due to a lack of studies.

However, these infants are not similar to preterm FGR infants, since the pathophysiology of small growth may be the consequence of limited intrauterine space and not of intrauterine malnutrition.

6. The Preterm FGR Infant

Preterm and term FGR infants should not be comparable, since they are different regarding their maturity, growth, and nutritional needs. It is unclear whether poor growth, catch-up growth, and early nutrition have similar effects in preterm and term FGR infants [53]. Data regarding the best feeding practices of preterm SGA and specifically preterm FGR infants are lacking. Considerations when feeding the preterm FGR infants are shown in Table 1.

Table 1. Considerations in nutritional management of preterm FGR infants.

Considerations in Nutritional Management of Preterm FGR Infants
• Optimal catch-up growth is essential for proper neurocognitive development
• Excessive catch-up growth may lead to adverse metabolic consequences later in life
• Increased nutrient deficits due to intrauterine malnutrition, prematurity, and morbidities in the early postnatal life
• Increased risk of NEC due to postnatal impaired gut function secondary to intrauterine malnutrition and a consequent reduction in gut perfusion
• Delayed feeding initiation due to fear of NEC
• Slow advancement of feeds, more time to reach full enteral feeds due to feeding intolerance
• Human milk is preferred over formula, since it was found to be protective against NEC and later adverse metabolic consequences

In their recent report, the ESPGHAN authors have increased the recommended energy for very preterm infants during hospitalization [54]. There are some concerns that even this increased amount of energy does not fit the needs of all preterm infants [55–58]. This may be the case, especially in SGA preterm infants with higher nutritional deficits whose needs may be different than those of preterm AGA infants. As already mentioned, regarding FGR and/or SGA infants, the ESPGHAN committee proposed the same nutritional management as for AGA infants due to the paucity of data, although initial weight loss is often less and acceptable up to 4–7% of birth weight [1,54]. There was no distinction between constitutionally SGA and FGR infants.

The goal Is to optimize enteral nutrition in preterm FGR neonates without increasing the risk of morbidities, such as NEC [2]. FGR infants are at increased risk of NEC due to postnatal impaired gut function secondary to intrauterine malnutrition and a consequent reduction in gut perfusion [4,16,32].

Another question in clinical practice is the optimal timing of starting enteral nutrition, especially in infants with abnormal Doppler studies. In these infants, delayed enteral feeding due to the fear of NEC can lead to additive nutrient deficits. For the immediate postnatal period for preterm SGA, if the abdominal examination is normal, Dutta et al. suggested starting feeding in the first day of life, with slow advancement of volumes at the lowest end of the range [59]. A randomized trial of preterm FGR infants (SGA preterm who had abnormal antenatal umbilical Doppler flows) found that an initiation of minimal enteral feeding in the first 5 days of life or less did not affect the incidence of NEC or feeding intolerance [60]. In another randomized trial of 404 infants younger than 35 weeks' gestation, it was shown that milk feed initiation on the second day of life led to earlier full milk feed achievement by 3 days compared to feed initiation on day 6, with no difference in NEC incidence. However, the group of preterm FGR infants younger than 29 weeks' gestation reached full enteral feeds at a median age of 9 days later than predicted from the study feeding regimen, and they also had an over three-fold increased incidence of NEC compared to older infants. Feeding intolerance occurred at a younger age, at lower milk volumes, and lasted longer in the group of infants younger than 29 weeks' gestation [61]. Similarly no difference in the incidence of NEC was observed in an RCT on preterm SGA infants that received minimal enteral feeding for five days compared to no enteral feeding [62]. Another randomized trial on 133 IUGR infants comparing the effects of an early versus late enteral feeding in preterm FGR infants had the same conclusion, since the onset of feeding did not affect the incidence of NEC or feeding intolerance [63].

Most of these RCTs were included in a recent Cochrane review. This review included 1551 very preterm or very low birth weight infants, half of which were FGR or had reversed end-diastolic flow velocities in the fetal aorta or umbilical artery. They found that there was no reduced risk in NEC or all-cause mortality, but there was only a slightly decreased risk of feed intolerance after the delayed introduction of progressive enteral feeds. However, this was low-certainty evidence [64].

Dutta et al. proposed in 2015 that an advancement of feeds should be extremely slow in preterm SGA babies with gestation < 29 weeks and absent/reversed end-diastolic umbilical flow. Specifically, they suggested that an advancement of volumes in the first 10 days of life should be at the lowest end of the range [59]. This is due to the results of a randomized trial that showed that these infants failed to tolerate even a slow advancement of feeds. The median volume of milk tolerated in the first 10 days was <20 mL/kg/day. The median age to reach full feeds (150 mL/kg/day) was 28 days compared to 19 days in the group of infants 29 to 34 + 6 weeks gestational age with abnormal antenatal Doppler studies [65]. This means that infants born < 29 weeks' gestation may have additional nutrient deficits, and therefore, they may need more aggressive nutrition later to catch-up.

The American Society for Parenteral and Enteral Nutrition guidelines recommended early minimal enteral feeding within the first two days of life and advancement of feeding volumes at 30 mL/kg/d in infants weighing $\geq$ 1000 g [66]. It remains under question whether this applies also to FGR preterm infants. The strength of the recommendation was weak; therefore, larger multicenter prospective trials are mandatory to answer questions regarding the initiation of enteral feeding and feeding volume advancement.

Human milk is preferred over formula [59]. In a retrospective study of 420 preterm SGA infants, human milk was associated with a decreased risk of NEC and late-onset sepsis [2]. Even in the very high-risk group of preterm infants < 29 weeks gestation, breast milk was protective against NEC [65]. A Cochrane review in preterm and LBW infants found that formula feeding led to greater weight gain, linear and head growth and a higher risk of NEC compared with donor breast milk. This evidence was of moderate certainty. There was no difference in mortality, long-term growth or neurological development [67].

As already mentioned, preterm FGR infants may accumulate nutrient deficits during the first days of life due to the higher risk of morbidities, the need for hospitalization, and the hesitation to start early feeding or to feeding intolerance. Cohorts of SGA preterm infants showed a high incidence of postnatal growth failure [2,17,68]. In a cohort of 1776 SGA infants, 97% of them remained SGA at 36 weeks' corrected age [17], and the same was shown in a smaller cohort of 104 preterm infants of whom 21% were SGA and remained SGA at 40 weeks postmenstrual age [68]. Growth restriction in preterm neonates was found to be inversely related to younger gestational age and weight at birth [69]. A small study of preterm SGA infants showed that an exclusive human milk-based diet led to weight gain equal to the AGA group during a follow-up period of 12–15 months with no increased adiposity or elevated insulin resistance at 2 years of age [70]. On the other hand, in a retrospective cohort of 420 preterm SGA infants, growth failure persisted at discharge in infants receiving either exclusive human milk or cow's milk diet [2].

Senterre et al., in their prospective observational study of preterm SGA infants, demonstrated that SGA infants were able to tolerate higher nutritional intakes during the first weeks of life and had higher weight gain compared to AGA. Preterm SGA were started with nutritional intakes of 40 $\pm$ 6 kcal/kg/day, while enteral feeds were introduced at a mean age of 2.9 ± 4.2 days. In the third week, the mean nutritional intake was 130 ± 17 kcal/kg/day and the enteral intake was 127 ± 55 mL/kg/day. Parenteral nutrition was discontinued at a mean age of 21.3 days [71]. The authors concluded that nutritional supply in the first days of life is essential to improve growth in the first week of life and to limit postnatal weight loss and growth restriction.

7. Conclusions

Available guidelines did not provide specific recommendations for SGA or FGR infants due to the paucity of studies. Prospective studies are mandatory to assess the optimal nutritional management of different groups of infants. Constitutional SGA infants, FRG infants and specifically preterm FGR and FGR infants of multiple pregnancies should be distinguished in future guidelines, and specific recommendations should be given for each group.

In conclusion, in preterm FGR infants, a balance should be kept between the optimal catch-up growth that is vital for normal neurologic development and excessive catch-up growth that may lead to the development of cardiovascular and metabolic disorders later in life. Preterm FGR infants have accumulative nutrient deficits due to prematurity, fetal malnutrition, comorbidities in the first days of life, delayed initiation of enteral feeding, slow advancement of feeds, and tolerance of lower feeding volumes. This is more evident in infants < 29 weeks' gestation. This means that they may need more aggressive nutrition later to catch up, since data indicate that many preterm SGA infants remain SGA at discharge. Breastfeeding is preferred over enriched infant formulas to reduce the risk of NEC and later metabolic adverse consequences.

Author Contributions: C.K. performed the literature search and drafted the manuscript. D.R. and F.B. contributed to literature search and drafting the work. A.S. and M.B. critically revised the manuscript. V.G. proposed the writing of the article, supervised, and critically revised the work. All authors have read and agreed to the published version of the manuscript.

Funding: This research received no external funding.

Institutional Review Board Statement: Not applicable.

Informed Consent Statement: Not applicable.

Data Availability Statement: Not applicable.

Conflicts of Interest: The authors declare no conflict of interest.

References

1. Supplementary Digital Content no.1. ESPGHAN Committee of Nutrition (CoN) Position Paper on Enteral Nutrition for Preterm Infants: Introduction, Methods and Limitations. Available online: http://links.lww.com/MPG/C974 (accessed on 6 April 2023).
2. Fleig, L.; Hagan, J.; Lee, M.L.; Abrams, S.A.; Hawthorne, K.M.; Hair, A.B. Growth outcomes of small for gestational age preterm infants before and after implementation of an exclusive human milk-based diet. *J. Perinatol.* **2021**, *41*, 1859–1864. [CrossRef] [PubMed]
3. Shah, M.D.; Shah, S.R. Nutrient deficiencies in the premature infant. *Pediatr. Clin. N. Am.* **2009**, *56*, 1069–1083. [CrossRef] [PubMed]
4. Dorling, J.; Kempley, S.; Leaf, A. Feeding growth restricted preterm infants with abnormal antenatal Doppler results. *Arch. Dis. Child. Fetal Neonatal Ed.* **2005**, *90*, F359–F363. [CrossRef] [PubMed]
5. Chan, P.Y.; Morris, J.M.; Leslie, G.I.; Kelly, P.J.; Gallery, E.D. The long-term effects of prematurity and intrauterine growth restriction on cardiovascular, renal, and metabolic function. *Int. J. Pediatr.* **2010**, *2010*, 280402. [CrossRef]
6. Martín-Calvo, N.; Goni, L.; Tur, J.A.; Martínez, J.A. Low birth weight and small for gestational age are associated with complications of childhood and adolescence obesity: Systematic review and meta-analysis. *Obes. Rev.* **2022**, *23* (Suppl. S1), e13380. [CrossRef]
7. Damhuis, S.E.; Ganzevoort, W.; Gordijn, S.J. Abnormal Fetal Growth: Small for Gestational Age, Fetal Growth Restriction, Large for Gestational Age: Definitions and Epidemiology. *Obstet. Gynecol. Clin. N. Am.* **2021**, *48*, 267–279. [CrossRef]
8. Maulik, D. Fetal growth restriction: The etiology. *Clin. Obstet. Gynecol.* **2006**, *49*, 228–235. [CrossRef]
9. Kesavan, K.; Devaskar, S.U. Intrauterine Growth Restriction: Postnatal Monitoring and Outcomes. *Pediatr. Clin. N. Am.* **2019**, *66*, 403–423. [CrossRef]

10. WHO. Expert Committee on Physical Status: The Use Interpretation of Anthropometry & World Health Organization. In *Physical Status: The Use of and Interpretation of Anthropometry, Report of a WHO Expert Committee*; World Health Organization: Geneva, Switzerland, 1995.
11. Clayton, P.E.; Cianfarani, S.; Czernichow, P.; Johannsson, G.; Rapaport, R.; Rogol, A. Management of the child born small for gestational age through to adulthood: A consensus statement of the International Societies of Pediatric Endocrinology and the Growth Hormone Research Society. *J. Clin. Endocrinol. Metab.* **2007**, *92*, 804–810. [CrossRef]
12. Lees, C.C.; Romero, R.; Stampalija, T.; Dall'Asta, A.; DeVore, G.A.; Prefumo, F.; Frusca, T.; Visser, G.H.A.; Hobbins, J.C.; Baschat, A.A.; et al. Clinical Opinion: The diagnosis and management of suspected fetal growth restriction: An evidence-based approach. *Am. J. Obstet. Gynecol.* **2022**, *226*, 366–378. [CrossRef]
13. Lee, A.C.; Kozuki, N.; Cousens, S.; Stevens, G.A.; Blencowe, H.; Silveira, M.F.; Sania, A.; Rosen, H.E.; Schmiegelow, C.; Adair, L.S.; et al. Estimates of burden and consequences of infants born small for gestational age in low and middle income countries with INTERGROWTH-21(st) standard: Analysis of CHERG datasets. *BMJ* **2017**, *358*, j3677. [CrossRef] [PubMed]
14. de Onis, M.; Blössner, M.; Villar, J. Levels and patterns of intrauterine growth retardation in developing countries. *Eur. J. Clin. Nutr.* **1998**, *52* (Suppl. S1), S5–S15. [PubMed]
15. He, H.; Miao, H.; Liang, Z.; Zhang, Y.; Jiang, W.; Deng, Z.; Tang, J.; Liu, G.; Luo, X. Prevalence of small for gestational age infants in 21 cities in China, 2014–2019. *Sci. Rep.* **2021**, *11*, 7500. [CrossRef] [PubMed]
16. Bernstein, I.M.; Horbar, J.D.; Badger, G.J.; Ohlsson, A.; Golan, A. Morbidity and mortality among very-low-birth-weight neonates with intrauterine growth restriction. The Vermont Oxford Network. *Am. J. Obstet. Gynecol.* **2000**, *182*, 198–206. [CrossRef]
17. Lemons, J.A.; Bauer, C.R.; Oh, W.; Korones, S.B.; Papile, L.A.; Stoll, B.J.; Verter, J.; Temprosa, M.; Wright, L.L.; Ehrenkranz, R.A.; et al. Very low birth weight outcomes of the National Institute of Child health and human development neonatal research network, January 1995 through December 1996. NICHD Neonatal Research Network. *Pediatrics* **2001**, *107*, E1. [CrossRef]
18. Fang, S. Management of preterm infants with intrauterine growth restriction. *Early Hum. Dev.* **2005**, *81*, 889–900. [CrossRef]
19. Ananth, C.V.; Vintzileos, A.M. Distinguishing pathological from constitutional small for gestational age births in population-based studies. *Early Hum. Dev.* **2009**, *85*, 653–658. [CrossRef]
20. Clausson, B.; Gardosi, J.; Francis, A.; Cnattingius, S. Perinatal outcome in SGA births defined by customised versus population-based birthweight standards. *BJOG* **2001**, *108*, 830–834. [CrossRef]
21. Mongelli, M.; Figueras, F.; Francis, A.; Gardosi, J. A customized birthweight centile calculator developed for an Australian population. *Aust. N. Z. J. Obstet. Gynaecol.* **2007**, *47*, 128–131. [CrossRef]
22. Figueras, F.; Figueras, J.; Meler, E.; Eixarch, E.; Coll, O.; Gratacos, E.; Gardosi, J.; Carbonell, X. Customised birthweight standards accurately predict perinatal morbidity. *Arch. Dis. Child. Fetal Neonatal Ed.* **2007**, *92*, F277–F280. [CrossRef]
23. Gardosi, J.; Chang, A.; Kalyan, B.; Sahota, D.; Symonds, E.M. Customised antenatal growth charts. *Lancet* **1992**, *339*, 283–287. [CrossRef]
24. Carberry, A.E.; Gordon, A.; Bond, D.M.; Hyett, J.; Raynes-Greenow, C.H.; Jeffery, H.E. Customised versus population-based growth charts as a screening tool for detecting small for gestational age infants in low-risk pregnant women. *Cochrane Database Syst. Rev.* **2014**, *2014*, Cd008549. [CrossRef]
25. Gordijn, S.J.; Beune, I.M.; Thilaganathan, B.; Papageorghiou, A.; Baschat, A.A.; Baker, P.N.; Silver, R.M.; Wynia, K.; Ganzevoort, W. Consensus definition of fetal growth restriction: A Delphi procedure. *Ultrasound Obstet. Gynecol.* **2016**, *48*, 333–339. [CrossRef]
26. Taine, M.; Charles, M.A.; Beltrand, J.; Rozé, J.C.; Léger, J.; Botton, J.; Heude, B. Early postnatal growth and neurodevelopment in children born moderately preterm or small for gestational age at term: A systematic review. *Paediatr. Perinat. Epidemiol.* **2018**, *32*, 268–280. [CrossRef]
27. Ibáñez, L.; Lopez-Bermejo, A.; Suárez, L.; Marcos, M.V.; Díaz, M.; de Zegher, F. Visceral adiposity without overweight in children born small for gestational age. *J. Clin. Endocrinol. Metab.* **2008**, *93*, 2079–2083. [CrossRef]
28. Jaquet, D.; Deghmoun, S.; Chevenne, D.; Collin, D.; Czernichow, P.; Lévy-Marchal, C. Dynamic change in adiposity from fetal to postnatal life is involved in the metabolic syndrome associated with reduced fetal growth. *Diabetologia* **2005**, *48*, 849–855. [CrossRef]
29. Woo Baidal, J.A.; Locks, L.M.; Cheng, E.R.; Blake-Lamb, T.L.; Perkins, M.E.; Taveras, E.M. Risk Factors for Childhood Obesity in the First 1,000 Days: A Systematic Review. *Am. J. Prev. Med.* **2016**, *50*, 761–779. [CrossRef] [PubMed]
30. Huang, Y.T.; Lin, H.Y.; Wang, C.H.; Su, B.H.; Lin, C.C. Association of preterm birth and small for gestational age with metabolic outcomes in children and adolescents: A population-based cohort study from Taiwan. *Pediatr. Neonatol.* **2018**, *59*, 147–153. [CrossRef] [PubMed]
31. Barker, D.J. The origins of the developmental origins theory. *J. Intern. Med.* **2007**, *261*, 412–417. [CrossRef]
32. Bozzetti, V.; Tagliabue, P.E. Enteral feeding of intrauterine growth restriction preterm infants: Theoretical risks and practical implications. *Pediatr. Med. Chir.* **2017**, *39*, 160. [CrossRef] [PubMed]
33. Tudehope, D.; Vento, M.; Bhutta, Z.; Pachi, P. Nutritional requirements and feeding recommendations for small for gestational age infants. *J. Pediatr.* **2013**, *162*, S81–S89. [CrossRef]
34. Milovanovic, I.; Njuieyon, F.; Deghmoun, S.; Chevenne, D.; Levy-Marchal, C.; Beltrand, J. Innate small babies are metabolically healthy children. *J. Clin. Endocrinol. Metab.* **2012**, *97*, 4407–4413. [CrossRef] [PubMed]
35. Karlberg, J.; Albertsson-Wikland, K. Growth in full-term small-for-gestational-age infants: From birth to final height. *Pediatr. Res.* **1995**, *38*, 733–739. [CrossRef]

36. Recio Linares, A.; Bezanilla López, C.; Barasoain Millán, A.; Domínguez Uribe-Echevarría, M.; García Rodríguez, C.; Torrejón López, M.; Pérez Fernández, E.; Botija Arcos, G.; Barrio Merino, A. Longitudinal study of the newborn small for gestational age. Growth recovery and conditioning factors. *Nutr. Hosp.* **2022**, *39*, 520–529. [CrossRef]
37. Campisi, S.C.; Carbone, S.E.; Zlotkin, S. Catch-Up Growth in Full-Term Small for Gestational Age Infants: A Systematic Review. *Adv. Nutr.* **2019**, *10*, 104–111. [CrossRef]
38. Castanys-Muñoz, E.; Kennedy, K.; Castañeda-Gutiérrez, E.; Forsyth, S.; Godfrey, K.M.; Koletzko, B.; Ozanne, S.E.; Rueda, R.; Schoemaker, M.; van der Beek, E.M.; et al. Systematic review indicates postnatal growth in term infants born small-for-gestational-age being associated with later neurocognitive and metabolic outcomes. *Acta Paediatr.* **2017**, *106*, 1230–1238. [CrossRef] [PubMed]
39. Singhal, A.; Cole, T.J.; Fewtrell, M.; Kennedy, K.; Stephenson, T.; Elias-Jones, A.; Lucas, A. Promotion of faster weight gain in infants born small for gestational age: Is there an adverse effect on later blood pressure? *Circulation* **2007**, *115*, 213–220. [CrossRef]
40. Singhal, A.; Kennedy, K.; Lanigan, J.; Fewtrell, M.; Cole, T.J.; Stephenson, T.; Elias-Jones, A.; Weaver, L.T.; Ibhanesebhor, S.; MacDonald, P.D.; et al. Nutrition in infancy and long-term risk of obesity: Evidence from 2 randomized controlled trials. *Am. J. Clin. Nutr.* **2010**, *92*, 1133–1144. [CrossRef] [PubMed]
41. Santiago, A.C.T.; Cunha, L.; Vieira, N.S.A.; Oliveira Moreira, L.M.; Oliveira, P.R.; Lyra, P.P.R.; Alves, C.A.D. Breastfeeding in children born small for gestational age and future nutritional and metabolic outcomes: A systematic review. *J. Pediatr.* **2019**, *95*, 264–274. [CrossRef] [PubMed]
42. Soto, N.; Bazaes, R.A.; Peña, V.; Salazar, T.; Avila, A.; Iñiguez, G.; Ong, K.K.; Dunger, D.B.; Mericq, M.V. Insulin sensitivity and secretion are related to catch-up growth in small-for-gestational-age infants at age 1 year: Results from a prospective cohort. *J. Clin. Endocrinol. Metab.* **2003**, *88*, 3645–3650. [CrossRef]
43. Leunissen, R.W.; Kerkhof, G.F.; Stijnen, T.; Hokken-Koelega, A. Timing and tempo of first-year rapid growth in relation to cardiovascular and metabolic risk profile in early adulthood. *JAMA* **2009**, *301*, 2234–2242. [CrossRef]
44. Lin, L.; Gamble, G.D.; Crowther, C.A.; Bloomfield, F.H.; Agosti, M.; Atkinson, S.A.; Biasini, A.; Embleton, N.D.; Fewtrell, M.S.; Lamy-Filho, F.; et al. Sex-Specific Effects of Nutritional Supplements for Infants Born Early or Small: An Individual Participant Data Meta-Analysis (ESSENCE IPD-MA) I-Cognitive Function and Metabolic Risk. *Nutrients* **2022**, *14*, 418. [CrossRef] [PubMed]
45. Groene, S.G.; Stegmeijer, K.J.J.; Tan, R.; Steggerda, S.J.; Haak, M.C.; Slaghekke, F.; Roest, A.A.W.; Heijmans, B.T.; Lopriore, E.; van Klink, J.M.M. Long-term effects of selective fetal growth restriction (LEMON): A cohort study of neurodevelopmental outcome in growth discordant identical twins in the Netherlands. *Lancet Child Adolesc. Health* **2022**, *6*, 624–632. [CrossRef]
46. National Institute for Health and Care Excellence. Guidelines. In *Twin and Triplet Pregnancy*; National Institute for Health and Care Excellence (NICE): London, UK, 2019.
47. Good clinical practice advice: Management of twin pregnancy. *Int. J. Gynaecol. Obstet.* **2019**, *144*, 330–337. [CrossRef] [PubMed]
48. Khalil, A.; Beune, I.; Hecher, K.; Wynia, K.; Ganzevoort, W.; Reed, K.; Lewi, L.; Oepkes, D.; Gratacos, E.; Thilaganathan, B.; et al. Consensus definition and essential reporting parameters of selective fetal growth restriction in twin pregnancy: A Delphi procedure. *Ultrasound Obstet. Gynecol.* **2019**, *53*, 47–54. [CrossRef] [PubMed]
49. Fox, N.S.; Rebarber, A.; Klauser, C.K.; Roman, A.S.; Saltzman, D.H. Intrauterine growth restriction in twin pregnancies: Incidence and associated risk factors. *Am. J. Perinatol.* **2011**, *28*, 267–272. [CrossRef] [PubMed]
50. Arbuckle, T.E.; Wilkins, R.; Sherman, G.J. Birth weight percentiles by gestational age in Canada. *Obstet. Gynecol.* **1993**, *81*, 39–48.
51. Secher, N.J.; Kaern, J.; Hansen, P.K. Intrauterine growth in twin pregnancies: Prediction of fetal growth retardation. *Obstet. Gynecol.* **1985**, *66*, 63–68.
52. Sukhwani, M.; Antolín, E.; Herrero, B.; Rodríguez, R.; de la Calle, M.; López, F.; Bartha, J.L. Management and perinatal outcome of selective intrauterine growth restriction in monochorionic pregnancies. *J. Matern. Fetal Neonatal Med.* **2021**, *34*, 3838–3843. [CrossRef]
53. Lapillonne, A.; Griffin, I.J. Feeding preterm infants today for later metabolic and cardiovascular outcomes. *J. Pediatr.* **2013**, *162*, S7–S16. [CrossRef]
54. Embleton, N.D.; Moltu, S.J.; Lapillonne, A.; van den Akker, C.H.P.; Carnielli, V.; Fusch, C.; Gerasimidis, K.; van Goudoever, J.B.; Haiden, N.; Iacobelli, S.; et al. Enteral Nutrition in Preterm Infants (2022): A Position Paper From the ESPGHAN Committee on Nutrition and Invited Experts. *J. Pediatr. Gastroenterol. Nutr.* **2022**, *76*, 248–268. [CrossRef]
55. Kosmeri, C.; Giapros, V.; Gounaris, A.; Sokou, R.; Siomou, E.; Rallis, D.; Makis, A.; Baltogianni, M. Are the current feeding volumes adequate for the growth of very preterm neonates? *Br. J. Nutr.* **2023**, 1–5. [CrossRef]
56. Gounaris, A.K.; Sokou, R.; Gounari, E.; Panagiotounakou, P.; Grivea, I.N. Post-natal growth of very preterm neonates. *Lancet Child Adolesc. Health* **2022**, *6*, e9–e10. [CrossRef]
57. Gounaris, A.; Sokou, R.; Theodoraki, M.; Gounari, E.; Panagiotounakou, P.; Antonogeorgos, G.; Ioakeimidis, G.; Parastatidou, S.; Konstantinidi, A.; Grivea, I.N. "Aggressive" Feeding of Very Preterm Neonates and Body Mass Index at School Age. *Nutrients* **2021**, *13*, 1901. [CrossRef]
58. Embleton, N.E.; Pang, N.; Cooke, R.J. Postnatal malnutrition and growth retardation: An inevitable consequence of current recommendations in preterm infants? *Pediatrics* **2001**, *107*, 270–273. [CrossRef]
59. Dutta, S.; Singh, B.; Chessell, L.; Wilson, J.; Janes, M.; McDonald, K.; Shahid, S.; Gardner, V.A.; Hjartarson, A.; Purcha, M.; et al. Guidelines for feeding very low birth weight infants. *Nutrients* **2015**, *7*, 423–442. [CrossRef]

60. Karagianni, P.; Briana, D.D.; Mitsiakos, G.; Elias, A.; Theodoridis, T.; Chatziioannidis, E.; Kyriakidou, M.; Nikolaidis, N. Early versus delayed minimal enteral feeding and risk for necrotizing enterocolitis in preterm growth-restricted infants with abnormal antenatal Doppler results. *Am. J. Perinatol.* **2010**, *27*, 367–373. [CrossRef]
61. Leaf, A.; Dorling, J.; Kempley, S.; McCormick, K.; Mannix, P.; Linsell, L.; Juszczak, E.; Brocklehurst, P. Early or delayed enteral feeding for preterm growth-restricted infants: A randomized trial. *Pediatrics* **2012**, *129*, e1260–e1268. [CrossRef] [PubMed]
62. van Elburg, R.M.; van den Berg, A.; Bunkers, C.M.; van Lingen, R.A.; Smink, E.W.; van Eyck, J.; Fetter, W.P. Minimal enteral feeding, fetal blood flow pulsatility, and postnatal intestinal permeability in preterm infants with intrauterine growth retardation. *Arch. Dis. Child. Fetal Neonatal Ed.* **2004**, *89*, F293–F296. [CrossRef] [PubMed]
63. Abdelmaaboud, M.; Mohammed, A. Early Versus Late Minimal Enteral Feeding in Weeks Preterm Growth-Restricted neonates with Abnormal Antenatal Doppler Studies. *J. Matern. Fetal Neonatal Med.* **2012**, 1–20. [CrossRef] [PubMed]
64. Young, L.; Oddie, S.J.; McGuire, W. Delayed introduction of progressive enteral feeds to prevent necrotising enterocolitis in very low birth weight infants. *Cochrane Database Syst. Rev.* **2022**, *1*, Cd001970. [CrossRef] [PubMed]
65. Kempley, S.; Gupta, N.; Linsell, L.; Dorling, J.; McCormick, K.; Mannix, P.; Juszczak, E.; Brocklehurst, P.; Leaf, A. Feeding infants below 29 weeks' gestation with abnormal antenatal Doppler: Analysis from a randomised trial. *Arch. Dis. Child. Fetal Neonatal Ed.* **2014**, *99*, F6–F11. [CrossRef] [PubMed]
66. Fallon, E.M.; Nehra, D.; Potemkin, A.K.; Gura, K.M.; Simpser, E.; Compher, C.; Puder, M.A.S.P.E.N. clinical guidelines: Nutrition support of neonatal patients at risk for necrotizing enterocolitis. *JPEN J. Parenter. Enter. Nutr.* **2012**, *36*, 506–523. [CrossRef] [PubMed]
67. Quigley, M.; Embleton, N.D.; McGuire, W. Formula versus donor breast milk for feeding preterm or low birth weight infants. *Cochrane Database Syst. Rev.* **2019**, *7*, Cd002971. [CrossRef]
68. Hair, A.B.; Hawthorne, K.M.; Chetta, K.E.; Abrams, S.A. Human milk feeding supports adequate growth in infants $\leq$ 1250 grams birth weight. *BMC Res. Notes* **2013**, *6*, 459. [CrossRef]
69. Clark, R.H.; Thomas, P.; Peabody, J. Extrauterine growth restriction remains a serious problem in prematurely born neonates. *Pediatrics* **2003**, *111*, 986–990. [CrossRef]
70. Visuthranukul, C.; Abrams, S.A.; Hawthorne, K.M.; Hagan, J.L.; Hair, A.B. Premature small for gestational age infants fed an exclusive human milk-based diet achieve catch-up growth without metabolic consequences at 2 years of age. *Arch. Dis. Child. Fetal Neonatal Ed.* **2019**, *104*, F242–F247. [CrossRef]
71. Senterre, T.; Rigo, J. Optimizing early nutritional support based on recent recommendations in VLBW infants and postnatal growth restriction. *J. Pediatr. Gastroenterol. Nutr.* **2011**, *53*, 536–542. [CrossRef]

nutrients

MDPI

Review

Knowledge Gaps and Current Evidence Regarding Breastfeeding Issues in Mothers with Chronic Diseases

Rozeta Sokou [1,2,*], Stavroula Parastatidou [3], Zoi Iliodromiti [2,*], Katerina Lampropoulou [4], Dionysios Vrachnis [5], Theodora Boutsikou [2], Aikaterini Konstantinidi [1] and Nicoletta Iacovidou [2]

[1] Neonatal Intensive Care Unit, "Agios Panteleimon" General Hospital of Nikea, 3 D.Mantouvalou Str., Nikea, 18454 Piraeus, Greece; kmaronia@gmail.com
[2] Neonatal Department, School of Medicine, National and Kapodistrian University of Athens, Aretaieio Hospital, 11528 Athens, Greece; theobtsk@gmail.com (T.B.); niciac58@gmail.com (N.I.)
[3] Neonatal Intensive Care Unit, "Elena Venizelou" Maternity Hospital, 11521 Athens, Greece; stavroula.parastatidou@gmail.com
[4] Neonatal Intensive Care Unit, School of Medicine, University of Ioannina, 45110 Ioannina, Greece; katerina.lambropoulou@yahoo.gr
[5] Endocrinology Unit, 2nd Department of Obstetrics and Gynecology, School of Medicine, National and Kapodistrian University of Athens, Aretaieio Hospital, 11528 Athens, Greece; dionisisvrachnis@gmail.com
* Correspondence: sokourozeta@yahoo.gr (R.S.); ziliodromiti@yahoo.gr (Z.I.)

Abstract: The prevalence of chronic maternal disease is rising in the last decades in the developed world. Recent evidence indicated that the incidence of chronic maternal disease ranges from 10 to 30% of pregnancies worldwide. Several epidemiological studies in mothers with chronic diseases have mainly focused on the risk for adverse obstetric outcomes. Evidence from these studies supports a correlation between maternal chronic conditions and adverse perinatal outcomes, including increased risk for preeclampsia, cesarean section, preterm birth, and admission in the Neonatal Intensive Care Unit (NICU). However, there is a knowledge gap pertaining to the management of these women during lactation. This review aimed at summarizing the available research literature regarding breastfeeding in mothers with chronic diseases. Adjusted and evidence-based support may be required to promote breastfeeding in women with chronic diseases; however, our comprehension of breastfeeding in this subpopulation is still unclear. The literature related to breastfeeding extends in various scientific areas and multidisciplinary effort is necessary to compile an overview of current evidence and knowledge regarding breastfeeding issues in mothers with chronic diseases.

Keywords: breastfeeding; maternal chronic disease; neonates; perinatal outcomes

1. Introduction

Breastfeeding is the best and most natural nutrition for infants. Through breastfeeding, infants are offered all the necessary nutrients and elements for their optimal growth and development. The World Health Organization, Unicef, and the American Academy of Pediatrics recommend exclusive breastfeeding for the first 6 months of life and continuation of breastfeeding (after introduction of solid foods at 6 months) until the first year of life and for as long as the mother and child desire [1–3]. There is indisputable evidence in the literature regarding breastfeeding benefits for the infant, the mother, the family, and the society, in general [4]. Maternal milk contains the ideal qualitative and quantitative composition for optimal neonatal growth. Breastfeeding contributes to the smooth physical and psychological development of the infant, conferring short-term as well as long-term benefits. First of all, breastfed infants have a decreased risk of childhood mortality [5–7]. Research has revealed that infants who have been breastfed for less than two months and those who are partially or not breastfed have a higher mortality risk compared to exclusively breastfed infants [8,9]. Breastfeeding for more than six months protects against obesity, diabetes, asthma, cardiac conditions, and increases final height [10–14]. Rich-Edwards et al. [14] investigated the association between breastfeeding and cardiac conditions and suggested that breastfed infants may present a lower risk of ischemic cardiovascular disease in adulthood. Additionally, breastfed children seem to have lower risk of developing certain types of childhood cancer, including leukemia and lymphomas [15,16]. Breastfeeding positively impacts cognitive, emotional, and social development of the infant [17,18]. Neonatal mortality and morbidity is reduced in breastfed neonates, in particular preterm newborns. Breastfeeding fortifies the immune system, promoting immune maturation and protecting infants against infections. Breastmilk interacts with gut microbiota and, to a degree, shapes microbiome colonization, with possible effects on long-term programming [19,20].

Breastfeeding contributes to the regular physical and psychological development of the infant, with short-term and long-term advantages. The majority of mothers are able to breastfeed and entitled to it, providing they are offered accurate information and are supported by family, healthcare system, and society.

The presence of a chronic disease is increasingly common in pregnant women, with a frequency of up to 10–30% [21,22]. The prevalence of chronic maternal disease is rising in the last decades in the developed world, with a reported increase from 4% in 1989 to 16% in 2013 [21]. This trend is possibly explained by the rise in disease rates in the general population, the increase in mean childbearing age of women, and the medical progress in assisted reproduction. Research in mothers with chronic diseases has mainly focused on their risk for adverse obstetric outcomes. Evidence from these studies supports a correlation between maternal chronic conditions and adverse perinatal outcomes, including increased risk for preeclampsia, cesarean section, preterm birth, and admission in the Neonatal Intensive Care Unit (NICU) [23–27]. However, there is a knowledge gap pertaining to the management of these women during lactation. The aim of this review was to summarize the available literature regarding breastfeeding in mothers with chronic diseases. Data from published studies are analyzed below and summarized in a relevant table in Supplementary Materials (Table S1).

2. Autoimmune Diseases and Breastfeeding

Advantages of breastfeeding in mothers with autoimmune diseases are outlined in the literature. The high prevalence of autoimmune conditions among women indicates the crucial role of gender and hormonal implication in the pathogenesis of these diseases. Evidence suggests a relationship between prolactin and autoimmune diseases, in particular systematic lupus erythematosus (SLE), rheumatoid arthritis (RA), and peripartum cardiomyopathy (PPCM) [28–33]. Prolactin is mainly produced in the pituitary gland and its role is not only to stimulate the growth of the mammary gland and the production of milk during lactation, but also to modify the maternal behavior. Genes coding for prolactin are located in chromosome 6, close to HLA-DRB1. Polymorphisms of the human prolactin gene may affect the pathogenesis of autoimmune conditions [29,34]. Elevated prolactin levels may interfere with B-cell tolerance through various mechanisms [28,35], while prolactin induces the expression of IL-2 receptor and the production of IFN-γ and IL-1 (Figure 1). It modifies the maturation of dendritic and thymus cells, leading to IFN-α production and enhancement of pro-B-cells generation.

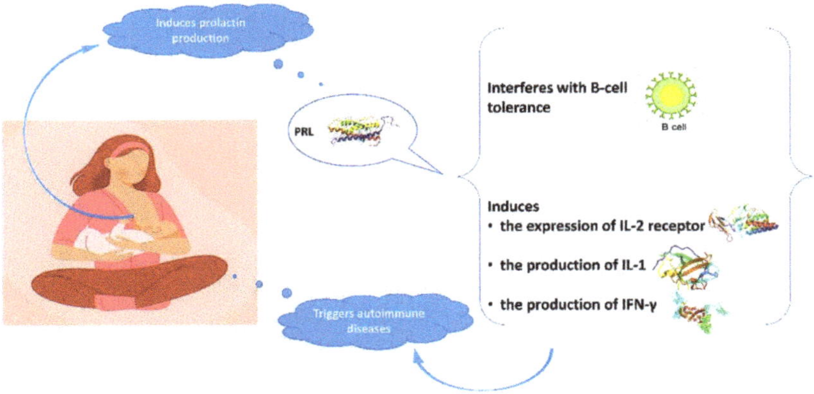

Figure 1. Interaction of prolactin with autoimmune system.

2.1. *Systematic Lupus Erythematosus and Breastfeeding*

Systematic lupus erythematosus (SLE) is a chronic, multisystemic, inflammatory disease of autoimmune etiology, commonly presented in young women of reproductive age. Prolactin has been found to be implicated in the pathogenesis of antiphospholipid syndrome and the observed impaired fertility [36–38]. Recently, Song et al. [31], in a meta-analysis, revealed a significantly positive correlation between prolactin and SLE activity. In a large, cohort study by Orbach et al. [39], SLE patients with hyperprolactinemia presented with significantly more episodes of pleuritis, pericarditis, and peritonitis, and had more frequently anemia and proteinuria compared to patients with normal prolactin levels. The authors concluded that dopamine agonists could be a potential treatment for SLE patients with hyperprolactinemia. In other studies, treatment with bromocriptine has reduced disease activity, and therapy cessation was associated with SLE flares [36,37]. Current evidence supports the benefits of treatment with bromocriptine in refractory SLE or in the prevention of flares after labor [37]. Conclusively, these findings question whether mothers with SLE should breastfeed.

Contrary to the numerous prospective and retrospective studies published on pregnancy outcomes of women with SLE [40,41], data regarding breastfeeding are currently scarce. Breastfeeding rates and duration seem to be decreased in SLE patients. Orefice et al. [42] in a cohort study reported that the vast majority of mothers with SLE (96.5%) were planning to breastfeed during pregnancy and 71.9% did breastfeed. However, half of these patients ceased breastfeeding after 3 months. Additionally, factors including cesarean section, preterm birth, intrauterine growth restriction (IUGR), and disease flares were positively correlated with non-breastfeeding. Also, a relationship between treatment with hydroxychloroquine (HCQ) and delayed breastfeeding cessation was reported for the first time. In subsequent studies, HCQ has shown reduction in disease relapse risk during and after pregnancy [43,44], decreased rates of recurrent neonatal lupus and improvement of labor outcome [45,46]. In another study, Noviani et al. reported that 49% of participating SLE patients decided to breastfeed [47]. This rate was not significantly affected by socioeconomic factors. Furthermore, disease activity after labor, full-term labor, breastfeeding education and planning were positively correlated with breastfeeding. Transfer of HCQ, azathioprine, methotrexate, and prednisone to maternal milk seems very limited and all drugs are compatible with breastfeeding [47]. Acevedo et al. [48] recorded reduced breastfeeding rates and duration in SLE patients: they breastfed their children half of the time that the mothers without SLE did (6 months vs. 12 months, respectively). The initiation of a new treatment was the main reason for breastfeeding cessation in spite of the fact that these drugs were low risk for breastfeeding. Breastfeeding duration could be improved by enhancing the level of information provided to patients. Complications during the postnatal period were mainly responsible for not initiation of breastfeeding.

HCQ is compatible with breastfeeding according to the American Academy of Pediatrics (AAP), and most SLE specialists recommend continuation of breastfeeding in SLE patients receiving antimalarial medicines [49,50]. Prednisone and ibuprofen in low doses are also acceptable options during pregnancy, while data on the use of other medicines for the treatment of SLE in pregnancy and lactation are limited. Current recommendations advocate for the initiation of HCQ when pregnancy is scheduled and the continuation of the drug throughout pregnancy and lactation [51].

2.2. *Rheumatoid Arthritis and Breastfeeding*

High prolactin levels may result either in autoimmune disease presentation in mothers with predisposition or in flares in patients with existing conditions [52]. Risk for RA onset increases during the postpartum period, particularly after the first pregnancy [53]. Women who developed RA within 12 months of the first pregnancy were five times more likely to have breastfed, while breastfeeding rates sharply declined in a subsequent pregnancy [54]. Barrett et al. [55] compared disease activity during and for 6 months after pregnancy between 49 patients who did not breastfeed, 38 who breastfed for the first time and 50 who had previous breastfeeding experience. Following adjustment for possible confounding factor, including treatment, patients who were breastfeeding for the first time showed increased disease activity 6 months after labor, indicated by self-reported symptoms, number of affected joints, and C-reactive protein levels, suggesting that this flare could be caused by breastfeeding. Brennan and Silman [54] investigated whether the presentation of RA after labor could be attributed to breastfeeding. Through a media campaign, the authors interviewed 187 women who presented RA within 12 months of labor and compared their breastfeeding history with that of 149 women of similar age selected from the patient registers of a nationwide group of general practitioners. In total, 88 women developed RA after their first pregnancy, and 80% of them breastfed. This rate was higher than the prevalence of breastfeeding (50%) in the 129 controls (adjusted odds ratio (aOR) 5.4, 95% confidence intervals (CI) 2.5–11.4). The risk for RA development was less increased following breastfeeding in a second (OR 2.0) and not increased in a third pregnancy (OR 0.6). More recently, Eudy et al. [56] in a cross-sectional study reported that most women with RA breastfed and were regularly receiving treatment during lactation. Disease activity seemed to worsen, in particular for the patients who did not receive treatment during lactation, while improvement was only observed in women who followed treatment during breastfeeding. Ince-Askan et al. [57] in a prospective cohort study concluded that only 4% of mothers with arthritis exclusively breastfed until 26 weeks compared to 25% of the general population.

2.3. *Idiopathic Inflammatory Bowel Diseases and Breastfeeding*

Idiopathic inflammatory bowel diseases (IBDs) are chronic intestinal disorders usually diagnosed during the second and third decades of life. The effect of pregnancy on the course of disease varies; the majority of patients remain in remission, while a few of them improve probably due to generalized immunosuppression during gestation. Contrarily, 1/3 of patients deteriorate [58,59]. Although the exact mechanisms explaining aggravation in pregnancy are not known, it is speculated that the cause may be the lack of maternal- fetal immunocompatibility [60]. Consequently, women with IBD may present with disease activation and need treatment at conception, pregnancy, or labor. Women with IBD are at increased risk for spontaneous abortions, preterm labor, and low birth weight neonates [59,61]. Some researchers suggest an increased risk of chromosomal disorders (although the role of disease activity relative to that of the drug exposures has not been elucidated) and adverse perinatal outcomes in patients with IBD [59,62]. Breastfeeding rates in women with IBD range among studies. Dotan et al. [62] reported that mothers with IBD breastfed less frequently. Approximately 1/3 of them did not breastfeed at all compared to 1/5 of healthy controls ($p < 0.005$), and short-term and long-term breastfeeding were also less common in mothers with IBD. Moreover, mothers who received treatment with immunomodulators and steroids had significantly lower breastfeeding rates in comparison to women who were only administered 5-ASA. In a study by Moffatt et al. [63], 83.3% of IBD patients began to breastfeed compared to 77.1% of the general population ($p > 0.05$). With regards to breastfeeding duration, 56.1% of IBD patients vs. 44.4% of the general population breastfed for more than 24 weeks ($p = 0.02$) [63]. The rate of disease flare during the first year after labor was 26% for breastfeeding and 29.4% for non-breastfeeding patients with Chron's disease (CD, $p = 0.76$) and 29.2% for breastfeeding vs. 44.4% ($p = 0.44$) for non-breastfeeding women with ulcerative colitis (UC). The risk for disease flare was independent of age, disease length, and socio-economic status. The authors concluded that IBD does not seem to reduce chances of breastfeeding. Lactation is not associated with increased risk of flares; contrarily, it could be protective during the first year after labor. Kane et al. [64] studied 122 women with IBD who were asymptomatic during pregnancy. Only 44% breastfed due to doctor recommendations, fear of drug interactions, and personal choice. Of those who breastfed, 43% presented postpartum disease flare. Non-adjusted OR for disease activity in women with breastfeeding history was 2.2 (95% CI 1.2–3.9, $p = 0.004$). After risk stratification by disease type, OR for UC was 0.89 (95% CI 0.29–2.7, $p > 0.05$), and for CD it was 3.8 (95% CI 1.9–7.4, $p < 0.05$). Following adjustment for treatment cessation, statistical significance of OR was not retained. These results indicate that a significant number of IBD patients do not breastfeed. A relationship between breastfeeding and disease activity may be owing to IBD treatment cessation.

Breastfeeding has been associated with prevention of IBD in children [62,65,66], a benefit which should be taken into serious consideration by mothers with IBD.

2.4. Multiple Sclerosis and Breastfeeding

Multiple sclerosis (MS) is an autoimmune inflammatory disease in which sclerotic plaques are formed in the central nervous system causing neuronal demyelination and damage. MS is usually encountered in women of childbearing age [67], and although disease modifying treatments (DMTs) reduce relapse rates, none of these treatments are recommended during pregnancy or breastfeeding [68–70].

MS relapse rates are decreased during the last trimester of pregnancy, but they rise during the first 3 months after labor, with up to 30% of patients relapsing [71]. Postpartum relapses are associated with high risk of disability [71] and deterioration of existing disability [72]. Women are frequently faced with the dilemma of breastfeeding or not breastfeeding and re-initiating DMT after labor. Despite the many observational studies, there is no consensus to date as to whether there is a relationship between breastfeeding and postpartum relapse control [72–75]. In 2012, a meta-analysis showed that non-breastfeeding women had double the risk of postpartum relapse than breastfeeding mothers [76]. However, there is great heterogeneity among studies included in this meta-analysis, and researchers did not assess whether disease activity before pregnancy affected the findings of the study or if the results were attributed to exclusive breastfeeding and its different hormonal impact from non-exclusive breastfeeding. Krysko et al. [70], in a 2021 systematic review and meta-analysis, demonstrated that breastfeeding was correlated with lower rate of postpartum MS relapses, with this beneficial effect being greater in cases of increased disease activity and exclusive breastfeeding. For a mother with MS, and possibly mobility problems, breastfeeding advantages may help improve her quality of life and health.

3. Epilepsy and Breastfeeding

Women with epilepsy often face unique problems and practical issues with pregnancy and lactation, and their breastfeeding rate tends to be low [77–79]. The main concern seems to be the possible risk to the child from the transfer of antiepileptic drugs (AED) in the maternal milk [80]. The 2009 guidelines on the management of pregnant women with epilepsy, issued by the American Academy of Neurology, highlight the lack of evidence regarding breastfeeding safety, which is stressful for both mothers and healthcare providers [81]. Reports of possible adverse events of AED, including suppression, irritability, hepatic dysfunction, or rash, in exposed infants are rare [82,83]. However, pharmacokinetic assessments are complex and published studies investigating AED concentrations in maternal milk and/or infant plasma are scarce [82]. Concerns have also been raised that the prolonged exposure to AED through breastfeeding might affect the developing brain, resulting in behavioral or mental disorders. Nevertheless, data from the Neurodevelopmental Effects of Antiepileptic Drugs (NEAD) indicated that breastfed children whose mothers received lamotrigine, carbamazepine, valproic acid, or phenytoin during pregnancy had higher intelligence quotient at 6 years compared to non-breastfed children [84]. Additionally, some women with epilepsy fear that breastfeeding increases sleep deprivation and possibly increases the risk of seizure episodes [79]. Studies have exhibited that mothers who breastfeed during the first 3 months tend to sleep more and less disturbed at night compared to non-breastfeeding mothers [85].

It seems that AED can be found in maternal milk; however, this exposure is limited compared to that of the transfer through placenta during pregnancy. Most AED are considered safe during lactation, and mothers with epilepsy should be encouraged to breastfeed [79]. Despite the recommendations in the literature, breastfeeding rates in mothers with epilepsy remain low [78].

4. Asthma and Breastfeeding

Asthma is the most common, severe, chronic respiratory disease, complicating 4% to 8% of pregnancies [86]. Approximately 1/3 of pregnant women suffer from asthma exacerbation during pregnancy, 1/3 remain stable, and 1/3 experience improvement [87]. This disease course variability is still under investigation [86,88].

There is evidence that asthma can negatively affect pregnancy outcome and that pregnancy may modify the clinical status of an asthmatic woman. Inadequately treated asthma may cause maternal hypoxemia, which can complicate pregnancy and labor outcome. Women with asthma are at increased risk of preterm labor, cesarean section, premature rupture of membranes, chorioamnionitis, placenta abruption, low birth weight neonate (the more compromised the pulmonary function, the lower the birth weight), extended hospital stay, and perinatal mortality [86,87]. The impact of breastfeeding in children of asthmatic mothers is unclear; some studies report a protective role against childhood asthma, while others report ambiguous results [89–91]. Meghan et al. [92], using data of 2773 infants from the Canadian Healthy Infant Longitudinal Development (CHILD), showed an inverse correlation between breastfeeding of asthmatic mothers and infant wheezing, independent of maternal smoking, education, and other risk factors (adjusted relative risk (aRR) 0.52, 95% CI 0.35–0.77 for $\geq$12 vs. <6 months of breastfeeding). Compared to non-breastfeeding, wheezing was reduced by 62% with exclusive breastfeeding, and by 37% with breastfeeding supplemented with solid foods at 6 months. Breastfeeding was not protective if supplemented with formula. Harvey et al. [89] studied the prevalence of wheezing, as reported by parents at 6 and 12 months of life. Breastfeeding for more than 6 months was associated with lower aRR at 6 months compared to no breastfeeding (aRR 0.54, 95% CI 0.30–0.96). Breastfeeding for more than 6 months was associated with lower risk for bronchiolitis and healthcare utilization in high-risk infants due to maternal asthma, both at 6 and at 12 months. The relationship between breastfeeding and asthma or recurrent wheezing varied depending on the age of the child, as well as the presence of maternal asthma or atopia in the child. In a study of 1246 children by Wright et al. [90], breastfeeding was correlated with a lower risk of recurrent wheezing during the first 2 years of life, but a higher risk of asthma and recurrent wheezing after the age of 6 years only for atopic children of asthmatic mothers.

Differences in concentrations and activation of leukocytes and cytokines have been described in the milk of mothers with and without asthma, differences which may alter the immunologic response of the infant. Although the specific mechanisms of immunologic alterations are yet to be elucidated, the relevant differences in the content of maternal milk may help explain the beneficial role of breastfeeding in children of asthmatic mothers [93].

Data demonstrate a lower breastfeeding initiation and duration and decreased rates of exclusive breastfeeding in women with asthma compared to those in the general population [94]. Breastfeeding rates tend to be lower in case of drug-treated asthma during pregnancy or postpartum [95].

Women with asthma should be assured that medical treatment is less dangerous for the fetus/infant than a severe exacerbation. Breastfeeding should continue in women receiving treatment, as only traces of the drugs are excreted in maternal milk. The decision to change a successful therapeutic regimen must be weighed against possible adverse effects of the drug continuation on the infant [96]. Breastfeeding does not impact the status of maternal asthma and, if appropriately controlled, asthma does not affect the duration of breastfeeding. Mothers should be encouraged to maintain a breastmilk stash that could be used in case of hospitalization or severe exacerbation which would obstruct breastfeeding.

5. Congenital Heart Disease (CHD) and Breastfeeding

Pregnancy is complicated by maternal CHD in 1–4% of cases. Data regarding worldwide prevalence of CHR in pregnancy are limited [97]. Sudden Adult Death Syndrome, PPCM, aortic dissection and myocardial infraction (MI) were the most common causes of maternal death in the UK during 2006–2008 [98,99]. The awareness of risk related to cardiovascular disease during gestation and the management of women with severe pre-existing cardiac conditions are vital for scheduling of pregnancy and monitoring for probable fetal and maternal morbidity and mortality [97]. Every treatment during pregnancy affects the mother as well as the fetus, and therefore the optimal management for both should be targeted. Scientific societies, including the American Heart Association (AHA), the American College of Cardiology (ACC), and the European Society of Cardiology (ESC), have published guidelines on the management of cardiac conditions during pregnancy [97]. Since there is lack of prospective or randomized clinical trials, recommendations and guidelines mainly correspond to level of evidence C [97]. Large registries and prospective trials are necessary for the enhancement of current knowledge. The ESC Registry of Pregnancy and Cardiac disease (ROPAC) and the EUROmediCAT registry of major congenital anomalies provide data on the epidemiology and exposure to medicines in pregnancy [100,101]. Due to progress in the diagnosis and surgical management of patients with CHD, the majority of these children grow up, and the number of pregnancies with underlying CHD is rising [102].

Hormonal changes cause significant hemodynamic alterations from the beginning of pregnancy, with increase in blood volume, heart rate, stroke volume, and cardiac output, and decrease in vascular resistance [103]. After labor, maternal blood volume decreases to gradually return to pre-gestation levels at 6 months postpartum. These hemodynamic adaptations may lead to cardiovascular events, including cardiac failure and arrythmias, in women with CHD [104].

Breastfeeding can also affect hemodynamic changes after labor; however, data on its impact on cardiac output or clinical course of patients with CHD are scarce. A study in rats exhibited significant increase in cardiac output in breastfed vs. non-breastfed animals [105]. Similarly, circulating blood volume and cardiac output were found increased during lactation in rabbits [106]. Lactating hormones, like prolactin and oxytocin, have been associated with aggravation of maternal cardiac diseases, including PPCM and aortic dissection in the context of Marfan syndrome [32,107]. Matsuzaka et al. [108] reported that women with CHD tend to opt for formula feeding from the first month postpartum. However, significant differences in postpartum cardiovascular events and levels of brain natriuretic peptide (BNP) associated with breastfeeding were not observed.

ESC does not recommend breastfeeding for women with severe cardiac disease (class of recommendation IIb). If a joint decision is made on continuation of breastfeeding (in patients with mild to moderate cardiac disease), watchful use of medicines and assessment of probable adverse effects on the infant are recommended [97].

Breastfeeding does not increase arterial blood pressure. Anti-hypertensive agents are excreted in breast milk, usually in low concentrations, with the exception of propranolol and nifedipine, the levels of which are similar to maternal plasma [97,109].

6. Sickle Cell Disease and Breastfeeding

Sickle cell disease (SCD) in pregnancy is associated with a sixfold increase in maternal mortality and increased risk of gestational hypertension, birth of a small for gestational age (SGA) neonate, preterm birth, and stillbirth [110]. The risk for obstetric complications and perinatal mortality is higher in pregnant women with SCD [111]. Complications related to the disease, including painful crises prepartum and postpartum, pulmonary complications, anemia, preeclampsia, and eclampsia, are also higher in women with SCD [112]. In developed countries, pregnancies with SCD are actively monitored and managed, with improved results [110]. In the United States, pregnancy-related complications have declined during the last decades, despite the still elevated maternal mortality and the occurrence of spontaneous abortions and perinatal deaths [112].

There is no evidence that lactation accelerates painful crises and patients with SCD should be encouraged to breastfeed [113]. Hydroxyurea is the licensed treatment for the management of SCD in adults and children over 9 months [114]. As an inhibitor of ribonucleotide reductase, it has a potential teratogen and mutational effect, and its use in pregnancy and lactation is contraindicated. Nevertheless, women with SCD have an increased risk of morbidity and mortality during pregnancy and after labor; therefore, cessation or modification of the optimal treatment could be harmful for both mothers and infants. In women who breastfeed every 2–3 h, levels of hydroxyurea in the milk are 3.4% of the relative infant dosage, which is below recommended safety levels. Also, if mothers with SCD pump and discard the milk after administration of hydroxyurea, the percentage of the drug transferred through breastmilk is further reduced by 50%. In this case, the infant will be exposed to a drug dose of <1 mg/kg/day, much lower than the doses of 20–30 mg/kg/day used for the treatment of infants with SCD [114,115]. Therefore, and due to the minimal amount of hydroxyurea transferred through human milk, it is safe for lactating mothers to receive hydroxyurea [114]. Patients with SCD may need opioid analgesics for effective pain management during pregnancy and lactation. Neonates of mothers on chronic analgesic treatment should be monitored for symptoms of abstinence syndrome [113]. In addition, as opioids are excreted in breastmilk, decision on their long-term administration must be individualized [113].

7. Thalassemia and Breastfeeding

Current therapeutic management of patients with thalassemia has improved their prognosis, survival and quality of life. Thus, pregnancies in women with thalassemia are increasing, and awareness of the specific risk factors is vital for the proper monitoring and management of these patients and their fetuses. Pregnancy with thalassemia is considered to be high risk, and follow-up by a team of specialists is required.

Low rates of breastfeeding in women with thalassemia could be explained by the necessity of re-initiation of treatments like chelates that are contraindicated during lactation [116,117]. Women with thalassemia who plan to breastfeed should begin deferoxamine (immediately after the 24 h infusion of deferoxamine postpartum). Deferoxamine is excreted in breastmilk but is not harmful for the neonate as it is not absorbed orally. Data on the safety of breastfeeding with other chelates are scarce [117].

8. Malignancies and Breastfeeding

Preservation of fertility following cancer has become feasible. Breastfeeding is also possible. In case of treatment, advantages of the drug over benefits of breastfeeding for the mother and the infant should be considered.

Reliable evidence regarding breastfeeding in women with a history of breast cancer is currently unavailable. Guidelines by the Society of Obstetricians and Gynecologists of

Canada (SOGC) state that women should be encouraged to breastfeed since there is no evidence that breastfeeding increases the risk of relapse or development of a novel tumor or that it endangers infant health [118]. According to a study published in *The Lancet*, the total incidence of breast cancer in developed countries could be reduced by half (2.7 from 6.3 per 100 women up to 70 years old) if women had the mean number of births and duration of breastfeeding common in developing countries [119,120]. Breastfeeding represents almost 2/3 of the estimated decrease in breast cancer prevalence [118]. The observed protection is related to hormonal changes during lactation, which delay menstruation and reduce exposure to estrogens that are associated with risk of breast cancer [121]. Additionally, during pregnancy and lactation, apoptosis of breast cells is frequent, helping remove cells with possible DNA defects and decreasing risk of breast cancer [121,122].

However, a recent systematic review by Bhurosy et al. [123] reported that breastfeeding is challenging among breast cancer survivors. Conservative surgical and irradiation therapy may reduce but not eliminate the ability of the affected breast to produce milk. Other issues faced by cancer survivors include uncertainty concerning breastfeeding, lack of support by doctors and family members, lack of access to a certified lactation consultant (IBCLS), nipple pain and discomfort. Social and clinical factors associated with successful breastfeeding include breastfeeding motivation, consultation and support by a multidisciplinary team of healthcare professionals, family members, or friends, the use of the other breast, and lactation enhancement with appropriate diet and galactagogues [123].

Patients with chronic myelogenous leukemia (CML) who achieve optimal response with tyrosine kinase inhibitors (TKIs) have high survival expectancy and concerns are raised regarding family planning. TKIs are potentially teratogenic, classified as pregnancy category D by the FDA, and their use in pregnancy is not recommended unless the treatment benefits outweigh the possible risks [124]. The suggestion for TKI cessation and breastfeeding for a short period of 2–5 days after labor is also acceptable [124,125].

Reduction in risk for breast and ovarian cancer is among the benefits of breastfeeding. Specialists who follow-up pregnant and lactating cancer survivors should be aware of the close monitoring necessary throughout this period [126]. Healthcare providers need to reassure women that breastfeeding has not proved to increase the risk of relapse. Galactagogues are often phytoestrogens in a concentrated form, which could promote oncogenesis or decrease the efficacy of hormonal therapy [127]. Domperidone and other drugs inducing prolactin release may be contraindicated due to an increased risk of breast cancer development with elevated prolactin [126,128].

9. Diabetes Mellitus and Breastfeeding

Preexisting diabetes mellitus (DM) type I or II affects 1–1.5% of all pregnancies and may lead to adverse maternal and neonatal outcomes [129]. Breastfeeding rates among women with preexisting DM are very low; relevant studies mainly include women with DM type I [129–131]. Both exclusive and any breastfeeding rates are lower in women with type I DM vs. non-diabetic mothers [132]. Herskin et al. [133] reported different rates of breastfeeding between women with DM type I and type II, both at hospital discharge (76% vs. 45%, respectively) and at 4 months after labor (49% vs. 23%, respectively). Decreased prevalence of breastfeeding may be due to increased morbidity, hospital practices that do not support exclusive breastfeeding, and issues with glycemic control of the mother. Initiation of breastfeeding is frequently challenging for women with DM because of high rates of pregnancy and labor complications, cesarean section and neonatal morbidity, including prematurity, respiratory distress, IUGR, and congenital anomalies [134–136]. Neonatal hypoglycemia could also affect the mode of feeding. Hypoglycemia is related to intrauterine hyperglycemia and subsequent fetal hyperinsulinism [137]. Moreover, early mother–child separation can hinder breastfeeding [138]. Establishment of stage II of lactogenesis is delayed by 24 h in mothers with DM type I; however, the milk production at 7 days after labor is similar to that of non-diabetic mothers [139]. Neonates of mothers with type I DM exhibit more immature breastfeeding reflex [140]. Early breastfeeding initiation could reduce neonatal borderline hypoglycemia and increase mean plasma glucose levels [141]. Maternal diet and insulin dosing should be closely monitored due to the postpartum change in glucose levels to ensure adequate control. Fluctuation of plasma glucose levels can delay production of breastmilk and lead to poor supply. Milk production depends on the proper development of breast during pregnancy. Insulin metabolism controls milk secretion, supporting mammary gland differentiation [142]. Insulin upregulates genes related to mammary epithelial cell (MEC) proliferation and downregulates genes responsible for MEC differentiation [143,144]. Insulin resistance may be associated with decreased secretory differentiation and subsequent reduced milk production [145]. The need for insulin of an exclusively breastfeeding mother is often reduced in up to 50% of pre-pregnancy requirements [146]. For infants of mothers with type I or II DM, breastfeeding possibly bears greater advantages. Breastfeeding protects against infectious diseases contributing to the infant's short-term immunity. Lately, a long-term protective effect of breastfeeding against obesity and type II DM has been confirmed [147–150]. Longer duration of breastfeeding correlated with lower incidence of type II DM in several studies globally [148–150]. Breastfeeding is estimated to reduce the risk of type II DM by up to 50% [151].

10. Thyroid Disorders and Breastfeeding

10.1. Hypothyroidism

Maternal hypothyroidism is not a contraindication for breastfeeding. Treatment with thyroxine continues throughout lactation. Thyroid hormones are essential for the normal development of the mammary gland and initiation of lactation. T4 and T3 levels are significantly correlated with milk production [152]. Thyroid insufficiency negatively impacts breastmilk supply [153]. In a study in rats, oxytocin levels and milk production were lower in breastfeeding mothers with hypothyroidism, while triglyceride concentration was also reduced in their milk [154].

10.2. Hyperthyroidism

During pregnancy and lactation, hyperthyroidism is usually managed with anti-thyroid drugs, which inhibit the synthesis of thyroid hormones. Treatment with radioactive iodine and surgical removal of the thyroid gland are reserved for cases refractory to medicines. Hyperthyroidism is not a contraindication for breastfeeding, but the drugs administered to the mother should be taken into consideration [155]. Based on the literature, both propylthiouracil and methimazole in moderate doses (<300 mg/day for propylthiouracil and 20–30 mg/day for methimazole) are safe during lactation, as their concentration in breastmilk is minimal [156]. The drugs are preferably taken in divided doses, immediately after breastfeeding, to avoid the period of maximum plasma drug levels [155,157]. Close clinical and laboratory monitoring of the mother and the child are necessary. Breastfeeding is contraindicated during treatment with radioactive iodine and for at least 4 weeks after cessation of the therapy [156].

10.3. Postpartum Thyroiditis

Postpartum thyroiditis is an autoimmune thyroid condition, presenting within the first year after labor, in women without clinical evidence of thyroid dysfunction before pregnancy. Its incidence is estimated at approximately 7% of women and varies depending on genetic background and iodine intake [158]. Women with type I DM are at increased risk of postpartum thyroiditis. The hyperthyroidic period presents 2–6 months after labor, often at 3 months, with 1/3 of affected women being asymptomatic. Otherwise, they could have issues with the care of the infant due to anxiety and nervousness [158]. Lactation is usually unaffected. The hypothyroidic period presents 3–12 months after labor, often at 8 months, with 20–64% of cases leading to permanent hypothyroidism. Symptoms like tiredness, loss of concentration, memory problems, constipation, lack of interest in the infant's care, and depression can easily be confused for postpartum depression in women who have recently given birth [159,160].

Traces of maternal thyroid hormones are excreted in breastmilk. Thyroxin concentration was measured at 0.83 μg/L, which does not have a significant impact on the status of infantile thyroid hormones [156]. In cases of other autoimmune diseases, hyperprolactinemia of lactation has been considered as a risk factor for disease exacerbation [161]. There are no data regarding the effect of breastfeeding on the presentation or exacerbation of thyroiditis [156].

11. Chronic Infectious Diseases and Breastfeeding

11.1. Human Immunodeficiency Virus (HIV) Infection and Breastfeeding

During the last decades, significant progress concerning mother-to-child transmission of HIV has been observed [162]. The virus is excreted in breastmilk and can be transmitted during lactation. Viral, maternal, and infant factors affect the risk of transmission. The viral load in the breastmilk is a determinant factor. Lifelong antiretroviral therapy is currently the gold standard for prevention of mother-to-child transmission in case of breastfeeding. In addition to maternal antiretroviral treatment, neonatal post-exposure neonatal prophylaxis is recommended. Initiation of antiretroviral therapy prior to pregnancy is optimal. If sustainably undetectable viral load has been achieved, the risk of transmission is estimated to be up to 1%. Elimination of this risk requires formula feeding and non-breastfeeding. In low- and middle-income countries, WHO recommends exclusive breastfeeding in HIV-infected adherent to therapy women for six months followed by complementary introduction of solid foods and continuation of breastfeeding for two years or longer [163]. In high-resources settings, most organizations encourage patient-centered, evidence-based counselling on infant feeding options [164].

Mothers with HIV should be offered constant access to antiretroviral treatment and continuous support in their decision to breastfeed. Close viral monitoring is necessary in lactating mothers to promptly identify any rise of viral load and appropriately modify treatment. Antiretroviral treatment is considered safe during pregnancy and lactation, as their excretion in breastmilk is negligible [165].

Women with HIV face additional barriers for exclusive breastfeeding, including disease-related stigma and the burden of a chronic condition, compared to HIV-uninfected mothers [166]. Exclusive breastfeeding is proposed by WHO as a strategy preventing mother-to-child transmission of HIV, adding to the other well-known benefits of breastfeeding. Results from a study in Kenya indicated that rates of breastfeeding initiation and exclusive breastfeeding at six months were higher among HIV-infected women compared to those of non-infected mothers [166].

11.2. Human T-Cell Lymphotropic Virus Type-I (HTLV-I) Infection and Breastfeeding

Breastfeeding has been reported to be the main source of vertical transmission of vertical transmission of HTLV-I accounted for approximately 95% of mother-to-child transmission cases [167,168]. A meta-analysis conducted by Boostani et al. [167] showed that a short period (less than 6 months) of breastfeeding does not increase the likelihood of mother-to-child transmission of HTLV-I infection, while breastfeeding of longer than 6 months greatly increases the rate of HTLV-I transmission. A recent meta-analysis [168] showed that there was no significant increase in the risk of mother-to-child transmission when breast-feeding lasted for ≤3 months compared with exclusively formula-fed infants (pooled relative risk (RR), 0.72; 95% confidence interval (CI), 0.30–1.77), but there was an almost threefold increase in risk when breastfeeding was carried out for up to 6 months (RR, 2.91, 95% CI, 1.69–5.03).

11.3. Hepatitis B Virus (HBV)-Infected Mothers and Breastfeeding

Vertical transmission of HBV is a prevalent cause of HBV spread, resulting in an estimated 50% of the global chronic infections [169]. Routine screening of pregnant women and universal active and passive immunization of neonates have decreased mother-to-child transmission by 95%. HBV has been detected in breastmilk and concerns for transmission through lactation have been raised and investigated. Numerous studies, even before the introduction of HBV vaccine, have not confirmed an increase in the risk of mother-to-child transmission. Therefore, WHO recommends breastfeeding in case of maternal chronic hepatitis B irrespective of the mother's disease status and availability of the vaccine [170]. A 2011 meta-analysis reported that despite infectiousness of breastmilk, breastfeeding is not associated with increased risk of infantile HBV infection [171]. This finding was consistent even in mothers with high infectivity, probably due to vaccine protection and transmission during delivery.

Antiviral treatment is recommended during pregnancy in selected cases of chronic HBV with high viral load in an attempt to minimize transmission during gestation and delivery [165]. Treatment may need to continue postnatally, during lactation. Nucleoside analogues are recommended during pregnancy; however, due to paucity of published studies, their safety during breastfeeding is not established [172]. It has been confirmed that fetuses in utero are exposed to significantly higher drug levels than infants through breastmilk. Additionally, the same medicines are recommended for use in lactating mothers with HIV. Cumulating evidence suggests that mothers with chronic HBV on antiviral therapy should be encouraged to breastfeed.

11.4. Hepatitis C Virus (HCV)-Infected Mothers and Breastfeeding

Infection with HCV remains a public health concern and its incidence among women of child-bearing age warrants screening during pregnancy. The risk of vertical transmission of HCV is estimated at 6%, rising to 10% in case of maternal HIV co-infection [173]. Although HCV is detected in breastmilk, avoidance of breastfeeding does not seem to reduce the risk of mother-to-child transmission [174]. Breastfeeding is recommended unless bleeding or cracked nipples are present. Nevertheless, HCV-infected women breastfeed at lower rates compared to the general population. Mothers with chronic HCV infection should be informed and supported during lactation.

Safety of direct-acting antiviral medicine used for the treatment of HCV has not been studied in lactating women [175]. Data from animal studies indicate that the drugs are excreted into breastmilk but have not demonstrated adverse effects on the offspring. Currently, until published evidence becomes available, these medicines are not recommended for use during pregnancy and lactation.

12. Discussion

Cumulative evidence suggests that women with chronic diseases present lower breastfeeding rates compared with healthy women. Both exclusive and any breastfeeding duration for women with preexisting DM is reduced compared to those of non-diabetic mothers [132,176,177]. Furthermore, women with polycystic ovary syndrome (PCOS) [178], IBD [64], arthritis [55], and epilepsy [78,79] breastfeed less often than non-affected women. Adjusted and evidence-based support may be required to promote breastfeeding in women with chronic diseases; however, our comprehension of breastfeeding in this subpopulation is still unclear. The literature related to breastfeeding extends in various scientific areas and multidisciplinary effort is necessary to compile an overview of current evidence and knowledge regarding breastfeeding issues in mothers with chronic diseases.

Scime et al. [179], in a cross-sectional study using data from the 2015/2016 Canadian Community Health Survey (CCHS), assessed the probable correlation between breastfeeding and chronic maternal diseases after adjustment for possible socio-demographic confounding factors. The prevalence of self-reported chronic diseases was 11.9% (95% CI 9.8–14.1); musculoskeletal problems and hypertension were the most common conditions. Another study, conducted in the USA in 2008 reported 26.6% of pregnant women suffering from a chronic physical or psychological disease, most frequently arthritis (6.3%), hypertension (5.7%) and asthma (5.0%) [180]. A recent population study in Denmark exhibited a 15.8% of pregnant women with chronic diseases [21]. Arterial hypertension remains the main cause of non-infectious morbidity in the general population [181], which is also reflected during pregnancy.

Women with chronic diseases seem to begin to breastfeed independently of the disease status. This can be explained by the high intrahospital postpartum support of breastfeeding. No correlation was found between pre-existing diabetes and initiation of breastfeeding (adjusted odds ratio (aOR) 0.9, 95% CI 0.9–1.0) after adjusting for maternal and obstetric complications [182] in a study from Ohio. Moffatt et al. [63] also reported that 83.3% of IBD patients vs. 77.1% of the general population began breastfeeding ($p > 0.05$). No relationship between PCOS and initiation of breastfeeding was recorded (aOR 0.9, 95% CI 0.6–1.4) [183]. Similarly, Scime et al. [179] highlighted comparable non-breastfeeding rates in women with (10.4%) and without (8.7%) chronic disease after adjustment for confounding factors (aOR 0.96, 95% CI 0.54–1.71). Women with chronic disease presented similar rates of early (<6 months) cessation of any breastfeeding (aOR 1.40, 95% CI 0.82–2.40), but a more than twofold risk of early cessation of exclusive breastfeeding (aOR 2.48, 95% CI 1.49–4.12) compared to healthy women. A Swedish prospective cohort study resulted in a significantly lower percentage of any breastfeeding at 6 months in women with type I DM compared to non-diabetic mothers (61.5% vs. 76.7%, respectively, $p = 0.025$), but no difference in exclusive breastfeeding at 6 months (44.4% vs. 40.5%, respectively, $p = 0.729$) [136]. Comparable rates of any breastfeeding for more than 24 weeks were also reported between women with and without IBD (56.1% vs. 44.4%, respectively, $p = 0.02$) [63].

The protective effect of breastfeeding is more powerful in case of exclusive nutrition with maternal milk and is reduced with other supplemental feeding [184]. Findings of various studies indicate that the presence of a chronic maternal disease may negatively impact exclusive, but not partial breastfeeding rates at 6 months [57,179]. A probable explanation for the lower exclusive breastfeeding percentages in mothers with chronic diseases lies in the possible delay of stage II lactogenesis due to the condition itself or the treatment [185,186]. Women with delayed milk production (more than 72 h after birth) are faced with a higher risk of early exclusive breastfeeding cessation compared to mothers without delayed milk production [187]. Labor via cesarean section or need for NICU admission of the neonate are more common among women with chronic diseases and could inhibit attempts to exclusive breastfeeding because of the early (or prolonged) mother-child separation and the maternal stress [188,189]. Disease activity may be dependent on the changes induced by lactation, including the fluctuations (as in endocrine conditions [146]) or recess (as in autoimmune conditions [63,74]) of symptoms, and could affect decisions on breastfeeding. Although very few drugs are contraindicated during breastfeeding, women often receive discouraging advice concerning safety of medicines in lactation [190,191]. Finally, mothers' desire to "regain a sense of physical fitness", tiredness and exhaustion from neonatal care, and the feeling of physical or psychological unrest can also contribute to breastfeeding cessation [192]. Mothers with chronic diseases are sensitive to the gift of health and would choose the optimal feeding mode with short-term and long-term benefits for their offspring at the beginning of their life.

13. Conclusions

In-depth knowledge of the pathology of systematic diseases and the characteristics of the recommended treatments is vital when lactation is considered. Mothers with chronic diseases should be offered the possibility to breastfeed their infants, along with the necessary information, education, and support for this endeavor.

In case the therapeutic approach of the mother requires a drug possibly harmful for the infant, the choice between the treatment and breastfeeding is imminent. The mother, together with the healthcare professionals, needs to weigh the advantages of breastfeeding over the drug for the maternal and neonatal health and relationship. Recent technological advancements have helped analyze human milk, allowing for a better understanding of the complex protective mechanisms with long-term consequences. Maternal decisions on breastfeeding are affected by multiple physiological, obstetric, and psychological factors. Further research is necessary for a more effective comprehension of these determinants and the optimal support of breastfeeding in mothers with chronic diseases. Studies indicate that mothers with chronic conditions may benefit from the appropriate care and support in the hospital and in the society that can contribute to the establishment and maintenance of exclusive breastfeeding.

Supplementary Materials: The following supporting information can be downloaded at: https://www.mdpi.com/article/10.3390/nu15132822/s1, Table S1: Characteristics of retrieved studies.

Author Contributions: Conceptualization, R.S. and Z.I.; methodology, R.S. and S.P.; data curation, R.S., K.L., A.K., S.P., T.B., N.I. and Z.I.; investigation, R.S.; writing—original draft preparation, R.S., S.P. and Z.I.; writing—review and editing, A.K., T.B., R.S., K.L., D.V., Z.I., S.P. and N.I. All authors have read and agreed to the published version of the manuscript.

Funding: This research received no external funding.

Institutional Review Board Statement: Not applicable.

Informed Consent Statement: Not applicable.

Data Availability Statement: Data are contained within the article.

Conflicts of Interest: The authors declare no conflict of interest.

References

1. American Association of Pediatrics; Eidelman, A.I.; Schanler, R.J.; Johnston, M.; Landers, S.; Noble, L.; Szucs, K.; Viehmann, L. Breastfeeding and the Use of Human Milk. *Pediatrics* **2012**, *129*, e827–e841. [CrossRef]
2. World Health Organization (WHO). Breastfeeding. Available online: https://www.who.int/health-topics/breastfeeding#tab=tab_1 (accessed on 20 July 2022).
3. UNICEF. Breastfeeding. Available online: https://data.unicef.org/topic/nutrition/breastfeeding/ (accessed on 20 July 2022).
4. Benefits of breastfeeding. Nutrition in clinical care: An official publication of Tufts University. *Nutr. Clin. Care* **2003**, *6*, 125–131.
5. Li, R.; Ware, J.; Chen, A.; Nelson, J.M.; Kmet, J.M.; Parks, S.E.; Morrow, A.L.; Chen, J.; Perrine, C.G. Breastfeeding and post-perinatal infant deaths in the United States, A national prospective cohort analysis. *Lancet Reg. Health Am.* **2022**, *5*, 100094. [CrossRef] [PubMed]
6. Sankar, M.J.; Sinha, B.; Chowdhury, R.; Bhandari, N.; Taneja, S.; Martines, J.; Bahl, R. Optimal breastfeeding practices and infant and child mortality: A systematic review and meta-analysis. *Acta Paediatr. (Oslo Nor. 1992)* **2015**, *104*, 3–13. [CrossRef]
7. Ware, J.L.; Chen, A.; Morrow, A.L.; Kmet, J. Associations Between Breastfeeding Initiation and Infant Mortality in an Urban Population. *Breastfeed. Med.* **2019**, *14*, 465–474. [CrossRef]
8. Bahl, R.; Frost, C.; Kirkwood, B.R.; Edmond, K.; Martines, J.; Bhandari, N.; Arthur, P. Infant feeding patterns and risks of death and hospitalization in the first half of infancy: Multicentre cohort study. *Bull. World Health Organ.* **2005**, *83*, 418–426.
9. Vennemann, M.M.; Bajanowski, T.; Brinkmann, B.; Jorch, G.; Yücesan, K.; Sauerland, C.; Mitchell, E.A. Does breastfeeding reduce the risk of sudden infant death syndrome? *Pediatrics* **2009**, *123*, e406–e410. [CrossRef]
10. Wisnieski, L.; Kerver, J.; Holzman, C.; Todem, D.; Margerison-Zilko, C. Breastfeeding and Risk of Metabolic Syndrome in Children and Adolescents: A Systematic Review. *J. Hum. Lact. Off. J. Int. Lact. Consult. Assoc.* **2018**, *34*, 515–525. [CrossRef]
11. Oddy, W.H. Breastfeeding, Childhood Asthma, and Allergic Disease. *Ann. Nutr. Metab.* **2017**, *70* (Suppl. S2), 26–36. [CrossRef] [PubMed]
12. Martin, R.M.; Smith, G.D.; Mangtani, P.; Frankel, S.; Gunnell, D. Association between breast feeding and growth: The Boyd-Orr cohort study. *Arch. Dis. Child. Fetal Neonatal Ed.* **2002**, *87*, F193. [CrossRef]
13. Mohammad, M.A.; Haymond, M.W. The magic of mother's milk. *Diabetes* **2012**, *61*, 3076–3077. [CrossRef]
14. Rich-Edwards, J.W.; Stampfer, M.J.; Manson, J.E.; Rosner, B.; Hu, F.B.; Michels, K.B.; Willett, W.C. Breastfeeding during Infancy and the Risk of Cardiovascular Disease in Adulthood. *Epidemiology* **2004**, *15*, 550–556. [CrossRef]
15. Su, Q.; Sun, X.; Zhu, L.; Yan, Q.; Zheng, P.; Mao, Y.; Ye, D. Breastfeeding and the risk of childhood cancer: A systematic review and dose-response meta-analysis. *BMC Med.* **2021**, *19*, 90. [CrossRef]
16. Amitay, E.L.; Keinan-Boker, L. Breastfeeding and Childhood Leukemia Incidence: A Meta-analysis and Systematic Review. *JAMA Pediatr.* **2015**, *169*, e151025. [CrossRef]
17. Meier, P.P.; Patel, A.L.; Bigger, H.R.; Rossman, B.; Engstrom, J.L. Supporting breastfeeding in the neonatal intensive care unit: Rush Mother's Milk Club as a case study of evidence-based care. *Pediatr. Clin. N. Am.* **2013**, *60*, 209–226. [CrossRef]
18. Intestinal Permeability in Preterm Infants by Feeding Type: Mother's Milk Versus Formula. *Breastfeed. Med.* **2009**, *4*, 11–15. [CrossRef] [PubMed]

19. Camacho-Morales, A.; Caba, M.; García-Juárez, M.; Caba-Flores, M.D.; Viveros-Contreras, R.; Martínez-Valenzuela, C. Breastfeeding Contributes to Physiological Immune Programming in the Newborn. *Front. Pediatr.* **2021**, *9*, 3. [CrossRef] [PubMed]
20. Dimitroglou, M.; Iliodromiti, Z.; Christou, E.; Volaki, P.; Petropoulou, C.; Sokou, R.; Boutsikou, T.; Iacovidou, N. Human Breast Milk: The Key Role in the Maturation of Immune, Gastrointestinal and Central Nervous Systems: A Narrative Review. *Diagnostics* **2022**, *12*, 2208. [CrossRef]
21. Jølving, L.R.; Nielsen, J.; Kesmodel, U.S.; Nielsen, R.G.; Beck-Nielsen, S.S.; Nørgård, B.M. Prevalence of maternal chronic diseases during pregnancy—A nationwide population based study from 1989 to 2013. *Acta Obstet. Et Gynecol. Scand.* **2016**, *95*, 1295–1304. [CrossRef] [PubMed]
22. Scime, N.V.; Lee, S.; Jain, M.; Metcalfe, A.; Chaput, K.H. A Scoping Review of Breastfeeding in Women with Chronic Diseases. *Breastfeed. Med.* **2021**, *16*, 851–862. [CrossRef]
23. Colstrup, M.; Mathiesen, E.R.; Damm, P.; Jensen, D.M.; Ringholm, L. Pregnancy in women with type 1 diabetes: Have the goals of St. Vincent declaration been met concerning foetal and neonatal complications? *J. Matern.-Fetal Neonatal Med.* **2013**, *26*, 1682–1686. [CrossRef]
24. Lekšić, G.; Baretić, M.; Ivanišević, M.; Jurišić-Eržen, D. Pregnancy in Patients with Type One Diabetes Mellitus Treated with Continuous Subcutaneous Insulin Infusion-Preconception Basal Insulin Dose as a Potential Risk Factor for Fetal Overgrowth? *Int. J. Environ. Res. Public Health* **2020**, *17*, 6566. [CrossRef] [PubMed]
25. Smyth, A.; Oliveira, G.H.; Lahr, B.D.; Bailey, K.R.; Norby, S.M.; Garovic, V.D. A systematic review and meta-analysis of pregnancy outcomes in patients with systemic lupus erythematosus and lupus nephritis. *Clin. J. Am. Soc. Nephrol. CJASN* **2010**, *5*, 2060–2068. [CrossRef]
26. Metcalfe, A.; Sabr, Y.; Hutcheon, J.A.; Donovan, L.; Lyons, J.; Burrows, J.; Joseph, K.S. Trends in Obstetric Intervention and Pregnancy Outcomes of Canadian Women With Diabetes in Pregnancy From 2004 to 2015. *J. Endocr. Soc.* **2017**, *1*, 1540–1549. [CrossRef] [PubMed]
27. Bramham, K.; Parnell, B.; Nelson-Piercy, C.; Seed, P.T.; Poston, L.; Chappell, L.C. Chronic hypertension and pregnancy outcomes: Systematic review and meta-analysis. *BMJ (Clin. Res. Ed.)* **2014**, *348*, g2301. [CrossRef]
28. Borba, V.V.; Zandman-Goddard, G.; Shoenfeld, Y. Prolactin and Autoimmunity. *Front. Immunol.* **2018**, *9*, 73. [CrossRef]
29. Buskila, D.; Shoenfeld, Y. Prolactin, bromocriptine and autoimmune diseases. *Isr. J. Med. Sci.* **1996**, *32*, 23–27. [PubMed]
30. Fojtikova, M.; Tomasová Studýnková, J.; Filkova, M.; Lacinova, Z.; Gatterova, J.; Pavelka, K.; Vencovský, J.; Šenolt, L. Elevated prolactin levels in patients with rheumatoid arthritis: Association with disease activity and structural damage. *Clin. Exp. Rheumatol. Incl Suppl.* **2010**, *28*, 849.
31. Song, G.G.; Lee, Y.H. Circulating prolactin level in systemic lupus erythematosus and its correlation with disease activity: A meta-analysis. *Lupus* **2017**, *26*, 1260–1268. [CrossRef]
32. Hilfiker-Kleiner, D.; Kaminski, K.; Podewski, E.; Bonda, T.; Schaefer, A.; Sliwa, K.; Forster, O.; Quint, A.; Landmesser, U.; Doerries, C.; et al. A cathepsin D-cleaved 16 kDa form of prolactin mediates postpartum cardiomyopathy. *Cell* **2007**, *128*, 589–600. [CrossRef]
33. Hilfiker-Kleiner, D.; Haghikia, A.; Berliner, D.; Vogel-Claussen, J.; Schwab, J.; Franke, A.; Schwarzkopf, M.; Ehlermann, P.; Pfister, R.; Michels, G.; et al. Bromocriptine for the treatment of peripartum cardiomyopathy: A multicentre randomized study. *Eur. Heart J.* **2017**, *38*, 2671–2679. [CrossRef] [PubMed]
34. Anaya, J.-M.; Shoenfeld, Y. Multiple autoimmune disease in a patient with Hyperprolactinemia. *Isr. Med. Assoc. J. IMAJ* **2005**, *7*, 740–741. [PubMed]
35. Saha, S.; Gonzalez, J.; Rosenfeld, G.; Keiser, H.; Peeva, E. Prolactin alters the mechanisms of B cell tolerance induction. *Arthritis Rheum.* **2009**, *60*, 1743–1752. [CrossRef] [PubMed]
36. Leaños-Miranda, A.; Cárdenas-Mondragón, G. Serum free prolactin concentrations in patients with systemic lupus erythematosus are associated with lupus activity. *Rheumatology* **2006**, *45*, 97–101. [CrossRef]
37. Qian, Q.; Liuqin, L.; Hao, L.; Shiwen, Y.; Zhongping, Z.; Dongying, C.; Fan, L.; Hanshi, X.; Xiuyan, Y.; Yujin, Y. The effects of bromocriptine on preventing postpartum flare in systemic lupus erythematosus patients from South China. *J. Immunol. Res.* **2015**, *2015*, 316965. [CrossRef]
38. Praprotnik, S.; Agmon-Levin, N.; Porat-Katz, B.S.; Blank, M.; Meroni, P.L.; Cervera, R.; Miesbach, W.; Stojanovich, L.; Szyper-Kravitz, M.; Rozman, B.; et al. Prolactin's role in the pathogenesis of the antiphospholipid syndrome. *Lupus* **2010**, *19*, 1515–1519. [CrossRef]
39. Orbach, H.; Zandman-Goddard, G.; Boaz, M.; Agmon-Levin, N.; Amital, H.; Szekanecz, Z.; Szucs, G.; Rovensky, J.; Kiss, E.; Doria, A.; et al. Prolactin and autoimmunity: Hyperprolactinemia correlates with serositis and anemia in SLE patients. *Clin. Rev. Allergy Immunol.* **2012**, *42*, 189–198. [CrossRef]
40. Bundhun, P.K.; Soogund, M.Z.; Huang, F. Impact of systemic lupus erythematosus on maternal and fetal outcomes following pregnancy: A meta-analysis of studies published between years 2001–2016. *J. Autoimmun.* **2017**, *79*, 17–27. [CrossRef]
41. Chen, Y.J.; Chang, J.C.; Lai, E.L.; Liao, T.L.; Chen, H.H.; Hung, W.T.; Hsieh, T.Y.; Huang, W.N.; Chen, Y.H.; Lin, C.H.; et al. Maternal and perinatal outcomes of pregnancies in systemic lupus erythematosus: A nationwide population-based study. *Semin. Arthritis Rheum.* **2020**, *50*, 451–457. [CrossRef]
42. Orefice, V.; Ceccarelli, F.; Pirone, C.; Galoppi, P.; Spinelli, F.R.; Alessandri, C.; Brunelli, R.; Perrone, G.; Conti, F. Breastfeeding in women affected by systemic lupus erythematosus: Rate, duration and associated factors. *Lupus* **2021**, *30*, 913–920. [CrossRef]

43. Eudy, A.M.; Siega-Riz, A.M.; Engel, S.M.; Franceschini, N.; Howard, A.G.; Clowse, M.E.B.; Petri, M. Effect of pregnancy on disease flares in patients with systemic lupus erythematosus. *Ann. Rheum. Dis.* **2018**, *77*, 855–860. [CrossRef] [PubMed]
44. Izmirly, P.M.; Costedoat-Chalumeau, N.; Pisoni, C.N.; Khamashta, M.A.; Kim, M.Y.; Saxena, A.; Friedman, D.; Llanos, C.; Piette, J.C.; Buyon, J.P. Maternal use of hydroxychloroquine is associated with a reduced risk of recurrent anti-SSA/Ro-antibody-associated cardiac manifestations of neonatal lupus. *Circulation* **2012**, *126*, 76–82. [CrossRef] [PubMed]
45. Leroux, M.; Desveaux, C.; Parcevaux, M.; Julliac, B.; Gouyon, J.B.; Dallay, D.; Pellegrin, J.L.; Boukerrou, M.; Blanco, P.; Lazaro, E. Impact of hydroxychloroquine on preterm delivery and intrauterine growth restriction in pregnant women with systemic lupus erythematosus: A descriptive cohort study. *Lupus* **2015**, *24*, 1384–1391. [CrossRef] [PubMed]
46. Guillotin, V.; Bouhet, A.; Barnetche, T.; Richez, C.; Truchetet, M.E.; Seneschal, J.; Duffau, P.; Lazaro, E. Hydroxychloroquine for the prevention of fetal growth restriction and prematurity in lupus pregnancy: A systematic review and meta-analysis. *Jt. Bone Spine* **2018**, *85*, 663–668. [CrossRef]
47. Noviani, M.; Wasserman, S.; Clowse, M.E. Breastfeeding in mothers with systemic lupus erythematosus. *Lupus* **2016**, *25*, 973–979. [CrossRef]
48. Acevedo, M.; Pretini, J.; Micelli, M.; Sequeira, G.; Kerzberg, E. Breastfeeding initiation, duration, and reasons for weaning in patients with systemic lupus erythematosus. *Rheumatol. Int.* **2017**, *37*, 1183–1186. [CrossRef]
49. Al-Herz, A.; Schulzer, M.; Esdaile, J.M. Survey of antimalarial use in lupus pregnancy and lactation. *J. Rheumatol.* **2002**, *29*, 700–706.
50. American Academy of Pediatrics Committee on Drugs. Transfer of drugs and other chemicals into human milk. *Pediatrics* **2001**, *108*, 776–789. [CrossRef]
51. Megan, E.B.C.; Amanda, M.E.; Stephen, B.; Gillian, S.-S.; Andrzej, K.; Rebecca, F.-B.; Dafna, D.G.; Yair, M.; Cecilia, N.; Abir, M.; et al. Hydroxychloroquine in the pregnancies of women with lupus: A meta-analysis of individual participant data. *Lupus Sci. Med.* **2022**, *9*, e000651. [CrossRef]
52. Clapp, C.; Ortiz, G.; García-Rodrigo, J.F.; Ledesma-Colunga, M.G.; Martínez-Díaz, O.F.; Adán, N.; Martínez de la Escalera, G. Dual Roles of Prolactin and Vasoinhibin in Inflammatory Arthritis. *Front. Endocrinol.* **2022**, *13*, 905756. [CrossRef]
53. Silman, A.; Kay, A.; Brennan, P. Timing of pregnancy in relation to the onset of rheumatoid arthritis. *Arthritis Rheum.* **1992**, *35*, 152–155. [CrossRef]
54. Brennan, P.; Silman, A. Breast-feeding and the onset of rheumatoid arthritis. *Arthritis Rheum.* **1994**, *37*, 808–813. [CrossRef] [PubMed]
55. Barrett, J.H.; Brennan, P.; Fiddler, M.; Silman, A. Breast-feeding and postpartum relapse in women with rheumatoid and inflammatory arthritis. *Arthritis Rheum.* **2000**, *43*, 1010–1015. [CrossRef]
56. Eudy, A.M.; McDaniel, G.; Clowse, M.E.B. Pregnancy in rheumatoid arthritis: A retrospective study. *Clin. Rheumatol.* **2018**, *37*, 789–794. [CrossRef]
57. Ince-Askan, H.; Hazes, J.M.W.; Dolhain, R. Breastfeeding among Women with Rheumatoid Arthritis Compared with the General Population: Results from a Nationwide Prospective Cohort Study. *J. Rheumatol.* **2019**, *46*, 1067–1074. [CrossRef]
58. Nielsen, O.H.; Andreasson, B.; Bondesen, S.; Jacobsen, O.; Jarnum, S. Pregnancy in Crohn's disease. *Scand. J. Gastroenterol.* **1984**, *19*, 724–732. [CrossRef]
59. Beaulieu, D.B.; Kane, S. Inflammatory bowel disease in pregnancy. *World J. Gastroenterol.* **2011**, *17*, 2696–2701. [CrossRef]
60. Kane, S.; Kisiel, J.; Shih, L.; Hanauer, S. HLA disparity determines disease activity through pregnancy in women with inflammatory bowel disease. *Am. J. Gastroenterol.* **2004**, *99*, 1523–1526. [CrossRef] [PubMed]
61. Mahadevan, U.; Sandborn, W.J.; Li, D.K.; Hakimian, S.; Kane, S.; Corley, D.A. Pregnancy outcomes in women with inflammatory bowel disease: A large community-based study from Northern California. *Gastroenterology* **2007**, *133*, 1106–1112. [CrossRef] [PubMed]
62. Dotan, I.; Alper, A.; Rachmilewitz, D.; Israeli, E.; Odes, S.; Chermesh, I.; Naftali, T.; Fraser, G.; Shitrit, A.B.-G.; Peles, V.; et al. Maternal inflammatory bowel disease has short and long-term effects on the health of their offspring: A multicenter study in Israel. *J. Crohn's Colitis* **2013**, *7*, 542–550. [CrossRef]
63. Moffatt, D.C.; Ilnyckyj, A.; Bernstein, C.N. A Population-Based Study of Breastfeeding in Inflammatory Bowel Disease: Initiation, Duration, and Effect on Disease in the Postpartum Period. *Off. J. Am. Coll. Gastroenterol. ACG* **2009**, *104*, 2517–2523. [CrossRef]
64. Kane, S.; Lemieux, N. The Role of Breastfeeding in Postpartum Disease Activity in Women with Inflammatory Bowel Disease. *Off. J. Am. Coll. Gastroenterol. ACG* **2005**, *100*, 102–105. [CrossRef]
65. Orholm, M.; Fonager, K.; Sørensen, H.T. Risk of ulcerative colitis and Crohn's disease among offspring of patients with chronic inflammatory bowel disease. *Am. J. Gastroenterol.* **1999**, *94*, 3236–3238. [CrossRef]
66. Koletzko, S.; Sherman, P.; Corey, M.; Griffiths, A.; Smith, C. Role of infant feeding practices in development of Crohn's disease in childhood. *BMJ: Br. Med. J.* **1989**, *298*, 1617. [CrossRef]
67. Bove, R.; Chitnis, T. The role of gender and sex hormones in determining the onset and outcome of multiple sclerosis. *Mult. Scler.* **2014**, *20*, 520–526. [CrossRef]
68. Bove, R.; Alwan, S.; Friedman, J.M.; Hellwig, K.; Houtchens, M.; Koren, G.; Lu, E.; McElrath, T.F.; Smyth, P.; Tremlett, H.; et al. Management of multiple sclerosis during pregnancy and the reproductive years: A systematic review. *Obstet. Gynecol.* **2014**, *124*, 1157–1168. [CrossRef]

69. Wundes, A.; Pebdani, R.N.; Amtmann, D. What do healthcare providers advise women with multiple sclerosis regarding pregnancy? *Mult. Scler. Int.* **2014**, *2014*, 819216. [CrossRef] [PubMed]
70. Krysko, K.M.; Rutatangwa, A.; Graves, J.; Lazar, A.; Waubant, E. Association Between Breastfeeding and Postpartum Multiple Sclerosis Relapses: A Systematic Review and Meta-analysis. *JAMA Neurol.* **2020**, *77*, 327–338. [CrossRef] [PubMed]
71. Vukusic, S.; Hutchinson, M.; Hours, M.; Moreau, T.; Cortinovis-Tourniaire, P.; Adeleine, P.; Confavreux, C. Pregnancy and multiple sclerosis (the PRIMS study): Clinical predictors of post-partum relapse. *Brain* **2004**, *127*, 1353–1360. [CrossRef] [PubMed]
72. Portaccio, E.; Ghezzi, A.; Hakiki, B.; Sturchio, A.; Martinelli, V.; Moiola, L.; Patti, F.; Mancardi, G.L.; Solaro, C.; Tola, M.R.; et al. Postpartum relapses increase the risk of disability progression in multiple sclerosis: The role of disease modifying drugs. *J. Neurol. Neurosurg. Psychiatry* **2014**, *85*, 845–850. [CrossRef] [PubMed]
73. Jesus-Ribeiro, J.; Correia, I.; Martins, A.I.; Fonseca, M.; Marques, I.; Batista, S.; Nunes, C.; Macário, C.; Almeida, M.C.; Sousa, L. Pregnancy in Multiple Sclerosis: A Portuguese cohort study. *Mult. Scler. Relat. Disord.* **2017**, *17*, 63–68. [CrossRef]
74. Hellwig, K.; Rockhoff, M.; Herbstritt, S.; Borisow, N.; Haghikia, A.; Elias-Hamp, B.; Menck, S.; Gold, R.; Langer-Gould, A. Exclusive Breastfeeding and the Effect on Postpartum Multiple Sclerosis Relapses. *JAMA Neurol.* **2015**, *72*, 1132–1138. [CrossRef]
75. Langer-Gould, A.; Smith, J.; Albers, K.; Wu, J.; Kerezsi, E.; McClearnen, K.; Leimpeter, A.; Van Den Eeden, S. Pregnancy-related relapses and breastfeeding in a contemporary multiple sclerosis cohort. *Neurology* **2019**, *94*, e1939–e1949. [CrossRef]
76. Pakpoor, J.; Disanto, G.; Lacey, M.V.; Hellwig, K.; Giovannoni, G.; Ramagopalan, S.V. Breastfeeding and multiple sclerosis relapses: A meta-analysis. *J. Neurol.* **2012**, *259*, 2246–2248. [CrossRef] [PubMed]
77. Meador, K.J.; Baker, G.A.; Browning, N.; Clayton-Smith, J.; Combs-Cantrell, D.T.; Cohen, M.; Kalayjian, L.A.; Kanner, A.; Liporace, J.D.; Pennell, P.B.; et al. Effects of breastfeeding in children of women taking antiepileptic drugs. *Neurology* **2010**, *75*, 1954–1960. [CrossRef] [PubMed]
78. Johnson, E.L.; Burke, A.E.; Wang, A.; Pennell, P.B. Unintended pregnancy, prenatal care, newborn outcomes, and breastfeeding in women with epilepsy. *Neurology* **2018**, *91*, e1031–e1039. [CrossRef]
79. Noe, K. Further Evidence Breastfeeding by Women With Epilepsy Is Safe: Are Mothers Getting the Message? *Epilepsy Curr.* **2020**, *20*, 141–143. [CrossRef]
80. Birnbaum, A.K.; Meador, K.J.; Karanam, A.; Brown, C.; May, R.C.; Gerard, E.E.; Gedzelman, E.R.; Penovich, P.E.; Kalayjian, L.A.; Cavitt, J.; et al. Antiepileptic Drug Exposure in Infants of Breastfeeding Mothers With Epilepsy. *JAMA Neurol.* **2020**, *77*, 441–450. [CrossRef] [PubMed]
81. Harden, C.L.; Pennell, P.B.; Koppel, B.S.; Hovinga, C.A.; Gidal, B.; Meador, K.J.; Hopp, J.; Ting, T.Y.; Hauser, W.A.; Thurman, D.; et al. Management issues for women with epilepsy--focus on pregnancy (an evidence-based review): III. Vitamin K, folic acid, blood levels, and breast-feeding: Report of the Quality Standards Subcommittee and Therapeutics and Technology Assessment Subcommittee of the American Academy of Neurology and the American Epilepsy Society. *Epilepsia* **2009**, *50*, 1247–1255. [CrossRef]
82. Veiby, G.; Bjørk, M.; Engelsen, B.A.; Gilhus, N.E. Epilepsy and recommendations for breastfeeding. *Seizure* **2015**, *28*, 57–65. [CrossRef]
83. Veiby, G.; Engelsen, B.A.; Gilhus, N.E. Early child development and exposure to antiepileptic drugs prenatally and through breastfeeding: A prospective cohort study on children of women with epilepsy. *JAMA Neurol.* **2013**, *70*, 1367–1374. [CrossRef] [PubMed]
84. Meador, K.J.; Baker, G.A.; Browning, N.; Cohen, M.J.; Bromley, R.L.; Clayton-Smith, J.; Kalayjian, L.A.; Kanner, A.; Liporace, J.D.; Pennell, P.B.; et al. Breastfeeding in children of women taking antiepileptic drugs: Cognitive outcomes at age 6 years. *JAMA Pediatr.* **2014**, *168*, 729–736. [CrossRef] [PubMed]
85. Doan, T.; Gardiner, A.; Gay, C.L.; Lee, K.A. Breast-feeding increases sleep duration of new parents. *J. Perinat. Neonatal Nurs.* **2007**, *21*, 200–206. [CrossRef]
86. Shebl, E.; Chakraborty, R.K. Asthma in Pregnancy. Available online: https://www.ncbi.nlm.nih.gov/books/NBK532283/ (accessed on 22 April 2023).
87. Popa, M.; Peltecu, G.; Gica, N.; Ciobanu, A.M.; Botezatu, R.; Gica, C.; Steriade, A.; Panaitescu, A.M. Asthma in Pregnancy. Review of Current Literature and Recommendations. *Maedica* **2021**, *16*, 80–87.
88. Gluck, J.C.; Gluck, P.A. The effect of pregnancy on the course of asthma. *Immunol. Allergy Clin. North Am.* **2006**, *26*, 63–80. [CrossRef] [PubMed]
89. Harvey, S.M.; Murphy, V.E.; Gibson, P.G.; Collison, A.; Robinson, P.; Sly, P.D.; Mattes, J.; Jensen, M.E. Maternal asthma, breastfeeding, and respiratory outcomes in the first year of life. *Pediatr. Pulmonol.* **2020**, *55*, 1690–1696. [CrossRef]
90. Wright, A.L.; Holberg, C.J.; Taussig, L.M.; Martinez, F.D. Factors influencing the relation of infant feeding to asthma and recurrent wheeze in childhood. *Thorax* **2001**, *56*, 192–197. [CrossRef]
91. Guilbert, T.W.; Stern, D.A.; Morgan, W.J.; Martinez, F.D.; Wright, A.L. Effect of breastfeeding on lung function in childhood and modulation by maternal asthma and atopy. *Am. J. Respir. Crit. Care Med.* **2007**, *176*, 843–848. [CrossRef]
92. Meghan, B.A.; Lorena, V.; Zihang, L.; David, D.; Padmaja, S.; Allan, B.B.; Piushkumar, J.M.; Stuart, E.T.; Diana, L.L.; Malcolm, R.S. Breastfeeding, maternal asthma and wheezing in the first year of life: A longitudinal birth cohort study. *Eur. Respir. J.* **2017**, *49*, 1602019. [CrossRef]
93. Dixon, D.L.; Forsyth, K.D. Leukocytes in expressed breast milk of asthmatic mothers. *Allergol. Et Immunopathol.* **2017**, *45*, 325–332. [CrossRef]

94. Jensen, M.E.; Harvey, S.M.; Gibson, P.G.; Murphy1, V.E. Breastfeeding rates and barriers in women with asthma. In Proceedings of the 46th Annual Scientific Meeting of the Nutrition Society of Australia, Perth, Australia, 29 November–2 December 2022.
95. Davies, G.; Jordan, S.; Thayer, D.; Tucker, D.; Humphreys, I. Medicines prescribed for asthma, discontinuation and perinatal outcomes, including breastfeeding: A population cohort analysis. *PLoS ONE* **2020**, *15*, e0242489. [CrossRef]
96. Chambers, C.D.; Krishnan, J.A.; Alba, L.; Albano, J.D.; Bryant, A.S.; Carver, M.; Cohen, L.S.; Gorodetsky, E.; Hernandez-Diaz, S.; Honein, M.A.; et al. The safety of asthma medications during pregnancy and lactation: Clinical management and research priorities. *J. Allergy Clin. Immunol.* **2021**, *147*, 2009–2020. [CrossRef]
97. Regitz-Zagrosek, V.; Roos-Hesselink, J.W.; Bauersachs, J.; Blomström-Lundqvist, C.; Cífková, R.; De Bonis, M.; Iung, B.; Johnson, M.R.; Kintscher, U.; Kranke, P.; et al. 2018 ESC Guidelines for the management of cardiovascular diseases during pregnancy. *Eur. Heart J.* **2018**, *39*, 3165–3241. [CrossRef]
98. Cantwell, R.; Clutton-Brock, T.; Cooper, G.; Dawson, A.; Drife, J.; Garrod, D.; Harper, A.; Hulbert, D.; Lucas, S.; McClure, J.; et al. Saving Mothers' Lives: Reviewing maternal deaths to make motherhood safer: 2006–2008. The Eighth Report of the Confidential Enquiries into Maternal Deaths in the United Kingdom. *BJOG Int. J. Obstet. Gynaecol.* **2011**, *118* (Suppl. S1), 1–203. [CrossRef]
99. Kurinczuk, J.J.; Draper, E.S.; Field, D.J.; Bevan, C.; Brocklehurst, P.; Gray, R.; Kenyon, S.; Manktelow, B.N.; Neilson, J.P.; Redshaw, M.; et al. Experiences with maternal and perinatal death reviews in the UK--the MBRRACE-UK programme. *BJOG: Int. J. Obstet. Gynaecol.* **2014**, *121* (Suppl. S4), 41–46. [CrossRef] [PubMed]
100. van Hagen, I.M.; Boersma, E.; Johnson, M.R.; Thorne, S.A.; Parsonage, W.A.; Escribano Subías, P.; Leśniak-Sobelga, A.; Irtyuga, O.; Sorour, K.A.; Taha, N.; et al. Global cardiac risk assessment in the Registry Of Pregnancy And Cardiac disease: Results of a registry from the European Society of Cardiology. *Eur. J. Heart Fail.* **2016**, *18*, 523–533. [CrossRef] [PubMed]
101. de Jonge, L.; Garne, E.; Gini, R.; Jordan, S.E.; Klungsoyr, K.; Loane, M.; Neville, A.J.; Pierini, A.; Puccini, A.; Thayer, D.S.; et al. Improving Information on Maternal Medication Use by Linking Prescription Data to Congenital Anomaly Registers: A EUROmediCAT Study. *Drug Saf.* **2015**, *38*, 1083–1093. [CrossRef]
102. Yucel, E.; DeFaria Yeh, D. Pregnancy in Women with Congenital Heart Disease. *Curr. Treat. Options Cardiovasc. Med.* **2017**, *19*, 73. [CrossRef]
103. Ouzounian, J.G.; Elkayam, U. Physiologic changes during normal pregnancy and delivery. *Cardiol. Clin.* **2012**, *30*, 317–329. [CrossRef]
104. Drenthen, W.; Boersma, E.; Balci, A.; Moons, P.; Roos-Hesselink, J.W.; Mulder, B.J.; Vliegen, H.W.; van Dijk, A.P.; Voors, A.A.; Yap, S.C.; et al. Predictors of pregnancy complications in women with congenital heart disease. *Eur. Heart J.* **2010**, *31*, 2124–2132. [CrossRef]
105. Chatwin, A.L.; Linzell, J.L.; Setchell, B.P. Cardiovascular changes during lactation in the rat. *J. Endocrinol.* **1969**, *44*, 247–254. [CrossRef]
106. Ota, K.; Peaker, M. Lactation in the rabbit: Mammary blood flow and cardiac output. *Q. J. Exp. Physiol. Cogn. Med. Sci.* **1979**, *64*, 225–238. [CrossRef]
107. Habashi, J.P.; MacFarlane, E.G.; Bagirzadeh, R.; Bowen, C.; Huso, N.; Chen, Y.; Bedja, D.; Creamer, T.J.; Rykiel, G.; Manning, M.; et al. Oxytocin antagonism prevents pregnancy-associated aortic dissection in a mouse model of Marfan syndrome. *Sci. Transl. Med.* **2019**, *11*, eaat4822. [CrossRef] [PubMed]
108. Matsuzaka, Y.; Aoki-Kamiya, C.; Yokouchi-Konishi, T.; Shionoiri, T.; Nakanishi, A.; Iwanaga, N.; Chishaki, A.; Kurosaki, K.; Ohuchi, H.; Yoshimatsu, J. Breastfeeding and postpartum outcomes among women with congenital heart disease. *Int. J. Cardiol. Congenit. Heart Dis.* **2021**, *4*, 100167. [CrossRef]
109. Beardmore, K.S.; Morris, J.M.; Gallery, E.D.M. Excretion of antihypertensive medication into human breast milk: A systematic review. *Hypertens Pregnancy* **2002**, *21*, 85–95. [CrossRef]
110. Oteng-Ntim, E.; Meeks, D.; Seed, P.T.; Webster, L.; Howard, J.; Doyle, P.; Chappell, L.C. Adverse maternal and perinatal outcomes in pregnant women with sickle cell disease: Systematic review and meta-analysis. *Blood* **2015**, *125*, 3316–3325. [CrossRef] [PubMed]
111. Early, M.L.; Eke, A.C.; Gemmill, A.; Lanzkron, S.; Pecker, L.H. Comparisons of Severe Maternal Morbidity and Other Adverse Pregnancy Outcomes in Pregnant People With Sickle Cell Disease vs Anemia. *JAMA Netw. Open* **2023**, *6*, e2254545. [CrossRef] [PubMed]
112. Early, M.L.; Eke, A.C.; Gemmill, A.; Lanzkron, S.; Pecker, L.H. Severe Maternal Morbidity and Mortality in Sickle Cell Disease in the National Inpatient Sample, 2012–2018. *JAMA Netw. Open* **2023**, *6*, e2254552. [CrossRef]
113. Phillips, C.; Boyd, M.P. Perinatal and Neonatal Implications of Sickle Cell Disease. *Nurs. Women's Health* **2017**, *21*, 474–487. [CrossRef]
114. Ware, R.E.; Marahatta, A.; Ware, J.L.; McElhinney, K.; Dong, M.; Vinks, A.A. Hydroxyurea Exposure in Lactation: A Pharmacokinetics Study (HELPS). *J. Pediatr.* **2020**, *222*, 236–239. [CrossRef]
115. McGann, P.T.; Niss, O.; Dong, M.; Marahatta, A.; Howard, T.A.; Mizuno, T.; Lane, A.; Kalfa, T.A.; Malik, P.; Quinn, C.T.; et al. Robust clinical and laboratory response to hydroxyurea using pharmacokinetically guided dosing for young children with sickle cell anemia. *Am. J. Hematol.* **2019**, *94*, 871–879. [CrossRef] [PubMed]
116. Petrakos, G.; Andriopoulos, P.; Tsironi, M. Pregnancy in women with thalassemia: Challenges and solutions. *Int. J. Womens Health.* **2016**, *8*, 441–451. [CrossRef]
117. Origa, R.; Comitini, F. Pregnancy in Thalassemia. *Mediterr. J. Hematol. Infect. Dis.* **2019**, *11*, e2019019. [CrossRef] [PubMed]

118. Di Mattei, V.E.; Perego, G.; Taranto, P.; Mazzetti, M.; Ferrari, F.; Derna, N.; Peccatori, F.A.; Mangili, G.; Candiani, M. Psychological issues in breast cancer survivors confronted with motherhood: Literature review and a call to action. *Front. Psychol.* **2023**, *14*, 1133204. [CrossRef]
119. Woodman, I. Breast feeding reduces risk of breast cancer, says study. *BMJ (Clin. Res. Ed.)* **2002**, *325*, 184. [CrossRef]
120. Breast cancer and breastfeeding: Collaborative reanalysis of individual data from 47 epidemiological studies in 30 countries, including 50302 women with breast cancer and 96973 women without the disease. *Lancet* **2002**, *360*, 187–195. [CrossRef] [PubMed]
121. do Carmo França-Botelho, A.; Ferreira, M.C.; França, J.L.; França, E.L.; Honório-França, A.C. Breastfeeding and its relationship with reduction of breast cancer: A review. *Asian Pac. J. Cancer Prev. APJCP* **2012**, *13*, 5327–5332. [CrossRef]
122. Lefrère, H.; Lenaerts, L.; Borges, V.F.; Schedin, P.; Neven, P.; Amant, F. Postpartum breast cancer: Mechanisms underlying its worse prognosis, treatment implications, and fertility preservation. *Int. J. Gynecol. Cancer Off. J. Int. Gynecol. Cancer Soc.* **2021**, *31*, 412–422. [CrossRef]
123. Bhurosy, T.; Niu, Z.; Heckman, C.J. Breastfeeding is Possible: A Systematic Review on the Feasibility and Challenges of Breastfeeding Among Breast Cancer Survivors of Reproductive Age. *Ann. Surg. Oncol.* **2021**, *28*, 3723–3735. [CrossRef]
124. Abruzzese, E.; Trawinska, M.M.; Perrotti, A.P.; De Fabritiis, P. Tyrosine kinase inhibitors and pregnancy. *Mediterr. J. Hematol. Infect. Dis.* **2014**, *6*, e2014028. [CrossRef]
125. Chelysheva, E.; Aleshin, S.; Polushkina, E.; Shmakov, R.; Shokhin, I.; Chilov, G.; Turkina, A. Breastfeeding in Patients with Chronic Myeloid Leukaemia: Case Series with Measurements of Drug Concentrations in Maternal Milk and Literature Review. *Mediterr. J. Hematol. Infect. Dis.* **2018**, *10*, e2018027. [CrossRef]
126. Johnson, H.M.; Mitchell, K.B. ABM Clinical Protocol #34: Breast Cancer and Breastfeeding. *Breastfeed. Med.* **2020**, *15*, 429–434. [CrossRef]
127. Duffy, C.; Cyr, M. Phytoestrogens: Potential benefits and implications for breast cancer survivors. *J. Women's Health* **2003**, *12*, 617–631. [CrossRef] [PubMed]
128. Wang, M.; Wu, X.; Chai, F.; Zhang, Y.; Jiang, J. Plasma prolactin and breast cancer risk: A meta- analysis. *Sci. Rep.* **2016**, *6*, 25998. [CrossRef]
129. Cordero, L.; Stenger, M.R.; Landon, M.B.; Nankervis, C.A. Exclusive breastfeeding among women with type 1 and type 2 diabetes mellitus. *BMC Pregnancy Childbirth* **2022**, *22*, 69. [CrossRef]
130. Simmons, D.; Conroy, C.; Thompson, C.F. In-hospital breast feeding rates among women with gestational diabetes and pregestational Type 2 diabetes in South Auckland. *Diabet. Med.* **2005**, *22*, 177–181. [CrossRef]
131. Soltani, H.; Arden, M. Factors associated with breastfeeding up to 6 months postpartum in mothers with diabetes. *J. Obstet. Gynecol. Neonatal Nurs. JOGNN* **2009**, *38*, 586–594. [CrossRef]
132. Sorkio, S.; Cuthbertson, D.; Bärlund, S.; Reunanen, A.; Nucci, A.M.; Berseth, C.L.; Koski, K.; Ormisson, A.; Savilahti, E.; Uusitalo, U.; et al. Breastfeeding patterns of mothers with type 1 diabetes: Results from an infant feeding trial. *Diabetes/Metab. Res. Rev.* **2010**, *26*, 206–211. [CrossRef] [PubMed]
133. Herskin, C.W.; Stage, E.; Barfred, C.; Emmersen, P.; Ladefoged Nichum, V.; Damm, P.; Mathiesen, E.R. Low prevalence of long-term breastfeeding among women with type 2 diabetes. *J. Matern. Neonatal Med.* **2016**, *29*, 2513–2518. [CrossRef] [PubMed]
134. Evers, I.M.; de Valk, H.W.; Visser, G.H. Risk of complications of pregnancy in women with type 1 diabetes: Nationwide prospective study in the Netherlands. *BMJ (Clin. Res. Ed.)* **2004**, *328*, 915. [CrossRef] [PubMed]
135. Jensen, D.M.; Damm, P.; Moelsted-Pedersen, L.; Ovesen, P.; Westergaard, J.G.; Moeller, M.; Beck-Nielsen, H. Outcomes in type 1 diabetic pregnancies: A nationwide, population-based study. *Diabetes Care* **2004**, *27*, 2819–2823. [CrossRef]
136. Sparud-Lundin, C.; Wennergren, M.; Elfvin, A.; Berg, M. Breastfeeding in women with type 1 diabetes: Exploration of predictive factors. *Diabetes Care* **2011**, *34*, 296–301. [CrossRef]
137. Ward Platt, M.; Deshpande, S. Metabolic adaptation at birth. *Semin. Fetal Neonatal Med.* **2005**, *10*, 341–350. [CrossRef] [PubMed]
138. Maternal, C.E.; Modder, J.; Acolet, D. *Diabetes in Pregnancy: Caring for the Baby After Birth: Findings of a National Enquiry: England, Wales and Northern Ireland*; CEMACH: London, UK, 2007.
139. Webster, J.; Moore, K.; McMullan, A. Breastfeeding outcomes for women with insulin dependent diabetes. *J. Hum. Lact.* **1995**, *11*, 195–200. [CrossRef] [PubMed]
140. Hummel, S.; Winkler, C.; Schoen, S.; Knopff, A.; Marienfeld, S.; Bonifacio, E.; Ziegler, A.G. Breastfeeding habits in families with Type 1 diabetes. *Diabet. Med.* **2007**, *24*, 671–676. [CrossRef]
141. Chertok, I.R.; Raz, I.; Shoham, I.; Haddad, H.; Wiznitzer, A. Effects of early breastfeeding on neonatal glucose levels of term infants born to women with gestational diabetes. *J. Hum. Nutr. Diet.* **2009**, *22*, 166–169. [CrossRef]
142. Suwaydi, M.A.; Wlodek, M.E.; Lai, C.T.; Prosser, S.A.; Geddes, D.T.; Perrella, S.L. Delayed secretory activation and low milk production in women with gestational diabetes: A case series. *BMC Pregnancy Childbirth* **2022**, *22*, 350. [CrossRef] [PubMed]
143. Neville, M.C.; Webb, P.; Ramanathan, P.; Mannino, M.P.; Pecorini, C.; Monks, J.; Anderson, S.M.; MacLean, P. The insulin receptor plays an important role in secretory differentiation in the mammary gland. *Am. J. Physiol. Endocrinol. Metab.* **2013**, *305*, E1103–E1114. [CrossRef]
144. Watt, A.P.; Lefevre, C.; Wong, C.S.; Nicholas, K.R.; Sharp, J.A. Insulin regulates human mammosphere development and function. *Cell Tissue Res.* **2021**, *384*, 333–352. [CrossRef] [PubMed]
145. Nommsen-Rivers, L.A. Does Insulin Explain the Relation between Maternal Obesity and Poor Lactation Outcomes? An Overview of the Literature. *Adv. Nutr.* **2016**, *7*, 407–414. [CrossRef]

146. Riviello, C.; Mello, G.; Jovanovic, L.G. Breastfeeding and the basal insulin requirement in type 1 diabetic women. *Endocr. Pract.* **2009**, *15*, 187–193. [CrossRef]
147. Gunderson, E.P. Breast-feeding and diabetes: Long-term impact on mothers and their infants. *Curr. Diabetes Rep.* **2008**, *8*, 279–286. [CrossRef]
148. Kaul, P.; Bowker, S.L.; Savu, A.; Yeung, R.O.; Donovan, L.E.; Ryan, E.A. Association between maternal diabetes, being large for gestational age and breast-feeding on being overweight or obese in childhood. *Diabetologia* **2019**, *62*, 249–258. [CrossRef]
149. Kim, H.N.; Jung, Y.A.; Kang, L.L.; Park, H.K.; Hwang, H.S.; Park, K.Y. Association between Breastfeeding and Prevalence of Diabetes in Korean Parous Women: The Korea National Health and Nutrition Examination Survey, 2010–2014. *Korean J. Fam. Med.* **2018**, *39*, 273–278. [CrossRef] [PubMed]
150. Laine, M.K.; Kautiainen, H.; Gissler, M.; Pennanen, P.; Eriksson, J.G. Impact of gestational diabetes mellitus on the duration of breastfeeding in primiparous women: An observational cohort study. *Int. Breastfeed. J.* **2021**, *16*, 19. [CrossRef]
151. Pereira, P.F.; Alfenas, R.d.C.G.; Araújo, R.M.A. Does breastfeeding influence the risk of developing diabetes mellitus in children? A review of current evidence. *J. De Pediatr.* **2014**, *90*, 7–15. [CrossRef] [PubMed]
152. Stuebe, A.M.; Meltzer-Brody, S.; Pearson, B.; Pedersen, C.; Grewen, K. Maternal neuroendocrine serum levels in exclusively breastfeeding mothers. *Breastfeed. Med.* **2015**, *10*, 197–202. [CrossRef] [PubMed]
153. Joshi, J.V.; Bhandarkar, S.D.; Chadha, M.; Balaiah, D.; Shah, R. Menstrual irregularities and lactation failure may precede thyroid dysfunction or goitre. *J. Postgrad. Med.* **1993**, *39*, 137–141. [PubMed]
154. Hapon, M.B.; Simoncini, M.; Via, G.; Jahn, G.A. Effect of hypothyroidism on hormone profiles in virgin, pregnant and lactating rats, and on lactation. *Reproduction* **2003**, *126*, 371–382. [CrossRef]
155. Alexander, E.; Pearce, E.; Brent, G.; Brown, R.; Chen, H.; Dosiou, C.; Grobman, W.; Laurberg, P.; Lazarus, J.H.; Mandel, S.J.; et al. 2017 Guidelines of the American Thyroid 339 Association for the Diagnosis and Management of Thyroid Disease During Pregnancy and the 340 Postpartum. *Thyroid* **2017**, *27*, 315–389. [CrossRef]
156. Amino, N.; Arata, N. Thyroid dysfunction following pregnancy and implications for breastfeeding. *Best Pract. Res. Clin. Endocrinol. Metab.* **2020**, *34*, 101438. [CrossRef]
157. Mandel, S.J.; Cooper, D.S. The use of antithyroid drugs in pregnancy and lactation. *J. Clin. Endocrinol. Metab.* **2001**, *86*, 2354–2359. [CrossRef] [PubMed]
158. Ide, A.; Amino, N.; Kudo, T.; Yoshioka, W.; Hisakado, M.; Nishihara, E.; Ito, M.; Fukata, S.; Nakamura, H.; Miyauchi, A. Comparative frequency of four different types of pregnancy-associated thyrotoxicosis in a single thyroid centre. *Thyroid. Res.* **2017**, *10*, 4. [CrossRef]
159. Bergink, V.; Pop, V.; Nielsen, P.; Agerbo, E.; Munk-Olsen, T.; Liu, X. Comorbidity of autoimmune thyroid disorders and psychiatric disorders during the postpartum period: A Danish nationwide register-based cohort study. *Psychol. Med.* **2018**, *48*, 1291–1298. [CrossRef]
160. Kuijpens, J.L.; Vader, H.L.; Drexhage, H.A.; Wiersinga, W.M.; van Son, M.J.; Pop, V.J. Thyroid peroxidase antibodies during gestation are a marker for subsequent depression postpartum. *Eur. J. Endocrinol.* **2001**, *145*, 579–584. [CrossRef]
161. Borba, V.V.; Zandman-Goddard, G.; Shoenfeld, Y. Prolactin and autoimmunity: The hormone as an inflammatory cytokine. *Best Pract. Res. Clin. Endocrinol. Metab.* **2019**, *33*, 101324. [CrossRef] [PubMed]
162. Njom Nlend, A.E. Mother-to-Child Transmission of HIV Through Breastfeeding Improving Awareness and Education: A Short Narrative Review. *Int. J. Women's Health* **2022**, *14*, 697–703. [CrossRef] [PubMed]
163. WHO. HIV/AIDS: Infant Feeding and Nutrition. Available online: https://www.who.int/news-room/questions-and-answers/item/hiv-aids-infant-feeding-and-nutrition (accessed on 16 June 2023).
164. Powell, A.M.; Knott-Grasso, M.A.; Anderson, J.; Livingston, A.; Rosenblum, N.; Sturdivant, H.; Byrnes, K.C.; Martel, K.; Sheffield, J.S.; Golden, W.C.; et al. Infant feeding for people living with HIV in high resource settings: A multi-disciplinary approach with best practices to maximise risk reduction. *Lancet Reg. Health Am.* **2023**, *22*, 100509. [CrossRef]
165. Ehrhardt, S.; Xie, C.; Guo, N.; Nelson, K.; Thio, C.L. Breastfeeding while taking lamivudine or tenofovir disoproxil fumarate: A review of the evidence. *Clin. Infect. Dis.* **2015**, *60*, 275–278. [CrossRef] [PubMed]
166. Tuthill, E.L.; Miller, J.D.; Collins, S.M.; Widen, E.M.; Onono, M.; Young, S.L. HIV infection, hunger, breastfeeding self-efficacy, and depressive symptoms are associated with exclusive breastfeeding to six months among women in western Kenya: A longitudinal observational study. *Int. Breastfeed. J.* **2020**, *15*, 4. [CrossRef]
167. Boostani, R.; Sadeghi, R.; Sabouri, A.; Ghabeli-Juibary, A. Human T-lymphotropic virus type I and breastfeeding; systematic review and meta-analysis of the literature. *Iran. J. Neurol.* **2018**, *17*, 174–179. [CrossRef] [PubMed]
168. Itabashi, K.; Miyazawa, T. Mother-to-Child Transmission of Human T-Cell Leukemia Virus Type 1: Mechanisms and Nutritional Strategies for Prevention. *Cancers* **2021**, *13*, 4100. [CrossRef]
169. Petrova, M.; Kamburov, V. Breastfeeding and chronic HBV infection: Clinical and social implications. *World J. Gastroenterol.* **2010**, *16*, 5042–5046. [CrossRef] [PubMed]
170. WHO. Prevention of Mother-to-Child Transmission of Hepatitis B Virus: Guidelines on Antiviral Prophylaxis in Pregnancy. Available online: https://apps.who.int/iris/bitstream/handle/10665/333391/9789240002708-eng.pdf (accessed on 16 June 2023).
171. Zheng, Y.; Lu, Y.; Ye, Q.; Xia, Y.; Zhou, Y.; Yao, Q.; Wei, S. Should chronic hepatitis B mothers breastfeed? a meta analysis. *BMC Public Health* **2011**, *11*, 502. [CrossRef] [PubMed]

172. Li, E.-M.; Xiao, L.-X.; Xu, Z.; Mo, Z.-S.; Li, J.-Q.; Mei, Y.-Y.; Lin, C.-S. Factors associated with non-compliance with breastfeeding recommendation: A retrospective survey in hepatitis B virus-infected mothers who had taken Nucleos(t)ide analogs during pregnancy. *BMC Pregnancy Childbirth* **2021**, *21*, 551. [CrossRef]
173. Benova, L.; Mohamoud, Y.A.; Calvert, C.; Abu-Raddad, L.J. Vertical transmission of hepatitis C virus: Systematic review and meta-analysis. *Clin. Infect. Dis.* **2014**, *59*, 765–773. [CrossRef]
174. Espinosa, C.M.; Niestrath, R.G. Low Breastfeeding Rates and Complex Barriers to Breastfeeding and Breast Milk Utilization in Hepatitis C Perinatally Exposed Infants. *Pediatrics* **2021**, *147*, 323–324. [CrossRef]
175. Freriksen, J.J.M.; van Seyen, M.; Judd, A.; Gibb, D.M.; Collins, I.J.; Greupink, R.; Russel, F.G.M.; Drenth, J.P.H.; Colbers, A.; Burger, D.M. Review article: Direct-acting antivirals for the treatment of HCV during pregnancy and lactation—Implications for maternal dosing, foetal exposure, and safety for mother and child. *Aliment. Pharmacol. Ther.* **2019**, *50*, 738–750. [CrossRef]
176. Finkelstein, S.A.; Keely, E.; Feig, D.S.; Tu, X.; Yasseen, A.S., 3rd; Walker, M. Breastfeeding in women with diabetes: Lower rates despite greater rewards. A population-based study. *Diabet. Med.* **2013**, *30*, 1094–1101. [CrossRef]
177. Cornish, J.; Tan, E.; Teare, J.; Teoh, T.G.; Rai, R.; Clark, S.K.; Tekkis, P.P. A meta-analysis on the influence of inflammatory bowel disease on pregnancy. *Gut* **2007**, *56*, 830–837. [CrossRef]
178. Vanky, E.; Isaksen, H.; Moen, M.H.; Carlsen, S.M. Breastfeeding in polycystic ovary syndrome. *Acta Obs. Gynecol. Scand.* **2008**, *87*, 531–535. [CrossRef] [PubMed]
179. Scime, N.V.; Patten, S.B.; Tough, S.C.; Chaput, K.H. Maternal chronic disease and breastfeeding outcomes: A Canadian population-based study. *J. Matern. Fetal Neonatal Med.* **2022**, *35*, 1148–1155. [CrossRef] [PubMed]
180. Chatterjee, S.; Kotelchuck, M.; Sambamoorthi, U. Prevalence of chronic illness in pregnancy, access to care, and health care costs: Implications for interconception care. *Women's Health Issues* **2008**, *18*, S107–S116. [CrossRef]
181. Mills, K.T.; Stefanescu, A.; He, J. The global epidemiology of hypertension. *Nat. Rev. Nephrol.* **2020**, *16*, 223–237. [CrossRef] [PubMed]
182. Kachoria, R.; Oza-Frank, R. Differences in breastfeeding initiation by maternal diabetes status and race, Ohio 2006–2011. *Matern. Child Health J.* **2014**, *18*, 2226–2235. [CrossRef]
183. Joham, A.E.; Nanayakkara, N.; Ranasinha, S.; Zoungas, S.; Boyle, J.; Harrison, C.L.; Forder, P.; Loxton, D.; Vanky, E.; Teede, H.J. Obesity, polycystic ovary syndrome and breastfeeding: An observational study. *Acta Obs. Gynecol. Scand.* **2016**, *95*, 458–466. [CrossRef]
184. Kramer, M.S.; Kakuma, R. Optimal duration of exclusive breastfeeding. *Cochrane Database Syst. Rev.* **2012**, *2012*, Cd003517. [CrossRef]
185. De Bortoli, J.; Amir, L.H. Is onset of lactation delayed in women with diabetes in pregnancy? A systematic review. *Diabet. Med.* **2016**, *33*, 17–24. [CrossRef]
186. Hurst, N.M. Recognizing and treating delayed or failed lactogenesis II. *J. Midwifery Women's Health* **2007**, *52*, 588–594. [CrossRef]
187. Brownell, E.; Howard, C.R.; Lawrence, R.A.; Dozier, A.M. Delayed onset lactogenesis II predicts the cessation of any or exclusive breastfeeding. *J. Pediatr.* **2012**, *161*, 608–614. [CrossRef] [PubMed]
188. Prior, E.; Santhakumaran, S.; Gale, C.; Philipps, L.H.; Modi, N.; Hyde, M.J. Breastfeeding after cesarean delivery: A systematic review and meta-analysis of world literature. *Am. J. Clin. Nutr.* **2012**, *95*, 1113–1135. [CrossRef] [PubMed]
189. Alves, E.; Rodrigues, C.; Fraga, S.; Barros, H.; Silva, S. Parents' views on factors that help or hinder breast milk supply in neonatal care units: Systematic review. *Arch. Dis. Childhood. Fetal Neonatal Ed.* **2013**, *98*, F511–F517. [CrossRef] [PubMed]
190. Spiesser-Robelet, L.; Brunie, V.; de Andrade, V.; Gagnayre, R. Knowledge, Representations, Attitudes, and Behaviors of Women Faced With Taking Medications While Breastfeeding: A Scoping Review. *J. Hum. Lact.* **2016**, *33*, 98–114. [CrossRef] [PubMed]
191. Spencer, B. Medications and Breastfeeding for Mothers With Chronic Illness. *J. Obstet. Gynecol. Neonatal Nurs. JOGNN* **2015**, *44*, 543–552. [CrossRef] [PubMed]
192. Thomas, H. Women's postnatal experience following a medically complicated pregnancy. *Health Care Women Int.* **2004**, *25*, 76–87. [CrossRef]

nutrients

MDPI

Review

An Update on Lung Function of Extremely and Very Preterm Infants in Later Life: The Role of Early Nutritional Interventions

Despina D. Briana * and Ariadne Malamitsi-Puchner

Neonatal Intensive Care Unit, 3rd Department of Pediatrics, National and Kapodistrian University of Athens Medical School, Chaidari, 12462 Athens, Greece
* Correspondence: dbriana@med.uoa.gr; Tel.: +30-210-583-2228

Abstract: Birth occurring at ≤32 weeks' gestation ("very preterm") or at ≤28 weeks' gestation ("extremely preterm") potentially poses considerable health problems for the neonate, including respiratory sequelae, not only during the immediate newborn period, but throughout childhood and into adulthood. With the progressive improvements in neonatal care, the survival of extremely preterm and very preterm neonates has improved substantially. However, a considerable percentage of these infants suffer dysfunctions that may trigger, at some stage later in life, the onset of respiratory morbidities. The interruption of the normal development of the respiratory tract caused by preterm birth, in combination with postnatal lung injury caused by various interventions, e.g., mechanical ventilation and oxygen therapy, increases the risk ofthe development of long-term respiratory deficits in survivors. Those infants that are most affected are those who develop chronic lung disease of prematurity (also called bronchopulmonary dysplasia, BPD), but impaired lung function can develop irrespective of BPD diagnosis. Apart from indicating abnormal lung function in survivors of extreme prematurity, recent long-term follow-up studies also emphasize the crucial role of early nutritional intake as an effective strategy, which promotes lung growth and repair. This article will update the associations between extremely/very preterm birth with long-term respiratory outcomes. It will also discuss the protective effect of nutritional interventions, focusing on recently published follow-up data.

Keywords: extremely preterm neonate; very preterm neonate; bronchopulmonary dysplasia; nutrition; respiratory sequelae; chronic obstructive pulmonary disease

1. Introduction

The continuous advances in perinatal care in the last few decades (including the use of antenatal steroids and surfactant treatment), in combination with the less aggressive ventilatory support practices, have resulted in the survival of an increasing number of infants born at gestational ages (GA) ≤ 32 weeks (very preterm) or ≤28 weeks (extremely preterm). Preterm birth results in the interruption of prenatal lung development during the canalicular and saccular/early alveolar stages [1]. Early exposure to infection and inflammation, as well as mechanical ventilation and hyperoxia may cause additional damage to the immature lung [2].

A large proportion of preterm infants will eventually develop bronchopulmonary dysplasia (BPD), which is considered one of the gravest sequelae of preterm birth [3]. The "old" BPD definition provided by Northway and associates [4] >50 years ago included the characteristics of inflammation, airway smooth muscle hypertrophy, emphysema, and parenchymal fibrosis as a result of exposure to high oxygen concentration and high ventilation pressures. Since then, the cohort of premature infants, the treatment strategies of neonates, and the consequent pulmonary damage have substantially changed. The improved rates of survival among more immature infants, thanks to modern perinatal care, have resulted in the occurrence of a new BPD phenotype (disrupted lung development), which has different disease pathogenesis compared to "old" BPD (acute lung injury) [5,6]. The "new" BPD phenotype is characterized by markedly more immature lung tissue, as well as impaired alveolarization (reduced, large, thin-walled alveoli), dysmorphic pulmonary microvessel growth and less fibrosis, as compared to the "old BPD" [7]. Lung immaturity, as well as the disruption of alveolarization and the microvascular development in BPD are clinically translated into abnormal gas exchange and lung mechanics [8]. This new type of chronic lung disease of prematurity poses an additional demanding task to clinicians and researchers besides preventing lung damage, i.e., preserving normal lung tissue development.

The exact definition of BPD has been the subject of debate and is currently influenced by the need for supplemental oxygen at 28 days of life, while the severity of the disease is determined by assessing ventilator support and the fraction of the necessary inspired oxygen at 36 weeks postmenstrual age [5,9,10]. Overall, about 30–68% of infants <28 weeks' GA develop BPD [3,11]. This incidence is inversely related to GA and remained unchanged (or even increased) among the most premature infants due to the significant reduction in mortality and the substantial increase in the total number of infants with significant prematurity [3,11]. Large variations in BPD incidence between NICUs reflect population differences and differences in clinical treatment practices [12].

Previous longitudinal pulmonary function and long-term follow-up studies reported that most extremely/very preterm neonates with BPD present with a low lung function trajectory [13,14] and an increased risk for the future development of a chronic obstructive pulmonary disease (COPD)-like phenotype [15–17]. Furthermore, former extremely/very premature infants are predisposed to the development of other respiratory morbidities than chronic lung disease, due to factors associated with prematurity [18]. These infants present with a higher incidence of lower respiratory tract infections requiring re-hospitalizations, impaired lung mechanics, and developmental abnormalities of the airways, leading to recurrent wheezing and asthma. These sequelae may occur from early infancy throughout childhood and until adulthood [18].

Long-term respiratory outcome studies of extremely/very preterm infants are in need of constant updates due to alterations in patient population, rapid advances in the areas of pulmonary physiology and pathophysiology, as well as improvements in perinatal care practices, including nutritional interventions. In this respect, recent follow-up data highlight the crucial role of nutrition in promoting favorable long-term pulmonary outcomes in extremely/very preterm-born infants [19,20].

In the present manuscript, we review the associations between extremely/very premature birth with long-term pulmonary outcomes, with particular emphasis on the most recent data on the topic, and discuss current evidence, which emphasizes the long-term beneficial effect of nutritional interventions on lung growth and repair.

2. Long-Term Pulmonary Outcomes of Extremely/Very Preterm Birth

The lung function of prematurely born infants may be compromised during childhood and adulthood; this applies, in particular, to extremely preterm infants, those experiencing BPD or those who have been exposed to mechanical ventilation during the newborn period [21]. As lung tissue grows postnatally, several parameters related to pulmonary volumes may improve. Nevertheless, pathological changes in pulmonary flows may persist throughout adolescence or into adult life [21].

2.1. Pulmonary Outcomes during Infancy

Several clinical/experimental studies document that preterm birth disrupts alveolarization, leading to a decrease in the gas exchange surface area of the lung and thereby causing BPD [7,8]. Furthermore, lung immaturity predisposes to respiratory morbidities other than BPD [18]. Recent data demonstrate that following preterm birth, the airway epithelium is both structurally and functionally impaired, with evidence of epithelial thickening in addition to increased inflammation and apoptosis [22].

Thus, primarily obstructive pulmonary abnormalities were demonstrated in extremely preterm-born infants receiving contemporary intensive care at term-equivalent age, compared with healthy full-term controls [23]. Irrespective of BPD, a strikingly abnormal pulmonary function was present at the term-equivalent age, although this was observed more intensely in the BPD group. It is, therefore, suggested that the evaluation of lung morbidity only by diagnosis of BPD or not, is probably not adequate in predicting future respiratory health [23].Similarly, in a multicenter, longitudinal birth cohort study, extremely low GA neonates receiving ambient air or on low-flow nasal cannula support had abnormal tidal breathing patterns, with no differences noted between infants with and without BPD [24]. Neither prebronchodilator nor postbronchodilator tidal breathing patterns were associated with post-discharge pulmonary disease [24]. The authors hypothesized that, besides altered respiratory mechanics, other factors (e.g., respiratory tract viral infections) [25] may be responsible for the occurrence of respiratory morbidities among preterms.

Infants born extremely/very preterm with BPD of either degree of severity were followed-up in a longitudinal cohort study to 6 and 18 months of postnatal age. Respiratory symptoms, such as recurrent/chronic cough and wheezing, were recorded [26]. Passive lung mechanics and whole-body plethysmography, as well as tidal and raised volume rapid thoraco-abdominal compression techniques, were used to examine respiratory function. Infants with BPD presented with reduced airway function and respiratory compliance. However, mild and moderate/severe BPD differed only in terms of lower respiratory compliance in the latter, possibly as a result of delayed or altered alveolar formulation. Thus, the value of the early classification of BPD severity in predicting future lung function is considered to be very limited [26].

Gonçalves et al. [27] reported an increased incidence of impaired respiratory function in very preterm infants of 6–12 months of corrected age compared with same-aged full-term ones, as evaluated by forced expiratory flows using the chest compression technique, and volumes using total body plethysmography. Compromised lung function was associated with the degree of prematurity, restricted fetal growth, mechanical respiratory support and recurrent episodes of wheezing during infancy [27].

2.2. Pulmonary Outcomes during Childhood

Those infants who survive prematurity are at risk ofaltered pulmonary function during childhood. Only a limited number of follow-up studies have investigated the trajectories of respiratory function in extremely/very preterm-born children and showed a considerable persistent lung function compromise, which warrants follow-up and treatment consideration [28,29].

An earlier follow-up study investigated whether very preterm birth, BPD, and the degree of BPD severity, are predictive of future lung function in school-aged children born in the modern era, which is characterized by antenatal corticosteroids use and surfactant administration [30]. Preterm children presented with significantly decreased spirometric flow-volume parameters, as well as alveolar diffusion capacity compared with children born at term. The diagnosis of BPD was related to a marked reduction in both spirometry and diffusion capacity. Furthermore, very preterm birth and moderate/severe BPD pose an additive reduction in spirometric parameters of individuals by school age [30]. Longitudinal data on lung function in a group of extremely premature children born in the post-surfactant era also confirmed a significant airflow limitation, especially striking in BPD survivors who also demonstrated an abnormal airway growth trajectory, followed by a reduction in pulmonary function between 8 and 12 years of age [31].

Oscillatory mechanics, spirometry, multiple breath nitrogen washout, and diffusing capacity of the lung for carbon monoxide were used to test pulmonary function at 9–11 years of age in children born at term and at ≤32 weeks of gestation in the contemporary era [32]. In addition, preterm children underwent chest computed tomography (CT) and had their respiratory symptoms recorded. Compared with term controls, preterm children presented with pulmonary obstruction and hyperinflation, in addition to abnormal peripheral lung mechanics. Abnormalities in lung structure were seen in 92% of preterm children and were associated with more intense respiratory obstruction and increased incidence of severe respiratory symptoms, probably implying active lung disease [32].

A population-based cohort of children born at 22–26 weeks GA and controls born at term between 2004 and 2007 were followed-up at 6½ years of age with spirometry and impulse oscillometry [33]. It was demonstrated that a large percentage of extremely preterm-born children have impaired airway mechanics and a marked obstructive reduction in pulmonary function. A total of 40% of extremely preterm children and 15% of controls exhibited asthma-like disease. Furthermore, half of the children born at 22–24 weeks GA demonstrated a lung function below the lower limits of normal. Interestingly, severe BPD contributed to pulmonary outcomes only marginally [33].

Similarly, an earlier meta-analysis of follow-up studies including infants born preterm at 24–36 weeks GA between 1964 and 2000 demonstrated average forced expiratory volume in 1 s (FEV1) reductions of 16% in those with mild BPD and 19% in those with moderate to severe BPD [14]. The marginally significant (or even non-significant) differences in pulmonary function according to the severity of BPD in these studies suggest that respiratory deficits during childhood are probably related to the degree of prematurity and that the BPD classification is likely of limited value for the prediction of future pulmonary function as evaluated by spirometric parameters [14].

A recent longitudinal cohort study documented data on lung structure and function, as well as respiratory symptoms throughout childhood in a very preterm cohort born in the contemporary era [34]. It was reported that preterm children with and without BPD have declining pulmonary function trajectories from 4 to 12 years of age, with greater reductions reported in children with BPD, ongoing respiratory symptoms, and bronchial wall thickening (on chest CT) indicative of inflammation. These children may be predisposed to developing lung disease later in life [34]. Furthermore, there is evidence suggesting that lung function does not improve over time in very preterm-born children diagnosed with the severe form of either "old" or "new" BPD. By contrast, FEV1 and forced vital capacity (FVC) deteriorate from childhood to adulthood [35]. In line with these findings, a very recent study aimed to outline alterations in pulmonary function in a contemporary observational group of children born preterm whowere subsequently followedup for post-prematurity respiratory disease with pulmonary function testings [36]. Very preterm-born children demonstrated worsening obstruction in pulmonary function throughout childhood [36].

2.3. *Pulmonary Outcomes in Adolescence and Young Adulthood*

Pulmonary function normally increases during childhood and adolescence, reaches a peak in the mid-20s, and then gradually decreases with age [37]. This trajectory is modulated by genetic factors, antenatal events, and exposure to multiple events early in life [38].

A meta-analysis of cohort studies, mainly conducted during the pre-surfactant era, demonstrated that infants born either very preterm or with very low birthweight are at increased risk of not reaching their full lung growth potential during adolescence and early adulthood, a finding which suggests an increased risk of COPD in later adulthood [39].

Similarly, long-term data obtained in the post-surfactant era showed that survivors born either at a GA less than 28 weeks or with abirthweight less than 1000 g (particularly those who had BPD) will not achieve the normal peak of expiratory airflow by their mid-20s [40]. The authors conclude that since nowadays many more infants who were either born at <28 weeks GA or with <1000 gbirthweight are surviving into adulthood since the 1990s, many of them will end up developing symptoms of airway obstruction later in life, especially those who experienced BPD [40].

A very recently published population-based study [41] reported lung function trajectories from 10 to 35 years of age in infants who were born extremely preterm. Persistent airflow obstruction was reported in early adult life and throughout the onset of the age-related decline from 25 to 35 years. Lung function after extremely preterm birth was tracked in parallel, but was significantly lower as compared to the trajectories of term-born from 10 to 35 years, including the starting age-related decline from 25 to 35 years. An existing but diminishing long-term importance of BPD was recorded, probably reflecting the recent improvements in perinatal care. However, 30% of these extremely preterm-born infants met the post-bronchodilator spirometry criteria for COPD compared with 5% of term-born infants ($p < 0.001$) [41].

Extremely preterm-born adolescents with "new" BPD presented with poorer lung function compared with extremely preterm-born adolescents without BPD or moderate–late preterm-born ones in a multicenter cross-sectional study [42]. Extremely preterm-born adolescents with BPD had markedly lower FEV_1 and FVC, as well as significantly higher bronchodilator response and air-trapping. However, BPD adolescents did not demonstrate a higher incidence of asthma symptoms or a poorer quality of life, probably indicating that progress in perinatal care has favored the predominance of milder forms of chronic lung disease of prematurity [42]. In accordance, recent data demonstrated lower FEV1 in adolescents with BPD born extremely/very preterm, as compared to those without BPD, with lower FEV1 values significantly related to BPD severity [43]. The results of spirometry and impulse oscillometry measurements in the BPD compared with the non-BPD group indicate airway obstruction including involvement of peripheral airways, probably implying a predisposition to COPD in adult life in the group with severe BPD [43].

In line with these results, a recent prospective follow-up study reported poorer lung function in adolescents and young adults born extremely premature who experienced BPD, as compared to those without a BPD diagnosis [44]. Interestingly, 16% of subjects without BPD presented with impaired pulmonary function, suggesting that prematurity by itself has a negative impact on lung function [44]. Similar results were reported in another study which showed that spirometric parameters were worse during adulthood in those born prematurely without BPD vs. term controls [45].

Impaired alveolar development blocks lung-diffusing capacity. Disruption of alveolar growth due to extremely preterm birth may lead to COPD in early adulthood [46]. One controlled population-based report published in 2022 documented the longitudinal development of lung-diffusing capacity after extremely preterm birth from mid-childhood to adulthood [47]. Two cohorts born at $\leq$28 weeks GA or birthweight $\leq$ 1000 g between 1982 and 1985, as well as between 1991 and 1992 were evaluated twice, at ages 18 and 25 years and 10 and 18 years, respectively, and were compared with matched controls born at term. Extremely preterm-born individuals had impaired lung-diffusing capacity. The deficits tracked below (but in parallel) to matched full-term control groups from mid-childhood to adulthood [47].

Finally, a study investigating the association between prematurity and lung function with COPD in the sixth decade of life showed that severe prematurity is related to obstructive lung function deficits (including COPD) into middle age and that this effect was further aggravated bysmoking [48].

Overall, there is a paucity of longitudinal respiratory follow-up data after extremely/very preterm birth in the surfactant era, but existing evidence raises considerable concerns about the long-term pulmonary status of survivors of extremely/very preterm birth. Declines in pulmonary function are persistently observed in extremely/very preterm individuals during childhood, adolescence and adulthood and, therefore, a close targeted life-long monitoring of lung health is warranted [28,29]. However, it should be noted that premature birth is not included in authoritative statements, as a risk factor for COPD [49]. Furthermore, few pulmonologists consider early life factors in their clinical practice [49].

2.4. Differences in Pulmonary Outcomes at the Turn of the Millennium

Studies comparing respiratory outcomes in extremely preterm individuals born from 1980 to 2000 produced conflicting results, with most studies reporting improvements which parallel the remarkable recent advances in perinatal care [14,41,50,51].

Kotecha et al. compared findings from studies of pulmonary function conducted in the pre- and post-surfactant era, in participants aged between 5 and 23 years. One interesting finding was that the mean FEV1 for subjects with BPD had improved over time from those born in the late 1960s to those born in the early 1990s, indicating that lung impairment during the neonatal period might be less severe with ongoing improvements in neonatal care practices [14]. Another study from Norway compared respiratory health in extremely preterm-born children between 1991–1992 and 1999–2000 and showed that small airway obstruction and bronchial hyperresponsiveness were still present in children born preterm at the turn of the millennium, but outcomes were better than for children born similarly preterm in 1991–1992, especially after BPD. These data imply that better neonatal care practices improve both survival and long-term pulmonary outcomes [50].However, in a subsequent longitudinal prospective follow-up of all survivors of extremely preterm births in Victoria, Australia, during three periods (namely, 1991–1992, 1997, and 2005), no significant reduction in oxygen dependence was seen at 36 weeks and no significant improvement in lung function during childhood was detected over time, despite a marked increase in the use of less invasive ventilation after birth [51].

Finally, a very recently published population-based study addressed possible cohort effects over a period of major advances in perinatal/neonatal care [41]. Spirometry was repeated in three population-based cohorts born at $\leq$28 weeks GA or with birthweight $\leq$ 1000 g during 1982–1985, 1991–1992 and 1999–2000, and in full-term controls matched for age and gender. The deficits of these cohorts compared with term-born infants decreased with each decade of birth from 1980 to 2000 [41].

3. Nutritional Interventions and Long-Term Pulmonary Outcomes

Prematurity is a predisposing factor for the development of lung disease. BPD is associated with high morbidity and mortality rates in survivors of severe prematurity [52]. Irrespective of BPD diagnosis, premature infants are characterized by lung immaturity at birth and deficient control of breathing [18]. They face adverse pulmonary conditions in the neonatal period and are at risk of pulmonary disorders both in the mid- as well as in the long-term, such as respiratory tract infections during infancy, recurrent wheezing and asthma during childhood and abnormalities of pulmonary function in adulthood [18]. Thus, it is imperative to identify how early exposures can be modified to decrease the risk of developing BPD or other respiratory pathology before disease progression becomes irreversible.

Compelling evidence suggests that the alveoli continue to be formed postnatally throughout childhood and adulthood. Thus, current research should focus on further elucidation of those mechanisms responsible for postnatal lung growth, as well as the development of strategies to stimulate lung regeneration [7,53,54]. In this context, nutritional interventions have been proposed to promote postnatal alveolarization and lung growth, offering a unique opportunity to improve respiratory outcomes [19,55,56].

Intrauterine malnutrition is a common prenatal risk factor for BPD development when preterm birth occurs [57,58]. Malnutrition may continue postnatally since extreme prematurity poses several difficulties in providing adequate nutrient and energy intake. Both intra- and extra-uterine malnutrition may have devastating effects on the developing lung [59]. A recent study documented that very preterm infants who developed BPD received a calorie/protein ratio below that recommended for optimal growth during the first 4 weeks of life [60]. A retrospective cohort of very low birthweight infants also showed markedly lower energy and lipid intake among those who developed BPD during the first week of life [61]. Interestingly, an energy intake of less than 1778.2 kJ/kg in this time-period was related to a twofold increase in the adjusted risk of developing BPD. The authors emphasize the potential crucial role of early inclusion of lipids in parenteral nutrition, in order to promote (in combination with optimal protein content) an adequate energy intake and, therefore, to reduce the incidence of BPD [61]. Further retrospective data suggest that high fluid and low caloric intake in extremely preterm infants during the first week of life are associated with BPD severity [62].

In accordance, several studies pointed out extrauterine growth restriction, secondary to postnatal insufficiency in nutrient and energy intake, as a key risk factor for the development of BPD [63,64]. Due to increased energy expenditure, infants with established BPD have increased and often unmet caloric needs, compared with infants without BPD, which continue after discharge from the hospital [65]. Therefore, older studies have documented extrauterine growth restriction in BPD infants up to 12 months of age [66,67]. Interestingly, recent prospective data demonstrated poorer growth of very low birthweight infants with BPD until 36 weeks of corrected age but catch up growth accomplished by three months of corrected age, probably due to the continued improvements in nutritional practices applied to BPD infants [68].

Compelling data suggest a strong association between early nutrition and long-term pulmonary outcomes. In a cross-sectional study of 4- to 8-year-old children who had been born prematurely and were diagnosed with BPD, undernutrition at the age of 2 years was documented as the only factor predisposing to the development of airway distension. It was concluded that nutritional status at 2 years of age in children who were diagnosed with BPD has a significant effect on respiratory outcomes in childhood [69].

Up to the early 2000s, nutritional policies, applied to hospitalized neonates born with severe prematurity, resulted in significant extrauterine growth restriction [70]. In 2002, Ziegler et al. introduced a new era in the nutrition of the preterm, by reporting that "aggressive" nutrition, with increased early provision of protein and calories, resulted in better growth [71]. Nutrition of very preterm infants should ensure optimal growth as reflected in increases in body weight and head circumference. However, a recent whole-population study comprising infants born below 32 weeks of gestation in England and Wales between 2008 and 2019 showed that early postnatal weight loss has decreased, and subsequent weight gain has increased, but the weight at 36 weeks postmenstrual age was consistently below the weight of babies born at full-term. Greater weight at 36 weeks postmenstrual age was dependent on enteral nutritional intake [72]. It seems that despite significant changes in feeding policies after 2000, extrauterine growth restriction in extremely/very preterm infants remains a considerable concern.

Current recommendations suggest an adequate nutritional strategy that includes early "aggressive" parenteral nutrition, while initiating trophic feeding and advancing to concentrated nutritive enteral feeding, i.e., providing high energy in low volume, as soon as possible [19]. Priority is given to fortified mother's own milk, followed by fortified donor milk and preterm enriched formulas with a high density of energy and nutrients. Although evidence regarding effectiveness is limited, functional nutrient supplements, such as vitamins, zinc and iron, with a potential protective role against lung damage, are being re-evaluated. Feedings highly enriched in energy and nutrients should be given after discharge, i.e., either fortified breastmilk or enriched formula [19]. Very recently, the European Society of Pediatric Gastroenterology, Hepatology, and Nutrition (ESPGHAN) Committee of Nutrition (CoN) published an expert consensus on recommendations for the nutritional management of preterm infants with a birth weight of <1800 g. The authors emphasize the absence of strong scientific evidence in various topic areas and the need for additional high-quality research, particularly studies that evaluate long-term outcomes [73].

Until this day, few recent long-term studies have studied the effect of the type of early nutrition on lung function in children born preterm, but they produced interesting results [20,74,75]. In this respect, very encouraging findings regarding the impact of intensive early neonatal nutritional support up to 40–44 weeks postmenstrual age ("aggressive nutrition") and early use of nasal continuous positive airway pressure (nCPAP) on pulmonary function of very preterm neonates at school age were recently reported [20]. This study documented no significant differences in FEV1 and FVC, as well as in the incidence of lower respiratory tract infections and associated re-hospitalization up to 8 years of age either between very preterm cases and full-term controls or between the two subgroups of preterm infants with and without BPD. It was concluded that "aggressive" nutrition and early use of early nCPAP and their beneficial effect on early postnatal growth probably contributed to normal respiratory function in the study population [20]. In a 6-year follow-up study, very preterm-born infants breastfed at hospital discharge were subsequently randomized to receive either unfortified or fortified maternal milk, whereas those infants that were not breastfed received a preterm formula until 4 months of corrected age [74]. Fractional exhaled nitric oxide, airway resistance and occlusion measurements with reversibility were performed at 6 years of age. The results of the study indicated that protein-enriched nutrition after discharge may improve lung function in very preterm-born children [74]. In a cohort study with a similar design, compared to exclusively breastfed, very preterm infants supplemented with human milk fortifier or fed exclusively a preterm formula for 4 months did not have an increased risk of developing recurrent wheezing during the 1st year of life [75]. Furthermore, a study comprising infants with BPD aged less than 36 months, demonstrated that a longer duration of breast milk intake is associated with a reduced risk of acute and chronic pulmonary morbidities, such as episodes of cough or chest congestion, a reduced need for systematic administration of steroids and fewer re-hospitalizations. The authors highlight the crucial role of prolonged breast milk consumption among preterm infants with a BPD diagnosis in terms of protection against respiratory morbidities [76].

Further long-term follow-up studies, with larger populations, are essential in order to elucidate the potential modification of lung function in relation to early nutrition and growth in extremely and very preterm-born children [77].Moreover, prospective research is urgently needed to investigate whether better extrauterine growth of extremely/very preterm infants achieved by application of the new ESPGHAN CoN consensus-based feeding policies [73] will positively influence their respiratory outcome, as relevant retrospective data have shown [20].

4. Conclusions

Although the respiratory consequences of preterm birth are well-known, they remain poorly understood. BPD remains the most frequent adverse outcome for infants born <30 weeks of GA and the most common chronic lung disease in infancy. Accumulative evidence indicates persistent abnormalities of lung function in survivors of extreme prematurity throughout childhood and into adulthood, irrespective of BPD diagnosis. Long-term follow-up studies suggest that extremely/very premature birth represents an important precursor of chronic obstructive pulmonary disease that needs to be identified by pulmonologists and targeted by researchers. Nutrient intake and nutritional practices seem to have a major impact not only on short-term respiratory morbidities, but also long-term pulmonary outcomes. Efforts should remain focused on the prevention of preterm labor, but novel research should also aim at promoting postnatal alveolarization and lung regeneration. In this context, further follow-up studies focusing on the effect of early nutrition on respiratory health and lung function outcomes of extremely/very preterm individuals are urgently needed.

Author Contributions: D.D.B. prepared the initial draft; A.M.-P. reviewed and revised the manuscript. All authors have approved the submitted version and agree to be personally accountable for the author's own contributions and for ensuring that questions related to the accuracy or integrity of any part of the work, even ones in which the author was not personally involved, are appropriately investigated, resolved, and documented in the literature. All authors have read and agreed to the published version of the manuscript.

Funding: This research received no external funding.

Institutional Review Board Statement: Not applicable.

Informed Consent Statement: Not applicable.

Data Availability Statement: Not applicable.

Conflicts of Interest: The authors declare no conflict of interest.

References

1. O'Reilly, M.; Sozo, F.; Harding, R. Impact of preterm birth and bronchopulmonary dysplasia on the developing lung: Long-term consequences for respiratory health. *Clin. Exp. Pharmacol. Physiol.* **2013**, *40*, 765–773. [CrossRef] [PubMed]
2. Balany, J.; Bhandari, V. Understanding the impact of infection, inflammation, and their persistence in the pathogenesis of bronchopulmonary dysplasia. *Front. Med.* **2015**, *2*, 90. [CrossRef] [PubMed]
3. Stoll, B.J.; Hansen, N.I.; Bell, E.F.; Shankaran, S.; Laptook, A.R.; Walsh, M.C.; Hale, E.C.; Newman, N.S.; Schibler, K.; Carlo, W.A.; et al. Neonatal outcomes of extremely preterm infants from the NICHD Neonatal Research Network. *Pediatrics* **2010**, *126*, 443–456. [CrossRef] [PubMed]
4. Northway, W.H., Jr.; Rosan, R.C.; Porter, D.Y. Pulmonary disease following respirator therapy of hyaline-membrane disease. Bronchopulmonary dysplasia. *N. Engl. J. Med.* **1967**, *276*, 357–368. [CrossRef]
5. Jobe, A.H.; Bancalari, E. Bronchopulmonary dysplasia. *Am. J. Respir. Crit. Care. Med.* **2001**, *163*, 1723–1729. [CrossRef]
6. Baraldi, E.; Filippone, M. Chronic lung disease after premature birth. *N. Engl. J. Med.* **2007**, *357*, 1946–1955. [CrossRef]
7. Baker, C.D.; Alvira, C.M. Disrupted lung development and bronchopulmonary dysplasia: Opportunities for lung repair and regeneration. *Curr. Opin. Pediatr.* **2014**, *26*, 306–314. [CrossRef]
8. Thébaud, B.; Goss, K.N.; Laughon, M.; Whitsett, J.A.; Abman, S.H.; Steinhorn, R.H.; Aschner, J.L.; Davis, P.G.; McGrath-Morrow, S.A.; Soll, R.F.; et al. Bronchopulmonary dysplasia. *Nat. Rev. Dis. Primers* **2019**, *5*, 78. [CrossRef]
9. Ehrenkranz, R.A.; Walsh, M.C.; Vohr, B.R.; Jobe, A.H.; Wright, L.L.; Fanaroff, A.A.; Wrage, L.A.; Poole, K. Validation of the National Institutes of Health consensus definition of bronchopulmonary dysplasia. *Pediatrics* **2005**, *116*, 1353–1360. [CrossRef]
10. Higgins, R.D.; Jobe, A.H.; Koso-Thomas, M.; Bancalari, E.; Viscardi, R.M.; Hartert, T.V.; Ryan, R.M.; Kallapur, S.G.; Steinhorn, R.H.; Konduri, G.G.; et al. Bronchopulmonary Dysplasia: Executive Summary of a Workshop. *J. Pediatr.* **2018**, *197*, 300–308. [CrossRef]
11. Costeloe, K.L.; Hennessy, E.M.; Haider, S.; Stacey, F.; Marlow, N.; Draper, E.S. Short term outcomes after extreme preterm birth in England: Comparison of two birth cohorts in 1995 and 2006 (the EPICure studies). *BMJ* **2012**, *345*, e7976. [CrossRef] [PubMed]
12. Guimarães, H.; Rocha, G.; Vasconcellos, G.; Proença, E.; Carreira, M.L.; Sossai, M.R.; Morais, B.; Martins, I.; Rodrigues, T.; Severo, M. Bronchopulmonary dysplasia: Clinical practices in five Portuguese neonatal intensive care units. *Rev. Port. Pneumol.* **2010**, *16*, 273–286. [CrossRef]
13. Doyle, L.W.; Faber, B.; Callanan, C.; Freezer, N.; Ford, G.W.; Davis, N.M. Bronchopulmonary dysplasia in very low birth weight subjects and lung function in late adolescence. *Pediatrics* **2006**, *118*, 108–113. [CrossRef] [PubMed]
14. Kotecha, S.J.; Edwards, M.O.; Watkins, W.J.; Henderson, A.J.; Paranjothy, S.; Dunstan, F.D.; Kotecha, S. Effect of preterm birth on later FEV1, a systematic review and meta-analysis. *Thorax* **2013**, *68*, 760–766. [CrossRef]
15. Gibson, A.M.; Reddington, C.; McBride, L.; Callanan, C.; Robertson, C.; Doyle, L.W. Lung function in adult survivors of very low birth weight, with and without bronchopulmonary dysplasia. *Pediatr. Pulmonol.* **2015**, *50*, 987–994. [CrossRef]
16. Carraro, S.; Filippone, M.; Da Dalt, L.; Ferraro, V.; Maretti, M.; Bressan, S.; El Mazloum, D.; Baraldi, E. Bronchopulmonary dysplasia: The earliest and perhaps the longest lasting obstructive lung disease in humans. *Early Hum. Dev.* **2013**, *89* (Suppl. S3), S3–S5. [CrossRef] [PubMed]
17. Vollsæter, M.; Røksund, O.D.; Eide, G.E.; Markestad, T.; Halvorsen, T. Lung function after preterm birth: Development from mid-childhood to adulthood. *Thorax* **2013**, *68*, 767–776. [CrossRef]
18. Bogdan, R.D.; Bohiltea, R.E.; Toma, A.I. Respiratory Follow Up of the Premature Neonates-Rationale and Practical Issues. *J. Clin. Med.* **2022**, *11*, 1746. [CrossRef]
19. Rocha, G.; Guimarães, H.; Pereira-da-Silva, L. The Role of Nutrition in the Prevention and Management of Bronchopulmonary Dysplasia: A Literature Review and Clinical Approach. *Int. J. Environ.Res. Public Health* **2021**, *18*, 6245. [CrossRef] [PubMed]
20. Panagiotounakou, P.; Sokou, R.; Gounari, E.; Konstantinidi, A.; Antonogeorgos, G.; Grivea, I.N.; Daniil, Z.; Gourgouliannis, K.I.; Gounaris, A. Very preterm neonates receiving "aggressive" nutrition and early nCPAP had similar long-term respiratory outcomes as term neonates. *Pediatr. Res.* **2019**, *86*, 742–748. [CrossRef]
21. Jain, D.; Feldman, A.; Sangam, S. Predicting Long-Term Respiratory Outcomes in Premature Infants: Is It Time to Move beyond Bronchopulmonary Dysplasia? *Children* **2020**, *7*, 283. [CrossRef] [PubMed]
22. Salaets, T.; Aertgeerts, M.; Gie, A.; Vignero, J.; de Winter, D.; Regin, Y.; Jimenez, J.; Vande Velde, G.; Allegaert, K.; Deprest, J.; et al. Preterm birth impairs postnatal lung development in the neonatal rabbit model. *Respir. Res.* **2020**, *21*, 59. [CrossRef] [PubMed]
23. Bentsen, M.H.; Markestad, T.; Øymar, K.; Halvorsen, T. Lung function at term in extremely preterm-born infants: A regional prospective cohort study. *BMJ Open* **2017**, *7*, e016868. [CrossRef]
24. Ren, C.L.; Feng, R.; Davis, S.D.; Eichenwald, E.; Jobe, A.; Moore, P.E.; Panitch, H.B.; Sharp, J.K.; Kisling, J.; Clem, C.; et al. Tidal Breathing Measurements at Discharge and Clinical Outcomes in Extremely Low Gestational Age Neonates. *Ann. Am. Thorac. Soc.* **2018**, *15*, 1311–1319. [CrossRef] [PubMed]
25. Pryhuber, G.S. Postnatal infections and immunology affecting chronic lung disease of prematurity. *Clin. Perinatol.* **2015**, *42*, 697–718. [CrossRef] [PubMed]
26. Thunqvist, P.; Gustafsson, P.; Norman, M.; Wickman, M.; Hallberg, J. Lung function at 6 and 18 months after preterm birth in relation to severity of bronchopulmonary dysplasia. *Pediatr. Pulmonol.* **2015**, *50*, 978–986. [CrossRef]
27. Gonçalves, D.M.M.; Wandalsen, G.F.; Scavacini, A.S.; Lanza, F.C.; Goulart, A.L.; Solé, D.; Dos Santos, A.M.N. Pulmonary function in former very low birth weight preterm infants in the first year of life. *Respir. Med.* **2018**, *136*, 83–87. [CrossRef]

28. Cheong, J.L.Y.; Doyle, L.W. An update on pulmonary and neurodevelopmental outcomes of bronchopulmonary dysplasia. *Semin. Perinatol.* **2018**, *42*, 478–484. [CrossRef]
29. Moschino, L.; Bonadies, L.; Baraldi, E. Lung growth and pulmonary function after prematurity and bronchopulmonary dysplasia. *Pediatr. Pulmonol.* **2021**, *56*, 3499–3508. [CrossRef]
30. Ronkainen, E.; Dunder, T.; Peltoniemi, O.; Kaukola, T.; Marttila, R.; Hallman, M. New BPD predicts lung function at school age: Follow-up study and meta-analysis. *Pediatr. Pulmonol.* **2015**, *50*, 1090–1098. [CrossRef]
31. Fortuna, M.; Carraro, S.; Temporin, E.; Berardi, M.; Zanconato, S.; Salvadori, S.; Lago, P.; Frigo, A.C.; Filippone, M.; Baraldi, E. Mid-childhood lung function in a cohort of children with "new bronchopulmonary dysplasia". *Pediatr. Pulmonol.* **2016**, *51*, 1057–1064. [CrossRef] [PubMed]
32. Simpson, S.J.; Logie, K.M.; O'Dea, C.A.; Banton, G.L.; Murray, C.; Wilson, A.C.; Pillow, J.J.; Hall, G.L. Altered lung structure and function in mid-childhood survivors of very preterm birth. *Thorax* **2017**, *72*, 702–711. [CrossRef] [PubMed]
33. Thunqvist, P.; Tufvesson, E.; Bjermer, L.; Winberg, A.; Fellman, V.; Domellöf, M.; Melén, E.; Norman, M.; Hallberg, J. Lung function after extremely preterm birth-A population-based cohort study (EXPRESS). *PediatrPulmonol* **2018**, *53*, 64–72. [CrossRef] [PubMed]
34. Simpson, S.J.; Turkovic, L.; Wilson, A.C.; Verheggen, M.; Logie, K.M.; Pillow, J.J.; Hall, G.L. Lung function trajectories throughout childhood in survivors of very preterm birth: A longitudinal cohort study. *Lancet. Child. Adolesc. Health* **2018**, *2*, 350–359. [CrossRef] [PubMed]
35. Cardoen, F.; Vermeulen, F.; Proesmans, M.; Moens, M.; De Boeck, K. Lung function evolution in children with old and new type bronchopulmonary dysplasia: A retrospective cohort analysis. *Eur. J. Pediatr.* **2019**, *178*, 1859–1866. [CrossRef] [PubMed]
36. Levin, J.C.; Sheils, C.A.; Gaffin, J.M.; Hersh, C.P.; Rhein, L.M.; Hayden, L.P. Lung function trajectories in children with post-prematurity respiratory disease: Identifying risk factors for abnormal growth. *Respir. Res.* **2021**, *22*, 143. [CrossRef]
37. Agusti, A.; Faner, R. Lung function trajectories in health and disease. *Lancet. Respir. Med.* **2019**, *7*, 358–364. [CrossRef]
38. Bush, A. Lung development and aging. *Ann. Am. Thorac. Soc.* **2016**, *13* (Suppl. S5), S438–S446. [CrossRef]
39. Doyle, L.W.; Andersson, S.; Bush, A.; Cheong, J.L.Y.; Clemm, H.; Evensen, K.A.I.; Gough, A.; Halvorsen, T.; Hovi, P.; Kajantie, E.; et al. Expiratory airflow in late adolescence and early adulthood in individuals born very preterm or with very low birthweight compared with controls born at term or with normal birthweight: A meta-analysis of individual participant data. *Lancet Respir. Med.* **2019**, *7*, 677–686. [CrossRef]
40. Doyle, L.W.; Irving, L.; Haikerwal, A.; Lee, K.; Ranganathan, S.; Cheong, J. Airway obstruction in young adults born extremely preterm or extremely low birth weight in the postsurfactant era. *Thorax* **2019**, *74*, 1147–1153. [CrossRef]
41. Bårdsen, T.; Røksund, O.D.; Benestad, M.R.; Hufthammer, K.O.; Clemm, H.H.; Mikalsen, I.B.; Øymar, K.; Markestad, T.; Halvorsen, T.; Vollsæter, M. Tracking of lung function from 10 to 35 years after being born extremely preterm or with extremely low birth weight. *Thorax* **2022**, *77*, 790–798. [CrossRef]
42. Pérez-Tarazona, S.; Rueda Esteban, S.; García-García, M.L.; Arroyas Sanchez, M.; de Mir Messa, I.; Acevedo Valarezo, T.; Mesa Medina, O.; Callejón Callejón, A.; Canino Calderín, E.M.; Albi Rodriguez, S.; et al. Respiratory outcomes of "new" bronchopulmonary dysplasia in adolescents: A multicenter study. *Pediatr. Pulmonol.* **2021**, *56*, 1205–1214. [CrossRef] [PubMed]
43. Um-Bergström, P.; Hallberg, J.; Thunqvist, P.; Berggren-Broström, E.; Anderson, M.; Adenfelt, G.; Lilja, G.; Ferrara, G.; Sköld, C.M.; Melén, E. Lung function development after preterm birth in relation to severity of Bronchopulmonary dysplasia. *BMC Pulm. Med.* **2017**, *17*, 97. [CrossRef]
44. Harris, C.; Morris, S.; Lunt, A.; Peacock, J.; Greenough, A. Influence of bronchopulmonary dysplasia on lung function in adolescents who were born extremely prematurely. *Pediatr. Pulmonol.* **2022**, *57*, 3151–3157. [CrossRef] [PubMed]
45. Hurst, J.R.; Beckmann, J.; Ni, Y.; Bolton, C.E.; McEniery, C.M.; Cockcroft, J.R.; Marlow, N. Respiratory and cardiovascular outcomes in survivors of extremely preterm birth at 19 years. *Am. J. Respir. Crit. Care. Med.* **2020**, *202*, 422–432. [CrossRef] [PubMed]
46. McGrath-Morrow, S.A.; Collaco, J.M. Bronchopulmonary dysplasia: What are its links to COPD? *Ther. Adv. Respir. Dis.* **2019**, *13*, 1753466619892492. [CrossRef]
47. Satrell, E.; Clemm, H.; Røksund, O.D.; Hufthammer, K.O.; Thorsen, E.; Halvorsen, T.; Vollsæter, M. Development of lung diffusion to adulthood following extremely preterm birth. *Eur. Respir. J.* **2022**, *59*, 2004103. [CrossRef]
48. Bui, D.S.; Perret, J.L.; Walters, E.H.; Lodge, C.J.; Bowatte, G.; Hamilton, G.S.; Thompson, B.R.; Frith, P.; Erbas, B.; Thomas, P.S.; et al. Association between very to moderate preterm births, lung function deficits, and COPD at age 53 years: Analysis of a prospective cohort study. *Lancet. Respir. Med.* **2022**, *10*, 478–484. [CrossRef]
49. GOLD. Global Strategy for the Diagnosis, Management, and Prevention of Chronic Obstructive Pulmonary Disease: 2020 Report Published in Fontana, WI, USA. 2020. Available online: www.goldcopd.org (accessed on 15 May 2023).
50. Vollsæter, M.; Skromme, K.; Satrell, E.; Clemm, H.; Røksund, O.; Øymar, K.; Markestad, T.; Halvorsen, T. Children Born Preterm at the Turn of the Millennium Had Better Lung Function Than Children Born Similarly Preterm in the Early 1990s. *PLoS ONE* **2015**, *10*, e0144243. [CrossRef]
51. Doyle, L.W.; Carse, E.; Adams, A.M.; Ranganathan, S.; Opie, G.; Cheong, J.L.Y.; Victorian Infant Collaborative Study Group. Ventilation in extremely preterm infants and respiratory function at 8 years. *N. Engl. J. Med.* **2017**, *377*, 329–337. [CrossRef]
52. Lignelli, E.; Palumbo, F.; Myti, D.; Morty, R.E. Recent advances in our understanding of the mechanisms of lung alveolarization and bronchopulmonary dysplasia. *Am. J. Physiol. Cell. Mol. Physiol.* **2019**, *317*, L832–L887. [CrossRef] [PubMed]

53. Narayanan, M.; Owers-Bradley, J.; Beardsmore, C.S.; Mada, M.; Ball, I.; Garipov, R.; Panesar, K.S.; Kuehni, C.E.; Spycher, B.D.; Williams, S.E.; et al. Alveolarization continues during childhood and adolescence: New evidence from helium-3 magnetic resonance. *Am. J. Respir. Crit. Care. Med.* **2012**, *185*, 186–191. [CrossRef] [PubMed]
54. Butler, J.P.; Loring, S.H.; Patz, S.; Tsuda, A.; Yablonskiy, D.A.; Mentzer, S.J. Evidence for adult lung growth in humans. *N. Engl. J. Med.* **2012**, *367*, 244–247. [CrossRef] [PubMed]
55. Poindexter, B.B.; Martin, C.R. Impact of Nutrition on Bronchopulmonary Dysplasia. *Clin. Perinatol.* **2015**, *42*, 797–806. [CrossRef]
56. Hwang, J.S.; Rehan, V.K. Recent Advances in Bronchopulmonary Dysplasia: Pathophysiology, Prevention, and Treatment. *Lung* **2018**, *196*, 129–138. [CrossRef]
57. Soudée, S.; Vuillemin, L.; Alberti, C.; Mohamed, D.; Becquet, O.; Farnoux, C.; Biran, V.; Baud, O. Fetal Growth Restriction Is Worse than Extreme Prematurity for the Developing Lung. *Neonatology* **2014**, *106*, 304–310. [CrossRef]
58. Rocha, G.; De Lima, F.F.; Machado, A.P.; Guimarães, H.; Proença, E.; Carvalho, C.; Martins, L.G.; Martins, T.; Freitas, A.; Dias, C.P.; et al. Small for gestational age very preterm infants present a higher risk of developing bronchopulmonary dysplasia. *J. Neonatal-Perinat. Med.* **2019**, *12*, 419–427. [CrossRef]
59. Groh-Wargo, S.; Sapsford, A. Enteral Nutrition Support of the Preterm Infant in the Neonatal Intensive Care Unit. *Nutr. Clin. Pract.* **2009**, *24*, 363–376. [CrossRef]
60. Milanesi, B.G.; Lima, P.A.; Villela, L.D.; Martins, A.S.; Gomes-Junior, S.C.S.; Moreira, M.E.L.; Méio, M.D.B.B. Assessment of early nutritional intake in preterm infants with bronchopulmonary dysplasia: A cohort study. *Eur. J. Nucl. Med. Mol. Imaging* **2021**, *180*, 1423–1430. [CrossRef]
61. Uberos, J.; Jimenez-Montilla, S.; Molina-Oya, M.; García-Serrano, J.L. Early energy restriction in premature infants and bronchopulmonary dysplasia: A cohort study. *Br. J. Nutr.* **2020**, *123*, 1024–1031. [CrossRef]
62. Al-Jebawi, Y.; Agarwal, N.; Groh Wargo, S.; Shekhawat, P.; Mhanna, M.J. Low caloric intake and high fluid intake during the first week of life are associated with the severity of bronchopulmonary dysplasia in extremely low birth weight infants. *J. Neonatal-Perinat. Med.* **2020**, *13*, 207–214. [CrossRef]
63. Natarajan, G.; Johnson, Y.R.; Brozanski, B.; Farrow, K.N.; Zaniletti, I.; Padula, M.A.; Asselin, J.M.; Durand, D.J.; Short, B.L.; Pallotto, E.K.; et al. Postnatal Weight Gain in Preterm Infants with Severe Bronchopulmonary Dysplasia. *Am. J. Perinatol.* **2013**, *31*, 223–230. [CrossRef] [PubMed]
64. Malikiwi, A.I.; Lee, Y.-M.; Davies-Tuck, M.; Wong, F.Y. Postnatal nutritional deficit is an independent predictor of bronchopulmonary dysplasia among extremely premature infants born at or less than 28 weeks gestation. *Early Hum. Dev.* **2019**, *131*, 29–35. [CrossRef]
65. Groothuis, J.R.; Makari, D. Definition and outpatient management of the very low-birth-weight infant with bronchopulmonary dysplasia. *Adv. Ther.* **2012**, *29*, 297–311. [CrossRef] [PubMed]
66. McLeod, G.; Simmer, K.; Benninger, H.; Mitoulas, L.; Doherty, D.; Sherriff, J. Preterm infants with chronic lung disease: Are protein and energy intakes after discharge sufficient for optimal growth? *J. Paediatr. ChildHealth.* **2011**, *47*, 127–133. [CrossRef]
67. Bertino, E.; Coscia, A.; Boni, L.; Rossi, C.; Martano, C.; Giuliani, F.; Fabris, C.; Spada, E.; Zolin, A.; Milani, S. Weight growth velocity of very low birth weight infants: Role of gender, gestational age and major morbidities. *Early Hum. Dev.* **2009**, *85*, 339–447. [CrossRef]
68. Lehtinen, A.; Korhonen, P.; Hyödynmaa, E.; Koivisto, A.M.; Peltola, T.; Hämäläinen, M.; Moilanen, E.; Tammela, O. Adipokines played a limited role in predicting temporary growth differences between very low birthweight infants with and without bronchopulmonary dysplasia. *Acta Paediatr.* **2017**, *106*, 1583–1588. [CrossRef]
69. Bott, L.; Béghin, L.; Devos, P.; Pierrat, V.; Matran, R.; Gottrand, F. Nutritional Status at 2 Years in Former Infants with Bronchopulmonary Dysplasia Influences Nutrition and Pulmonary Outcomes During Childhood. *Pediatr. Res.* **2006**, *60*, 340–343. [CrossRef]
70. Lemons, J.A.; Bauer, C.R.; Oh, W.; Korones, S.B.; Papile, L.A.; Stoll, B.J.; Verter, J.; Temprosa, M.; Wright, L.L.; Ehrenkranz, R.A.; et al. Very low birth weight outcomes of the National Institute of Child health and human development neonatal research network, January 1995 through December 1996. NICHD Neonatal Research Network. *Pediatrics* **2001**, *107*, E1. [CrossRef]
71. Ziegler, E.E.; Thureen, P.J.; Carlson, S.J. Aggressive nutrition of the very low birthweight infant. *Clin. Perinatol.* **2002**, *29*, 225–244. [CrossRef] [PubMed]
72. Greenbury, S.F.; Angelini, E.D.; Ougham, K.; Battersby, C.; Gale, C.; Uthaya, S.; Modi, N. Birthweight and patterns of postnatal weight gain in very and extremely preterm babies in England and Wales, 2008–19: A cohort study. *Lancet Child. Adolesc. Health.* **2021**, *5*, 719–728. [CrossRef] [PubMed]
73. Embleton, N.D.; Moltu, S.J.; Lapillonne, A.; van den Akker, C.H.P.; Carnielli, V.; Fusch, C.; Gerasimidis, K.; van Goudoever, J.B.; Haiden, N.; Iacobelli, S.; et al. Enteral Nutrition in Preterm Infants (2022): A Position Paper From the ESPGHAN Committee on Nutrition and Invited Experts. *J. Pediatr. Gastroenterol. Nutr.* **2023**, *76*, 248–268. [CrossRef] [PubMed]
74. Toftlund, L.H.; Agertoft, L.; Halken, S.; Zachariassen, G. Improved lung function at age 6 in children born very preterm and fed extra protein post-discharge. *Pediatr. Allergy Immunol.* **2019**, *30*, 47–54. [CrossRef] [PubMed]
75. Zachariassen, G.; Faerk, J.; Esberg, B.H.; Fenger-Gron, J.; Mortensen, S.; Christesen, H.T.; Halken, S. Allergic diseases among very preterm infants according to nutrition after hospital discharge. *Pediatr. Allergy Immunol.* **2011**, *22*, 515–520. [CrossRef] [PubMed]

76. Kim, L.Y.; McGrath-Morrow, S.A.; Collaco, J.M. Impact of breast milk on respiratory outcomes in infants with bronchopulmonary dysplasia. *Pediatr. Pulmonol.* **2019**, *54*, 313–318. [CrossRef]
77. Bauer, S.E.; Vanderpool, C.P.B.; Ren, C.; Cristea, A.I. Nutrition and growth in infants with established bronchopulmonary dysplasia. *Pediatr. Pulmonol.* **2021**, *56*, 3557–3562. [CrossRef]

nutrients

MDPI

Article

Breastfeeding in Neonates Admitted to an NICU: 18-Month Follow-Up

Rozeta Sokou [1,2,*], Stavroula Parastatidou [1], Georgios Ioakeimidis [1], Evangelia-Filothei Tavoulari [1], Athanasia Makrogianni [1], Elina Isaakidou [1], Nicoletta Iacovidou [2] and Aikaterini Konstantinidi [1]

1 Neonatal Intensive Care Unit, "Agios Panteleimon" General Hospital of Nikea, 3 D. Mantouvalou Str., Nikea, 18454 Piraeus, Greece
2 Neonatal Department, Aretaieio Hospital, School of Medicine, National and Kapodistrian University of Athens, 11528 Athens, Greece
* Correspondence: sokourozeta@yahoo.gr; Tel.: +30-2132077346 or +30-2132077000

Abstract: Introduction: The admission of neonates to Neonatal Intensive Care Units (NICUs) has been identified as a primary inhibiting factor in the establishment of breastfeeding. The aims of this study were to (1) estimate the prevalence and duration of breastfeeding in infants/toddlers who had been admitted to an NICU in Greece and (2) to investigate factors, associated with the NICU stay, which affected the establishment and maintenance of breastfeeding in infants/toddlers previously admitted to the NICU. Materials and methods: Data for this cohort study were retrieved from interviews with mothers of infants/toddlers who had been admitted to our NICU as neonates during the period of 2017–2019. Interviews were conducted based on a questionnaire regarding the child's nutrition from birth to the day of the interview, including previous maternal experience with breastfeeding. Information related to the prenatal period, gestation age, delivery mode, duration of NICU stay, and neonatal feeding strategies during their hospital stay were recorded. Results: The response rate to the telephone interviews was 57%, resulting in 279 mother–infant pairs being included in this study. The results showed that 78.1% of children received maternal milk during their first days of life. Of all infants, 58.1% were exclusively breastfed during their first month, with a gradual decrease to 36.9% and 19.4% by the end of the third and sixth months of life, respectively. The prevalence of breastfed children reached 14.7% and 7.5% at the ages of twelve and eighteen months, respectively. In the multivariate analysis, prematurity emerged as an independent prognostic factor for the duration of exclusive and any breastfeeding (aHR 1.64, 95% CI: 1.03–2.62; and 1.69, 95% CI: 1.05–2.72, respectively; $p < 0.05$). Additionally, the nationality of the mother, NICU breastfeeding experience, the administration of maternal milk during neonatal hospital stay, and previous breastfeeding experience of the mother were independent prognostic factors for the duration of breastfeeding. Conclusions: Although breastfeeding is a top priority in our NICU, the exclusive-breastfeeding rates at 6 months were quite low for the hospitalized neonates, not reaching World Health Organization (WHO) recommendations. Mothers/families of hospitalized neonates should receive integrated psychological and practical breastfeeding support and guidance.

Keywords: breastfeeding; neonates; preterm neonates; breastfeeding support; lactation; hospitalized neonates

1. Introduction

For optimal health outcomes, the World Health Organization recommends exclusive breastfeeding for the first 6 months of life, followed by the appropriate introduction of complementary foods with continued breastfeeding to two years and beyond [1–3].

Multiple recent publications report the short-term and long-term advantages of maternal milk for preterm neonates. Maternal milk contains the optimal immunologic, antioxidative, and growth factors for various neonatal systems [4].

Feeding with human milk (HM) from the neonate's own mother reduces the risk for short-term and long-term morbidity and, subsequently, the cost of care of ill preterm and full-term neonates [5]. Regarding preterm neonates, higher HM doses are correlated with a lower risk of enteral feeding intolerance, late sepsis, chronic pulmonary disease, retinopathy of prematurity, neurocognitive impairment, and less hospital re-admissions by the ages of 18–30 months [6–16].

Almost 10–12% of neonates born in the United States are preterm, and admission to NICUs is necessary for many of them [17]. Approximately 10% of full-term neonates require more-advanced-than-usual medical care, and a large proportion of them is also admitted to NICUs. Hospitalized neonates represent a population with a higher risk of adverse short-term and long-term outcomes than healthy full-term neonates [18–20]. Admission to NICU has been suggested as a primary inhibiting factor in establishing breastfeeding, with neonates admitted to NICUs presenting lower rates of breastfeeding than healthy neonates [21–25]. Probable causes of this phenomenon include the separation of the mother and the neonate; the stress and anxiety of the mother, which may result in depressive disorder; and the clinical status of the mother and/or the neonate [26–29]. Until now, in Greece, the direct impact of postnatal mother–neonate separation in establishing and maintaining breastfeeding in neonates admitted to NICUs is largely unknown and needs to be further investigated.

The aims of this study were to (1) assess the prevalence and duration of breastfeeding in infants/toddlers who had been admitted to a Greek NICU and (2) to assess the probable effect of certain factors associated with the NICU stay on the rate, establishment, and duration of breastfeeding in infants/toddlers previously admitted to the NICU.

2. Materials and Methods

Data for this retrospective study were collected from interviews with mothers of infants/toddlers who were admitted to our NICU as neonates during 2017–2019. This research study followed the STROBE checklist (Supplementary Table S1).

2.1. Definitions

Exclusive Breastfeeding (EBF): The Infant Only Receives Maternal Milk and No Other Liquids, with the Exception of Vitamins, Rehydration Solutions, Minerals, and Medicines

The vast majority of neonates hospitalized in NICUs receive parenteral nutrition during the first days of life. In this study, the breastfeeding status was assessed following the achievement of full enteral feeding. Maternal milk during NICU stay was fortified in very-low-birthweight neonates; however, these neonates were included in the exclusively breastfed group if they had not received any formula milk.

Any Breastfeeding (BF): Breastfeeding, Either Exclusive or Partial Breastfeeding, Supplemented with Formula Milk or Other Foods.

2.2. Breastfeeding Support and Promotion in NICU

The NICU of General Hospital "Agios Panteleimon" is a perinatal center of the 2nd Health District, which includes West Attica areas and the Aegean Sea islands. A high percentage of the neonates admitted to our NICU are transferred from remote areas, with a significant impact on breastfeeding availability and establishment in this population. Maternal milk is valuable for the care/treatment provided in an NICU; therefore, the establishment of breastfeeding in hospitalized neonates is a primary target of our NICU. With all neonatal admissions, as soon as possible following birth, parents are informed by appropriately educated personnel on the advantages of breastfeeding, on ways to maintain lactation, and on the storage and transfer conditions of maternal milk. Relevant information materials with detailed instructions are handed out to the parents upon the admission of their neonate. When the maternal–neonatal state allows it, skin-to-skin contact is recommended and encouraged (twice daily for at least thirty minutes). All mothers are educated and supported to breastfeed throughout the day, provided this is permitted by the neonatal state, safely and successfully, under the supervision of experienced personnel.

2.3. Inclusion Criteria

All neonates born during the time period from January 2017 until December 2019 who were admitted to our NICU were included in this study.

2.4. Exclusion Criteria

Neonates of families residing in refugee camps were excluded from the study due to difficulties in communication (in the Greek or English language) with the mother/father and problems with the completion of the questionnaire.

Neonates with congenital anomalies directly affecting enteral feeding, neonates for whom breastfeeding was absolutely contraindicated, and all the neonates who died in the NICU were excluded from the study.

2.5. Measurement

A structured questionnaire was created in order to retrieve data with regards to the nutrition of the child from birth to the interview, as well as maternal breastfeeding experience previous to this child. The percentage of breastfed infants, the percentage of exclusively breastfed infants, and the percentage of infants who were still breastfed at three, six, nine, twelve, and >eighteen months of age were documented. Furthermore, data regarding demographic characteristics of the mothers, previous breastfeeding experience, the timing of solid foods introduction, and breastfeeding experience during the NICU stay of the neonate were recorded (questionnaire data are presented in detail in the Supplementary Materials). Information on the prenatal period, gestation length, delivery mode, the duration of hospital stay, and the feeding of the neonates during their hospital stay was retrieved from medical records.

2.6. Questionnaire Design

The questionnaire was designed to allow us to estimate the basic breastfeeding frequency indexes suggested by the WHO [2].

The questionnaire was pilot-tested in 21 mothers to determine the time needed for completion, the degree of participant comprehension, and the sequence of questions. Subsequently, the questionnaire was revised based on pilot testing.

2.7. Interview

Contact details were retrieved through the medical files from the admission of neonates to the NICU. The study primarily included data from interviews with mothers. In case the mother did not speak Greek, the father could answer the interview questions in the presence of the mother. A telephone interview was conducted when the study infants were older than twelve months (March 2021–May 2021). The interview duration was approximately six to ten minutes.

The study was conducted according to the guidelines of the Declaration of Helsinki and was approved by the Institutional Review Board of Nikeaia General Hospital "Agios Panteleimon" (3/11, 22 January 2020). The interview was conducted following the verbal consent of the parent. Recruitment data are presented in a flow diagram (Figure 1).

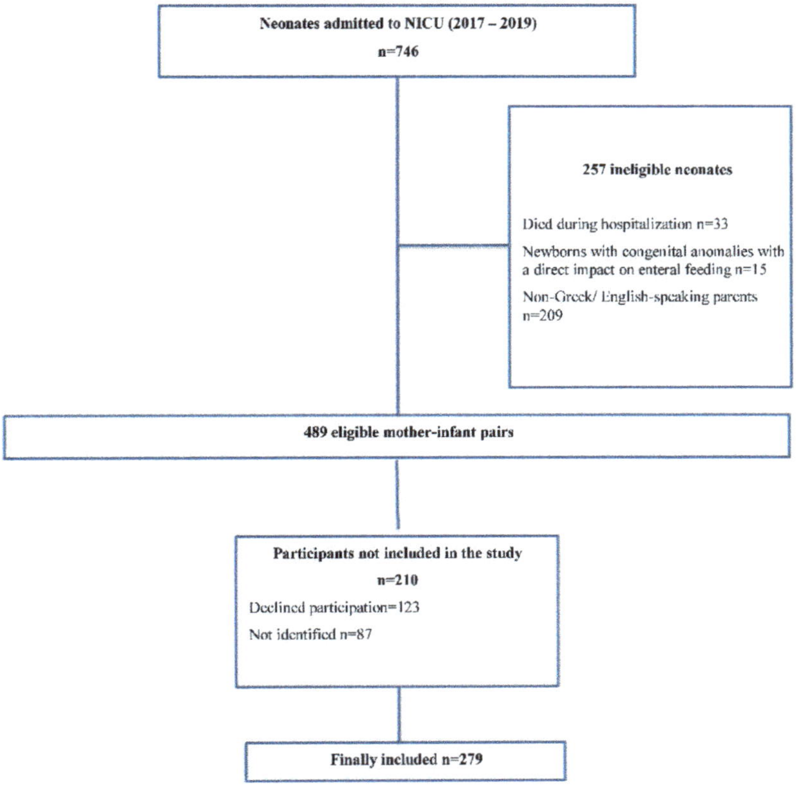

Figure 1. Flow chart of the study population.

2.8. Statistical Analysis

Before comparing the independent groups, data distribution was examined for the determination of the most appropriate analysis. Initially, data were visually assessed by comparing their histograms with the normal probability curve; then, the Kolmogorov–Smirnov test for normality was performed. Both assessments demonstrated that the data were not normally distributed. For the descriptive statistics of quantitative variables, median values and interquartile range were used. Absolute (N) and relative (%) frequencies were used to describe qualitative variables. The non-parametric Mann–Whitney U test was applied for the comparison of the quantitative variables (which were non-normally distributed) between two groups. For the comparison among more than two groups, the non-parametric Kruskal–Wallis criterion was used. The duration of breastfeeding was assessed using the Kaplan–Meier survival estimator, with the cessation of exclusive and any breastfeeding being considered as the final events for the analysis. Infants who were breastfed at the end of the study period were labeled as censored. The duration of breastfeeding was defined as the number of months until the cessation of breastfeeding or from birth until the final date of follow-up. A Cox proportional hazards regression analysis was applied for the investigation of the simultaneous effect of several risk factors on the duration of breastfeeding. Covariate effects were considered using hazard ratios (HRs) and their 95% confidence intervals. A significance level of 0.05 was set (two-tailed significance levels). The SPSS 22.0 statistical program (IBM SPSS Statistics for Windows, Version 22.0. Armonk, NY, USA: IBM Corp.) was used for the statistical analyses.

3. Results

3.1. Descriptive Results

The response rate to the telephone interviews was 57%, resulting in 279 mother–infant pairs being included in this study. A total of 255 mothers responded, 24 of whom had given birth to twins. Of all participating neonates, 56.3% were full-term, and 66.3% had been delivered via cesarean section; in total, 31.5% were inborn, while 68.5% were outborn. The median birthweight of our sample of infants was 2.700 g (1.960–3.250 g), and the median gestational age was 37 (34–38) weeks. Of the participating neonates, 25 (9%) were very-low-birthweight neonates; a total of 43 (15.4%) had a gestational age < 32 weeks, and 79 neonates (28.3%) were late preterm. A total of 21 neonates (7.5%) presented intrauterine growth restriction (IUGR), and 137 neonates (49.1%) had respiratory distress syndrome; in total, 67 neonates (24%) suffered from perinatal hypoxia, and 12 (4.3%) neonates were admitted for surgical purposes. Forty-two (15%) of the admitted neonates presented early-onset sepsis. Most of the participating mothers were Greek (72.4%), followed by Albanians (17.9%). The median length of stay in the NICU was 12 (7–23) days. The median time (months) to the initiation of infant formula or solids was 1 (0–5) and 6 (5–6) respectively. Permanent residents of Attica accounted for 60.2% of our sample. Nearly half of the participants (42.7%) had previous breastfeeding experience, and only 4.7% had attended breastfeeding classes. Of the participating mothers, 144 (51.6%) were primigravidae, while 135 were multigravidae. Among the multigravid mothers, 119 (88.1%) had breastfeeding experience with a previous child. Detailed demographic characteristics' data are presented in Table 1.

Table 1. Characteristics of the study population and median duration of any and exclusive breastfeeding (in months).

				Duration of Any Breastfeeding (Months)		Duration of Exclusive Breastfeeding (Months)	
				Median (IQR)	***p*-Value**	**Median (IQR)**	***p*-Value**
GA (weeks)		37	34–38	2 (1–6)		1 (0–5)	
BW (g)		2.700	1.960–3.250				
Nationality, N and %	Greek	202	72.4%	2 (0–60	0.001	1 (0–4)	0.008
	Albanian	50	17.9%	4.5 (1–12)		2.5 (0–6)	
	Other Balkan nationality *	8	2.9%	4 (1.25–21)		2 (0–5)	
	Indian	5	1.8%	9 (6–19)		5 (1.5–6)	
	Arab	7	5%	12 (0–120		6 (0–12)	
Permanent Residence, N and %	Attica	168	60.2%	2 (1–6.75)	0.998	1 (0–50	0.422
	Mainland Greece	70	25.1%	2 (0.75–6)		1.5 (0–5)	
	Islands	41	14.7%	2 (1–7.5)		2 (0–5)	
Delivery mode, N %	Vaginal	94	33.7%	3 (0.75–8.25)	0.421	1.5 (0–5)	0.125
	Cesarean section	185	66.3%	2 (1–6)		1 (0–4)	
Outborn, N and %	Yes	88	31.5%	2 (0–6)	0.24	1 (0–4.75)	0.214
	No	191	68.5%	2 (0–6)		1 (0–5)	
Maternal milk in NICU, N and %	No	78	28%	0 (0–2)	0.000	0 (0–0.25)	0.000
	Yes	201	72%	4 (1–8.0)		2 (0–6)	
NICU breastfeeding, N and %	No	135	48.6%	1 (0–3)	0.000	0 (0–2)	0.000
	Yes	143	51.4%	6 (2.0–12)		3 (1–6)	

Table 1. *Cont.*

				Duration of Any Breastfeeding (Months)		Duration of Exclusive Breastfeeding (Months)	
				Median (IQR)	*p*-Value	Median (IQR)	*p*-Value
Breastfeeding classes, N and %	No	266	95.3%	2 (1–6)	0.19	1 (0.5)	0.327
	Yes	13	4.7%	3 (1–16.5)		2 (1–5)	
Older child, N and %	No	145	51.6%	2 (0.5–6)	0.116	1 (0–5)	0.197
	Yes	136	48.4%	3 (1–8)		1 (0–5)	
Previous breastfeeding experience, N and %	No	160	57.3%	2 (0–6)	0.000	1 (0–4)	0.041
	Yes	119	42.7%	4 (1–8)		2 (0–5)	

Abbreviations: GA, gestational age; BW, birthweight; IQR, interquartile range; * Bulgarian and Romanian nationalities.

3.2. Prevalence of Breastfeeding

3.2.1. Exclusive Breastfeeding

The prevalence of exclusively breastfed infants was 58.1% for the first month of life and reduced to 36.9% by the end of the third month. By the end of the sixth month, only 19.4% of the infants were exclusively breastfed, with a gradual drop during the next months to reach 2.2% by the end of the eight month.

3.2.2. Any Breastfeeding

The breastfeeding rate during the first month of life was quite high, reaching 78.1% and remaining at 47.7% until the completed third month of life. During the next months, a gradual decrease in breastfeeding prevalence was observed, reaching 32.6% by the end of the sixth month. The percentages of breastfed infants at the ages of nine, twelve, and eighteen months were 17.9%, 14.7%, and 7.5%, respectively.

A shorter duration of exclusive breastfeeding was observed for preterm neonates compared with full-term neonates, and this difference was statistically significant (p-value < 0.05). The clinical characteristics of the study neonates are presented in Table 2.

Table 2. Clinical characteristics of preterm and full-term study neonates.

	Term Neonates (N = 157)				Preterm Neonates (N = 122)				
	Mean	Median	Percentile 25	Percentile 95	Mean	Median	Percentile 25	Percentile 95	*p*-Value
GA	38	38	38	40	33	33	32	36	0.000
BW	3294	3190	2820	4000	1948	1950	1620	2850	0.000
Hospital stay (days)	11	8	6	32	32	21	14	115	0.000
Duration of any breastfeeding (months)	6	3	1	25	3	2	0	12	0.000
Duration of exclusive breastfeeding (months)	3	2	0	6	2	1	0	6	0.002

Abbreviations: GA, gestational age; BW, birthweight.

The data from the Kaplan–Meier survival analysis of breastfed preterm and full-term neonates are presented in Table 3.

Table 3. Data on breastfeeding preterm and full-term neonates.

Means and Medians for Survival Time—Breastfeeding Duration (Months)									
Neonates	**Mean**				**Median**				***p*-Value**
	Estimate	Std. Error	95% Confidence Interval Lower Bound	95% Confidence Interval Upper Bound	Estimate	Std. Error	95% Confidence Interval Lower Bound	95% Confidence Interval Upper Bound	
Full-term neonates	6.875	0.703	5.497	8.253	3	0.597	1.831	4.169	0.00
Preterm neonates	3.416	0.44	2.553	4.279	2	0.22	1.569	2.431	
Overall	5.35	0.45	4.468	6.233	2	0.283	1.446	2.554	
Means and Medians for Survival Time—Exclusive-Breastfeeding Duration (Months)									
Full-term neonates	2.99	0.232	2.534	3.445	3	0.641	1.743	4.257	0.002
Preterm neonates	1.75	0.203	1.352	2.148	1	.	.	.	
Overall	2.441	0.162	2.124	2.758	1	0.277	0.457	1.543	

The rates of exclusive breastfeeding and any breastfeeding at selected ages are provided in detail in Figures 2 and 3 for preterm and full-term groups.

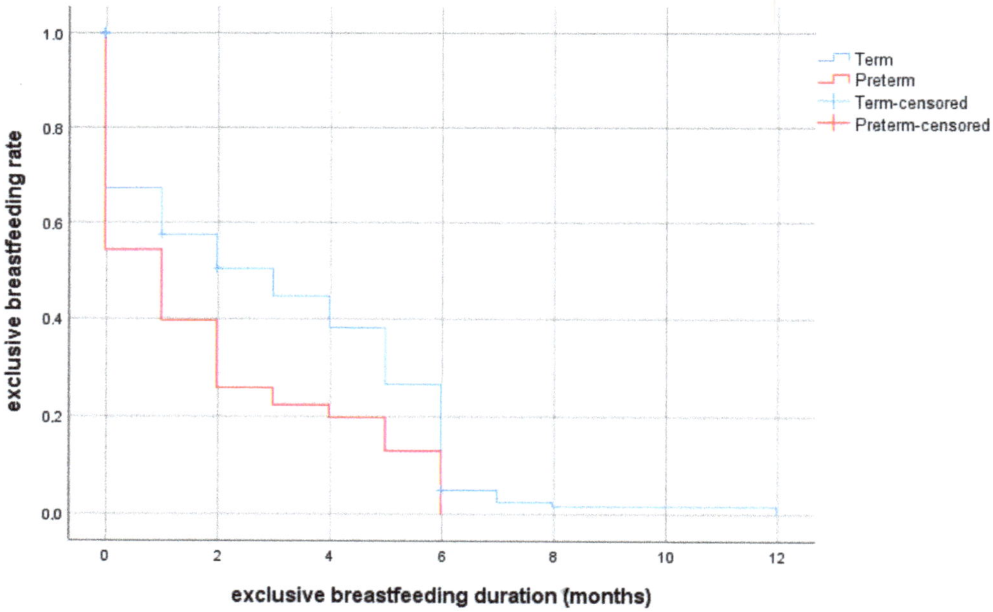

Figure 2. Probability of exclusive breastfeeding depending on duration (months, discrete survival curves) according to prematurity.

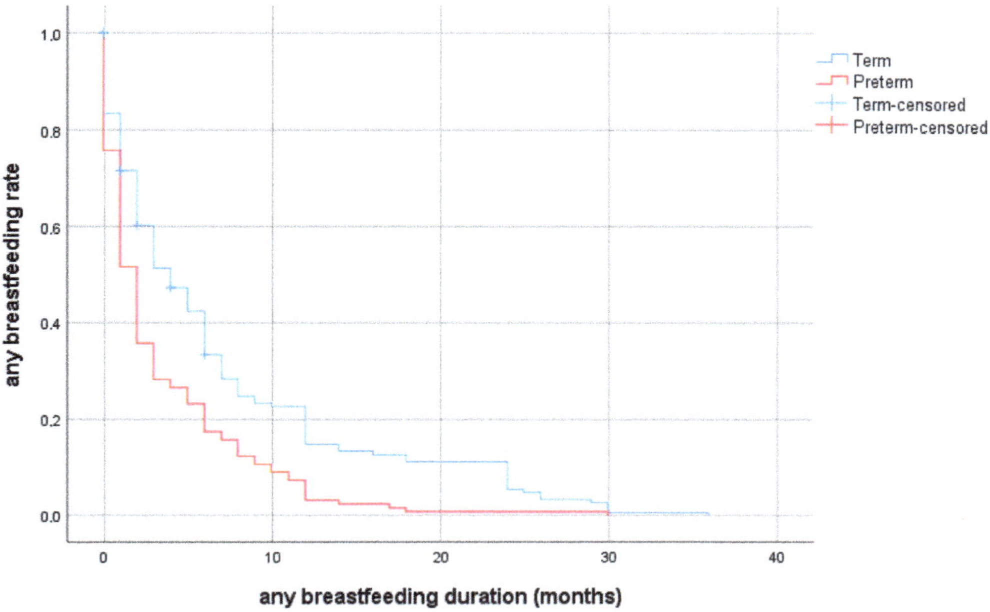

Figure 3. Probability of any breastfeeding depending on duration (months, discrete survival curves) according to prematurity.

The statistical analyses (Table 1) indicated that neonates of Greek-origin mothers had significantly shorter breastfeeding duration than neonates of mothers of other nationalities. Neonates who had received maternal milk during their NICU stay or had been breastfed in the NICU and those whose mothers had previous breastfeeding experience or had attended breastfeeding classes had been breastfed for significantly longer than the remaining neonates. The delivery mode (cesarean section) and transportation of the neonate affected the duration of breastfeeding, as a shorter duration of exclusive and any breastfeeding was observed in these neonates, but not at a statistically significant degree ($p > 0.05$). A multivariable analysis was conducted to investigate the impact of various factors on the duration of exclusive and any breastfeeding. The duration (in months) of exclusive breastfeeding and the duration of any breastfeeding were the dependent variables, while gestational age, delivery mode, nationality (categorized as Greek and other), inborn/outborn, permanent residence, prematurity, hospital stay, previous breastfeeding experience, feeding with maternal milk during hospital stay, breastfeeding experience in the NICU, and maternal attendance of breastfeeding classes were the independent variables. The multivariable analysis indicated prematurity as an independent prognostic factor for the duration of exclusive and any breastfeeding, with preterm neonates presenting a higher hazard ratio of earlier breastfeeding cessation than full-term neonates (aHR 1.64, 95% CI:1.026–2.62; and 1.69, 95% CI:1.054–2.72, respectively; $p < 0.05$). Furthermore, NICU breastfeeding experience, maternal-milk administration during hospital stay, and previous breastfeeding experience were positively and strongly correlated with breastfeeding duration, as a lower hazard ratio of breastfeeding discontinuation was noted ($p < 0.05$). The attendance of breastfeeding classes by the mother was an independent prognostic factor strongly associated with the duration of breastfeeding (aHR 0.41, 95% CI: 0.218–0.77; $p = 0.006$) but did not seem to affect the duration of exclusive breastfeeding (aHR 0.76, 95% CI: 0.424–1.375; $p = 0.37$). The multivariable analysis did not reveal any statistically significant effect on the duration of exclusive or any breastfeeding for the remaining factors under investigation (Tables 4 and 5).

Table 4. Prognostic factors associated with duration of exclusive breastfeeding (Cox proportional hazards regression analysis, N = 279).

Variable in the Equation	Duration of Exclusive Breastfeeding					
	B	SE	*p*-Value	aHR	95.0% CI	
					Lower	Upper
Preterm	0.494	0.239	0.04	1.64	1.026	2.62
Hospital stay (days)	0.003	0.003	0.32	1.00	0.997	1.01
Previous breastfeeding experience	−0.192	0.08	0.02	0.83	0.705	0.97
Maternal milk in NICU	−0.485	0.191	0.01	0.62	0.424	0.90
Breastfeeding in NICU	−0.429	0.171	0.01	0.65	0.466	0.91
Breastfeeding classes	−0.27	0.3	0.37	0.76	0.424	1.375
Gravida (<I)	0.253	0.225	0.26	1.29	0.829	2.001
GA (weeks)	0.064	0.047	0.18	1.07	0.972	1.169
BW (g)	0.00	0.00	1.00	1.00	1	1
Nationality (non-Greek)	−0.343	0.161	0.03	0.71	0.518	0.973
Permanent residence (Attica)	−0.069	0.09	0.44	0.93	0.782	1.112
Delivery mode (caesarian section)	0.098	0.141	0.49	1.10	0.837	1.453

Abbreviations: B, beta coefficient; CI, confidence interval; SE, standard error; aHR, adjusted hazard ratio; GA, gestational age; BW, birthweight.

Table 5. Prognostic factors associated with duration of any breastfeeding (Cox proportional hazards regression analysis, N = 279).

Variable	Breastfeeding Duration					
	B	SE	*p*-Value	aHR	95.0% CI	
					Lower	Upper
Preterm	0.527	0.242	0.03	1.694	1.054	2.722
Hospital stay (days)	0.003	0.003	0.425	1.003	0.996	1.009
Previous breastfeeding experience	−0.228	0.088	0.009	0.796	0.67	0.945
Maternal milk in NICU	−0.753	0.198	0.000	0.471	0.319	0.694
Breastfeeding in NICU	−0.58	0.173	0.001	0.56	0.399	0.785
Breastfeeding classes	−0.893	0.322	0.006	0.41	0.218	0.77
Gravida (<I)	0.088	0.244	0.718	1.092	0.677	1.763
GA (weeks)	0.042	0.048	0.385	1.042	0.949	1.145
BW (gr)	0.00	0.00	0.495	1	1	1
Nationality (non-Greek)	−0.457	0.16	0.004	0.633	0.463	0.866
Permanent residence (Attica)	−0.028	0.092	0.763	0.973	0.813	1.164
Delivery mode (cesarean section)	0.28	0.145	0.053	1.324	0.997	1.757

Abbreviations: B, beta coefficient; CI, confidence interval; SE, standard error; aHR, adjusted hazard ratio; GA, gestational age; BW, birthweight.

4. Discussion

Breastfeeding practices in Greece have not been thoroughly investigated. This study assesses breastfeeding status in a Greek NICU, contributing to the recognition of factors that affect the prevalence, establishment, and maintenance of breastfeeding in neonates admitted to the NICU. The percentage of exclusive breastfeeding at the first and sixth months of age in our study was lower than that recommended by the WHO [2] and CDC [30]. This was consistent with findings of previous studies [22,31,32]. The exclusive-breastfeeding rates in our study infants were similar to the respective rates of the general Greek population [31,32]. Maternal nationality, breastfeeding during NICU stay, maternal-milk administration during NICU stay, and maternal experience of breastfeeding older children were significantly positively correlated with the duration of breastfeeding. Prematurity, on the other hand, was inversely correlated with breastfeeding duration, which is consistent with data from other countries [5,33].

In our cohort, the prevalence of exclusively breastfed infants during the first month of life was 58.1%. Dritsakou et al. [34] recruited 161 healthy pregnant women who attended prenatal breastfeeding classes and assessed the effect of maternal diet, personal traits, and the intention to breastfeed on the breastfeeding duration of neonates admitted to a Greek NICU. The authors reported that 81% of the study neonates were exclusively breastfed at discharge.

There is published evidence that preterm neonates tend to breastfeed less and for a shorter period of time than full-term neonates [35,36], and our findings are also in accordance with this. Consistently with previous studies [33,37], prematurity emerged as an adverse factor for exclusive and any breastfeeding in our study neonates. Preterm neonates are generally transferred to the NICU immediately after birth and are separated from their mothers, which results in the late initiation of breastfeeding [38]. The lower the gestational age is, the longer the neonate's hospital stay is. Most preterm neonates below 34 weeks need to be fed via nasogastric tube due to sucking–swallowing incoordination. Neonates with respiratory distress, face anomalies, and central neural system disorders also require tube feeding, and the pumping of breast milk is necessary in these cases. The advantages of feeding preterm neonates with maternal milk, and especially colostrum, are paramount. However, and despite the significant efforts by the mothers and healthcare providers in NICUs, only around 30% of mothers giving birth to extremely low birthweight neonates manage to exclusively support the newborn with their milk during the first days of life [39,40]. The inability to ensure the required amount of milk to exclusively support the neonate is a primary aggravating factor for the psychology of the mother and may lead to the cessation of breastfeeding [41]. Medical personnel should focus on preterm and ill neonates, educating mothers to monitor daily lactation by completing a lactation diary, and intervene if needed for the optimization and promotion of breastfeeding in these neonates. The transfer of maternal milk by mothers and their families in order to feed the neonates during their NICU stay was associated with higher prevalence and duration of exclusive breastfeeding. Formula-feeding preterm neonates in the NICU was shown to affect the duration of exclusive breastfeeding following discharge [33]. In a national study in Denmark, it was observed that when mothers were allowed to visit and feed their preterm neonates in the NICU with a feeding cup or spoon, the hospital stay of these neonates was decreased. Moreover, mothers of neonates who had breastfed during their hospital stay continued breastfeeding for longer after discharge [42,43]. According to our findings, maternal-milk administration during hospital stay and breastfeeding experience in the NICU were prognostic independent variables for the duration of exclusive and any breastfeeding. Studies in multicultural societies demonstrated that refugees of any national group tended to maintain breastfeeding for longer than native mothers, even after the adjustment for socio-economic and demographic factors [44,45]. In our study population, the mother's nationality was found to be an independent confounding factor for the duration of breastfeeding, with Greek mothers ceasing breastfeeding earlier than mothers of any other nationality. Previous breastfeeding experience was positively correlated with the duration of breastfeeding. In a large study in the Netherlands [46], a similar correlation was noted, although shortly after birth, firstborn children were more likely to be breastfed. This finding may be attributed to the fact that the reasons that led to the breastfeeding of the older child still existed for the younger newborn. In addition, the mother is more confident, has already practiced breastfeeding, and may be more knowledgeable regarding its advantages. It is well established that breastfeeding classes/seminars bear multiple benefits for both the mother and the neonate, as they offer, before labor, important information on the process and advantages of breastfeeding, leading to its successful initiation and establishment [47,48]. Despite the low rate in our sample, the attendance of breastfeeding classes seemed to have a positive effect on the duration of breastfeeding.

Multiple studies have investigated risk factors for breastfeeding practices. A Lancet series in 2016 reported a wide range of historical, socioeconomical, cultural, and personal prognostic factors for breastfeeding practices [49]. There is evidence that cesarean section has a negative impact on the initiation and duration of breastfeeding, especially if it has been performed under general or spinal anesthesia [50,51]. This finding was attributed to the lower maternal prolactin levels, the post-operative pain and, particularly, to the delayed contact of the mother with the neonate. The labor mode was not associated with the duration of breastfeeding in our study. That could have been due to the fact that both preterm and full-term neonates who had been admitted to the NICU had failed to achieve the early skin-to-skin contact with their mothers and that the initiation of breastfeeding was delayed compared with healthy neonates.

Recent studies focused on the association of inhibiting neighborhood factors on the duration of breastfeeding. It was reported that the dependence on public transportation and long distance commuting to the NICU negatively affected the frequency of maternal visits and the pumping and transport of maternal milk [52,53]. A large proportion of our NICU hospitalized neonates are transferred from distant areas of the country; however, neonatal transfer and permanent residence did not seem to impact the establishment of breastfeeding in our study. This could be explained by the practices of supporting and promoting neonatal feeding with maternal milk that are applied in our NICU.

Maternal milk is the ideal nutrition for neonates and infants, protecting against infections and facilitating long-term health. Furthermore, it is a crucial element of public health, especially for preterm neonates (gestational age < 37 weeks) [54]. Breastfeeding bears immunological, nutritional, and neurodevelopmental benefits for preterm neonates. It is protective against necrotizing enterocolitis, bronchopulmonary dysplasia, and late sepsis [55–58]. Maternal-milk effects are dose-dependent. The quantity of maternal milk consumed by a neonate is inversely correlated with risk of death and necrotizing enterocolitis during the first 2 weeks of life [10]. Studies showed that high HM doses during the first 14–28 days of life are associated with a lower risk of various adverse outcomes in the NICU [7,10–12]. A research line indicated that it is the presence of bovine products (and not just the absence of feeding with HM) that negatively impacts intestinal permeability and colonization, rendering the association between HM and neonatal morbidity more complicated [6,16,59,60]. However, accumulating evidence suggests that bioactive HM components provide specific protection against morbidity through various mechanisms during different hospitalization periods in the NICU. Moreover, breastfeeding plays an important role on cognitive development, leading to a productive adulthood. Maternal milk includes long-chain polyunsaturated fatty acids, which promote brain growth. Research demonstrated that early visual acuity and cognitive functions are better developed in breastfed children [59,61,62]. Breastfeeding also appears to have a positive impact on infants' emotional well-being. It helps establish mother–infant bonding, due to skin-to-skin contact, which allows the infant to smell, touch, and feel their mother. Breastfeeding is pivotal for both the mother and the infant, as their developing bond is critical for the individual and reflects on the whole family. It has been shown that breastfed infants have closer and more intimate relationships with other family members. All in all, breastfeeding contributes to the smooth emotional and social development of the infant [28,60]. NICU admission of the neonate results in physical and psychologic separation from the mother, a key factor responsible for the failure of breastfeeding [63]. Rooming-in is extremely fortifying for breastfeeding because it contributes to the development of a communication code, providing peace, protection, and safety to the neonate. Breastfeeding plays an important role in the prognosis of preterm and ill neonates. In addition to the optimal nutrition that covers their substantial needs for growth and development, breastfeeding is also therapeutic for preterm neonates [64]. Data on the benefits of HM use in NICUs are intriguing, yet the incorporation of this evidence in practices, policies, procedures, and parental educational materials is limited. HM feeding is still under-prioritized over other therapeutic interventions implemented in the NICUs. Scarce information and lactation induction practices for the optimization of breastfeeding are available to healthcare professionals in NICUs and to the families of the neonates [5].

This study had a few limitations. The study design did not contain extensive data on the feeding status of the infant and/or the timing of breastfeeding initiation during their NICU stay. In addition, other important factors possibly affecting the duration of breastfeeding following the discharge of the neonate, including maternal age, educational level, and socio-economic status, were not recorded. Feedback on the duration of breastfeeding was provided by parents, making information bias possible; for example, mothers could have responded based on social expectations rather than their actual experience. The questionnaire was not validated in an extended Greek breastfeeding population. Sample size was only 279 mother–infant pairs. The breastfeeding practices of participants in this study may not be representative of regional or national practices. Probable systematic bias deriving from these limitations should be taken into account. Further large-scale, well-designed studies are necessary before the generalization of these study results.

5. Conclusions

Although breastfeeding support is a top priority in our NICU, the breastfeeding rates at six months for previously hospitalized infants were quite low compared with the standards set by the WHO. NICUs should promote breastfeeding, providing mothers/families with psychological support and comprehensive guidance on breastfeeding practices. The NICU environment is appropriate for educational interventions, as mothers are in close contact with healthcare professionals and have frequent access to lactation consultants and other breastfeeding resources. To better leverage this opportunity for the promotion of breastfeeding, healthcare professionals should identify mothers at a high risk of early breastfeeding cessation. Subsequently, educational and supportive interventions would need to be adjusted to overcome the obstacles impeding this subpopulation from breastfeeding. Evidence-based quality indicators are required for the comparative assessment of HM administration. The establishment of procedures that protect breastfeeding and the incorporation of lactation technologies that facilitate milk transportation are essential. An NICU is more than a treatment center for neonates; it is a living environment for newborns and their parents, with a focus on family-centered care.

Supplementary Materials: The following supporting information can be downloaded at: https://www.mdpi.com/article/10.3390/nu14183841/s1, Table S1: STROBE Statement—checklist of study.

Author Contributions: Conceptualization, R.S.; methodology, R.S. and A.K.; software, A.K. and R.S.; validation, R.S.; formal analysis, R.S.; data curation, R.S., S.P., A.K., G.I., A.M., E.-F.T., S.P., E.I. and N.I.; writing—original draft preparation, R.S. and S.P.; writing—review and editing, R.S., E.-F.T., A.K., S.P., G.I., E.I., A.M. and N.I.; visualization, R.S.; supervision. R.S.; project administration, R.S. All authors have read and agreed to the published version of the manuscript.

Funding: This research study received no external funding.

Institutional Review Board Statement: The study was conducted according to the guidelines of the Declaration of Helsinki and approved by the Institutional Review Board of Nikea General Hospital "Agios Panteleimon" (3/11, 22 January 2020).

Informed Consent Statement: Parental informed consent was obtained for all neonates involved in the study.

Data Availability Statement: The data presented in this study are available on request from the corresponding author.

Conflicts of Interest: The authors declare no conflict of interest.

References

1. Section on Breastfeeding; Eidelman, A.I.; Schanler, R.J.; Johnston, M.; Landers, S.; Noble, L.; Szucs, K.; Viehmann, L. Breastfeeding and the Use of Human Milk. *Pediatrics* **2012**, *129*, e827–e841. [CrossRef]
2. WHO. Breastfeeding. 2022. Available online: https://www.who.int/health-topics/breastfeeding#tab=tab_1 (accessed on 20 July 2022).
3. UNICEF. Breastfeeding. 2022. Available online: https://data.unicef.org/topic/nutrition/breastfeeding/ (accessed on 20 July 2022).
4. Dimitroglou, M.; Iliodromiti, Z.; Christou, E.; Volaki, P.; Petropoulou, C.; Sokou, R.; Boutsikou, T.; Iacovidou, N. Human Breast Milk: The Key Role in the Maturation of Immune, Gastrointestinal and Central Nervous Systems: A Narrative Review. *Diagnostics* **2022**, *12*, 2208. [CrossRef]
5. Meier, P.P.; Patel, A.L.; Bigger, H.R.; Rossman, B.; Engstrom, J.L. Supporting Breastfeeding in the Neonatal Intensive Care Unit: Rush Mother's Milk Club as a Case Study of Evidence-Based Care. *Pediatric Clin. N. Am.* **2013**, *60*, 209–226. [CrossRef] [PubMed]
6. Taylor, S.N.; Basile, L.A.; Ebeling, M.; Wagner, C.L. Intestinal permeability in preterm infants by feeding type: Mother's milk versus formula. *Breastfeed. Med.* **2009**, *4*, 11–15. [CrossRef] [PubMed]
7. Furman, L.; Taylor, G.; Minich, N.; Hack, M. The effect of maternal milk on neonatal morbidity of very low-birth-weight infants. *Arch. Pediatrics Adolesc. Med.* **2003**, *157*, 66–71. [CrossRef] [PubMed]
8. Schanler, R.J.; Shulman, R.J.; Lau, C. Feeding strategies for premature infants: Beneficial outcomes of feeding fortified human milk versus preterm formula. *Pediatrics* **1999**, *103*, 1150–1157. [CrossRef]
9. Schanler, R.J.; Lau, C.; Hurst, N.M.; Smith, E.O. Randomized trial of donor human milk versus preterm formula as substitutes for mothers' own milk in the feeding of extremely premature infants. *Pediatrics* **2005**, *116*, 400–406. [CrossRef]
10. Meinzen-Derr, J.; Poindexter, B.; Wrage, L.; Morrow, A.L.; Stoll, B.; Donovan, E.F. Role of human milk in extremely low birth weight infants' risk of necrotizing enterocolitis or death. *J. Perinatol.* **2009**, *29*, 57–62. [CrossRef]
11. Sisk, P.M.; Lovelady, C.A.; Gruber, K.J.; Dillard, R.G.; O'Shea, T.M. Human milk consumption and full enteral feeding among infants who weigh $\leq$ 1250 grams. *Pediatrics* **2008**, *121*, e1528–e1533. [CrossRef]
12. Sisk, P.M.; Lovelady, C.A.; Dillard, R.G.; Gruber, K.J.; O'Shea, T.M. Early human milk feeding is associated with a lower risk of necrotizing enterocolitis in very low birth weight infants. *J. Perinatol.* **2007**, *27*, 428–433. [CrossRef]
13. Vohr, B.R.; Poindexter, B.B.; Dusick, A.M.; McKinley, L.T.; Wright, L.L.; Langer, J.C.; Poole, W.K. Beneficial effects of breast milk in the neonatal intensive care unit on the developmental outcome of extremely low birth weight infants at 18 months of age. *Pediatrics* **2006**, *118*, e115–e123. [CrossRef]
14. Vohr, B.R.; Poindexter, B.B.; Dusick, A.M.; McKinley, L.T.; Higgins, R.D.; Langer, J.C.; Poole, W.K. Persistent beneficial effects of breast milk ingested in the neonatal intensive care unit on outcomes of extremely low birth weight infants at 30 months of age. *Pediatrics* **2007**, *120*, e953–e959. [CrossRef] [PubMed]
15. Hylander, M.A.; Strobino, D.M.; Pezzullo, J.C.; Dhanireddy, R. Association of human milk feedings with a reduction in retinopathy of prematurity among very low birthweight infants. *J. Perinatol.* **2001**, *21*, 356–362. [CrossRef] [PubMed]
16. Sullivan, S.; Schanler, R.J.; Kim, J.H.; Patel, A.L.; Trawöger, R.; Kiechl-Kohlendorfer, U.; Chan, G.M.; Blanco, C.L.; Abrams, S.; Cotten, C.M.; et al. An exclusively human milk-based diet is associated with a lower rate of necrotizing enterocolitis than a diet of human milk and bovine milk-based products. *J. Pediatrics* **2010**, *156*, 562–567.e1. [CrossRef] [PubMed]
17. Dimes, M.O. March of Dimes 2021 Report Card Reveals Slight Drop in Preterm Birth Rate First Time in Six Years Nation Keeps C- Grade. Available online: https://www.marchofdimes.org/news/march-of-dimes-2021-report-card.aspx (accessed on 20 July 2022).
18. Wang, L.; Du, K.N.; Zhao, Y.L.; Yu, Y.J.; Sun, L.; Jiang, H.B. Risk Factors of Nosocomial Infection for Infants in Neonatal Intensive Care Units: A Systematic Review and Meta-Analysis. *Med. Sci. Monit.* **2019**, *25*, 8213–8220. [CrossRef] [PubMed]
19. Sauve, R.; Lee, S.K. Neonatal follow-up programs and follow-up studies: Historical and current perspectives. *Paediatr. Child Health* **2006**, *11*, 267–270.
20. Naomi F Lauriello, G.P.A., Ted Rosenkrantz. Follow-Up of the NICU Patient. Available online: https://emedicine.medscape.com/article/1833812-overview (accessed on 27 August 2022).
21. Colaizy, T.T.; Morriss, F.H. Positive effect of NICU admission on breastfeeding of preterm US infants in 2000 to 2003. *J. Perinatol.* **2008**, *28*, 505–510. [CrossRef]
22. Gertz, B.; DeFranco, E. Predictors of breastfeeding non-initiation in the NICU. *Matern. Child Nutr.* **2019**, *15*, e12797. [CrossRef]
23. Laborie, S.; Abadie, G.; Denis, A.; Touzet, S.; Fischer Fumeaux, C.J. A Positive Impact of an Observational Study on Breastfeeding Rates in Two Neonatal Intensive Care Units. *Nutrients* **2022**, *14*, 1145. [CrossRef]
24. Bonet, M.; Blondel, B.; Agostino, R.; Combier, E.; Maier, R.F.; Cuttini, M.; Khoshnood, B.; Zeitlin, J. Variations in breastfeeding rates for very preterm infants between regions and neonatal units in Europe: Results from the MOSAIC cohort. *Arch. Dis. Child.-Fetal Neonatal Ed.* **2011**, *96*, F450. [CrossRef]
25. Bonnet, C.; Blondel, B.; Piedvache, A.; Wilson, E.; Bonamy, A.E.; Gortner, L.; Rodrigues, C.; van Heijst, A.; Draper, E.S.; Cuttini, M.; et al. Low breastfeeding continuation to 6 months for very preterm infants: A European multiregional cohort study. *Matern. Child Nutr.* **2019**, *15*, e12657. [CrossRef] [PubMed]

26. Foligno, S.; Finocchi, A.; Brindisi, G.; Pace, A.; Amadio, P.; Dall'Oglio, I.; Portanova, A.; Rossi, P.; Dotta, A.; Salvatori, G. Evaluation of Mother's Stress during Hospitalization Can Influence the Breastfeeding Rate. Experience in Intensive and Non Intensive Departments. *Int. J. Environ. Res. Public Health* **2020**, *17*, 1298. [CrossRef] [PubMed]
27. Purdy, I.B.; Singh, N.; Le, C.; Bell, C.; Whiteside, C.; Collins, M. Biophysiologic and social stress relationships with breast milk feeding pre- and post-discharge from the neonatal intensive care unit. *J. Obstet. Gynecol. Neonatal Nurs.* **2012**, *41*, 347–357. [CrossRef]
28. Krol, K.M.; Grossmann, T. Psychological effects of breastfeeding on children and mothers. *Bundesgesundheitsblatt Gesundh. Gesundh.* **2018**, *61*, 977–985. [CrossRef]
29. Lau, C. Breastfeeding Challenges and the Preterm Mother-Infant Dyad: A Conceptual Model. *Breastfeed. Med.* **2018**, *13*, 8–17. [CrossRef] [PubMed]
30. CDC. Breastfeeding Report Card. 2020. Available online: https://www.cdc.gov/breastfeeding/data/reportcard.htm (accessed on 24 July 2022).
31. Tigka, M.; Metallinou, D.; Nanou, C.; Iliodromiti, Z.; Lykeridou, K. Frequency and Determinants of Breastfeeding in Greece: A Prospective Cohort Study during the COVID-19 Pandemic. *Children* **2022**, *9*, 43. [CrossRef]
32. Iliodromiti, Z.; Zografaki, I.; Papamichail, D.; Stavrou, T.; Gaki, E.; Ekizoglou, C.; Nteka, E.; Mavrika, P.; Zidropoulos, S.; Panagiotopoulos, T.; et al. Increase of breast-feeding in the past decade in Greece, but still low uptake: Cross-sectional studies in 2007 and 2017. *Public Health Nutr.* **2020**, *23*, 961–970. [CrossRef] [PubMed]
33. Jiang, X.; Jiang, H. Factors associated with post NICU discharge exclusive breastfeeding rate and duration amongst first time mothers of preterm infants in Shanghai: A longitudinal cohort study. *Int. Breastfeed. J.* **2022**, *17*, 34. [CrossRef]
34. Dritsakou, K.; Massara, P.; Skourlis, N.; Liosis, G.; Skouroliakou, M. Maternal diet and breastfeeding duration of infants after NICU hospitalization in Greece: A cohort study. *J. Matern.-Fetal Neonatal Med.* **2016**, *30*, 2398–2403. [CrossRef]
35. ABM clinical protocol #10: Breastfeeding the late preterm infant (34(0/7) to 36(6/7) weeks gestation) (first revision June 2011). *Breastfeed. Med.* **2011**, *6*, 151–156. [CrossRef]
36. Jonsdottir, R.B.; Jonsdottir, H.; Orlygsdottir, B.; Flacking, R. A shorter breastfeeding duration in late preterm infants than term infants during the first year. *Acta Paediatr.* **2021**, *110*, 1209–1217. [CrossRef] [PubMed]
37. Perrella, S.L.; Williams, J.; Nathan, E.A.; Fenwick, J.; Hartmann, P.E.; Geddes, D.T. Influences on breastfeeding outcomes for healthy term and preterm/sick infants. *Breastfeed. Med.* **2012**, *7*, 255–261. [CrossRef] [PubMed]
38. Hamze, L.; Mao, J.; Reifsnider, E. Knowledge and attitudes towards breastfeeding practices: A cross-sectional survey of postnatal mothers in China. *Midwifery* **2019**, *74*, 68–75. [CrossRef]
39. Arslanoglu, S.; Moro, G.E.; Ziegler, E.E.; The WAPM Working Group on Nutrition. Optimization of human milk fortification for preterm infants: New concepts and recommendations. *J. Perinat. Med.* **2010**, *38*, 233–238. [CrossRef]
40. Dvorak, B.; Fituch, C.C.; Williams, C.S.; Hurst, N.M.; Schanler, R.J. Increased epidermal growth factor levels in human milk of mothers with extremely premature infants. *Pediatric Res.* **2003**, *54*, 15–19. [CrossRef] [PubMed]
41. Jónsdóttir, R.B.; Jónsdóttir, H.; Skúladóttir, A.; Thorkelsson, T.; Flacking, R. Breastfeeding progression in late preterm infants from birth to one month. *Matern. Child Nutr.* **2020**, *16*, e12893. [CrossRef]
42. Maastrup, R.; Hansen, B.M.; Kronborg, H.; Bojesen, S.N.; Hallum, K.; Frandsen, A.; Kyhnaeb, A.; Svarer, I.; Hallström, I. Factors Associated with Exclusive Breastfeeding of Preterm Infants. Results from a Prospective National Cohort Study. *PLoS ONE* **2014**, *9*, e89077. [CrossRef]
43. Bakker, L.; Jackson, B.; Miles, A. Oral-feeding guidelines for preterm neonates in the NICU: A scoping review. *J. Perinatol.* **2021**, *41*, 140–149. [CrossRef]
44. Singh, G.K.; Kogan, M.D.; Dee, D.L. Nativity/immigrant status, race/ethnicity, and socioeconomic determinants of breastfeeding initiation and duration in the United States, 2003. *Pediatrics* **2007**, *119* (Suppl. 1), S38–S46. [CrossRef]
45. Kana, M.A.; Rodrigues, C.; Fonseca, M.J.; Santos, A.C.; Barros, H. Effect of maternal country of birth on breastfeeding practices: Results from Portuguese GXXI birth cohort. *Int. Breastfeed. J.* **2018**, *13*, 15. [CrossRef]
46. Lanting, C.I.; Van Wouwe, J.P.; Reijneveld, S.A. Infant milk feeding practices in the Netherlands and associated factors. *Acta Paediatr.* **2005**, *94*, 935–942. [CrossRef] [PubMed]
47. Lumbiganon, P.; Martis, R.; Laopaiboon, M.; Festin, M.R.; Ho, J.J.; Hakimi, M. Antenatal breastfeeding education for increasing breastfeeding duration. *Cochrane Database Syst. Rev.* **2012**, Cd006425. [CrossRef]
48. Lumbiganon, P.; Martis, R.; Laopaiboon, M.; Festin, M.R.; Ho, J.J.; Hakimi, M. Antenatal breastfeeding education for increasing breastfeeding duration. *Cochrane Database Syst. Rev.* **2016**, *12*, Cd006425. [CrossRef]
49. Rollins, N.C.; Bhandari, N.; Hajeebhoy, N.; Horton, S.; Lutter, C.K.; Martines, J.C.; Piwoz, E.G.; Richter, L.M.; Victora, C.G. Why invest, and what it will take to improve breastfeeding practices? *Lancet* **2016**, *387*, 491–504. [CrossRef]
50. Leung, G.M.; Lam, T.H.; Ho, L.M. Breast-feeding and its relation to smoking and mode of delivery. *Obstet. Gynecol.* **2002**, *99*, 785–794. [CrossRef]
51. Kamath, B.D.; Todd, J.K.; Glazner, J.E.; Lezotte, D.; Lynch, A.M. Neonatal outcomes after elective cesarean delivery. *Obstet. Gynecol.* **2009**, *113*, 1231–1238. [CrossRef]
52. Latva, R.; Lehtonen, L.; Salmelin, R.K.; Tamminen, T. Visits by the family to the neonatal intensive care unit. *Acta Paediatr.* **2007**, *96*, 215–220. [CrossRef]

53. Sisk, P.; Quandt, S.; Parson, N.; Tucker, J. Breast milk expression and maintenance in mothers of very low birth weight infants: Supports and barriers. *J. Hum. Lact.* **2010**, *26*, 368–375. [CrossRef]
54. Størdal, K.; Lundeby, K.M.; Brantsæter, A.L.; Haugen, M.; Nakstad, B.; Lund-Blix, N.A.; Stene, L.C. Breast-feeding and Infant Hospitalization for Infections: Large Cohort and Sibling Analysis. *J. Pediatric Gastroenterol. Nutr.* **2017**, *65*, 225–231. [CrossRef]
55. Victora, C.G.; Bahl, R.; Barros, A.J.; França, G.V.; Horton, S.; Krasevec, J.; Murch, S.; Sankar, M.J.; Walker, N.; Rollins, N.C. Breastfeeding in the 21st century: Epidemiology, mechanisms, and lifelong effect. *Lancet* **2016**, *387*, 475–490. [CrossRef]
56. Hair, A.B.; Peluso, A.M.; Hawthorne, K.M.; Perez, J.; Smith, D.P.; Khan, J.Y.; O'Donnell, A.; Powers, R.J.; Lee, M.L.; Abrams, S.A. Beyond Necrotizing Enterocolitis Prevention: Improving Outcomes with an Exclusive Human Milk-Based Diet. *Breastfeed. Med.* **2016**, *11*, 70–74. [CrossRef] [PubMed]
57. McGuire, W.; Anthony, M.Y. Donor human milk versus formula for preventing necrotising enterocolitis in preterm infants: Systematic review. *Arch. Dis. Child.-Fetal Neonatal Ed.* **2003**, *88*, F11–F14. [CrossRef] [PubMed]
58. Chawanpaiboon, S.; Vogel, J.P.; Moller, A.B.; Lumbiganon, P.; Petzold, M.; Hogan, D.; Landoulsi, S.; Jampathong, N.; Kongwattanakul, K.; Laopaiboon, M.; et al. Global, regional, and national estimates of levels of preterm birth in 2014: A systematic review and modelling analysis. *Lancet Glob. Health* **2019**, *7*, e37–e46. [CrossRef]
59. Amiel Castro, R.; Glover, V.; Ehlert, U.; O'Connor, T.G. Breastfeeding, prenatal depression and children's IQ and behaviour: A test of a moderation model. *BMC Pregnancy Childbirth* **2021**, *21*, 62. [CrossRef]
60. Poton, W.L.; Soares, A.L.G.; Oliveira, E.R.A.; Gonçalves, H. Breastfeeding and behavior disorders among children and adolescents: A systematic review. *Rev. Saude Publica* **2018**, *52*, 9. [CrossRef]
61. Liu, S.; Ye, S.; Wang, Q.; Cao, Y.; Zhang, X. Breastfeeding and myopia: A cross-sectional study of children aged 6–12 years in Tianjin, China. *Sci. Rep.* **2018**, *8*, 10025. [CrossRef]
62. AlThuneyyan, D.A.; AlGhamdi, F.F.; AlZain, R.N.; AlDhawyan, Z.S.; Alhmly, H.F.; Purayidathil, T.S.; AlGindan, Y.Y.; Abdullah, A.A. The Effect of Breastfeeding on Intelligence Quotient and Social Intelligence Among Seven- to Nine-Year-Old Girls: A Pilot Study. *Front. Nutr.* **2022**, *9*, 726042. [CrossRef]
63. Treherne, S.C.; Feeley, N.; Charbonneau, L.; Axelin, A. Parents' Perspectives of Closeness and Separation With Their Preterm Infants in the NICU. *J. Obstet. Gynecol. Neonatal Nurs.* **2017**, *46*, 737–747. [CrossRef]
64. Del Ciampo, L.A.; Del Ciampo, I.R.L. Breastfeeding and the Benefits of Lactation for Women's Health. *Rev. Bras. Ginecol. Obs.* **2018**, *40*, 354–359. [CrossRef]

nutrients

MDPI

Article

Muscle Function, Body Composition, Insulin Sensitivity and Physical Activity in Adolescents Born Preterm: Impact of Gestation and Vitamin D Status

Claire L. Wood [1,2], Robert Tinnion [3], Kieren G. Hollingsworth [2], Michael I. Trenell [2], Mark S. Pearce [4], Tim D. Cheetham [1,2,†] and Nicholas D. Embleton [3,4,*]

1 Department of Paediatric Endocrinology, Royal Victoria Infirmary, Newcastle upon Tyne NE1 4LP, UK
2 Translational and Clinical Research Institute, Faculty of Medical Sciences, Newcastle University, Newcastle upon Tyne NE2 4HH, UK
3 Newcastle Neonatal Service, Royal Victoria Infirmary, Newcastle Hospitals NHS Foundation Trust, Newcastle upon Tyne NE1 4LP, UK
4 Population Health Sciences Institute, Faculty of Medical Sciences Newcastle University, Newcastle upon Tyne NE1 4LP, UK
* Correspondence: nicholas.embleton@ncl.ac.uk
† Joint senior author.

Abstract: Whilst several studies have explored adolescent metabolic and cognitive function after preterm birth, few have explored muscle function and physical activity. We set out to examine the relationship between gestational age and muscle metabolism in a cohort of adolescents who were born preterm. Participants were recruited from the Newcastle preterm birth growth study cohort. They did not have severe neurological disease and were not on daily medication. Participants underwent an assessment of oxidative muscle function using phosphorus magnetic resonance spectroscopy that included the half-time for recovery of equilibrium of phosphocreatine, $\tau_{1/2}$PCr. In addition, we measured key variables that might affect muscle function including physical activity levels determined by 3-day accelerometry, body composition using air displacement plethysmography, insulin sensitivity using the homeostatic model assessment/Matsuda index and serum vitamin D concentrations. 60 adolescents (35F) median age 15.6 years (range 12.1–18.8) with a median gestation of 31 weeks (range 24 to 34 weeks) underwent a single assessment. Males were more active and spent less time in sedentary mode. Time spent in light activity was associated with insulin sensitivity (IS) (Matsuda Index; $p < 0.05$) but there were no strong correlations between activity levels and gestational age. Greater fat mass, waist circumference and body mass index were all associated with lower IS. Gestational age was negatively associated with adjusted measures of oxidative muscle function ($\tau_{1/2}$PCr). In a stepwise multivariate linear regression model, gestational age at birth was the most significant predictor of oxidative muscle function ($p = 0.005$). Higher serum vitamin D levels were also associated with faster phosphocreatine recovery time ($p = 0.045$). Oxidative function in the skeletal muscle of adolescents born preterm is associated with gestational age and vitamin D concentrations. Our study suggests that being born preterm may have a long-term impact on muscle metabolism.

Keywords: preterm; muscle; vitamin D

1. Introduction

Preterm birth is associated with an increased risk of adverse outcomes in later life [1] with higher rates of obesity, type 2 diabetes (T2DM), cardiovascular disease, and other features of the metabolic syndrome [2]. The mechanisms are likely to be complex and may include epigenetic effects as well as effects on organogenesis with altered tissue development [1]. Prematurity may also impact on skeletal muscle development and function, which is important because skeletal muscle oxidative function is a key component of metabolic health [3]. Preterm delivery results in less time spent in the muscle-conditioning intra-uterine environment and can also be associated with lower rates of physical exercise in later life [4]. Insulin resistance in adults with T2DM is more common following preterm birth and limits the availability of glucose to the mitochondria with studies using phosphorus magnetic resonance spectroscopy (^{31}P-MRS) showing this can compromise skeletal muscle function [5]. Gentle regular exercise does not appear to improve substrate delivery in adults with T2DM but enhances insulin sensitivity by increasing lipolysis in skeletal muscle [6]. Changes in organogenesis, conditioning and subsequent use of skeletal muscle following preterm birth may therefore be important determinants of metabolic health outcomes. This is important because targeted exercise can reduce obesity in teenagers including those born preterm and offers potential strategies for reversing or ameliorating the adverse effects of preterm birth.

^{31}P-MRS is a non-invasive technique for assessment of organ structure and metabolite concentrations. The concentration of phosphorus nuclei (^{31}P) in chemically distinct compounds within muscle, including high energy metabolites such as PCr and ATP, can be quantified using a clinical MRI scanner with modified hardware. The use of a graded exercise apparatus to perform plantar flexion exercises can be used to deplete PCr stores while ATP homeostasis is preserved. Cessation of exercise permits oxidative phosphorylation of ATP and recovery of PCr concentrations. The rate of recovery to baseline PCr concentrations within muscle (denoted as $\tau_{1/2}$PCr) is used as a measure of mitochondrial oxidative function.

Vitamin D is as steroid hormone partly acquired through dietary sources but mainly generated by UV light passing through the skin and converting 7-dehydrocholesterol to vitamin D3. This then undergoes hydroxylation in the liver and then kidney to produce 1,25 dihydroxyvitamin D3. Effects of vitamin D are mediated throughout the body by vitamin D receptors in both bone and non-skeletal tissues such as muscle. Vitamin D deficiency in adults has been shown to have an impact on mitochondrial oxidative function when measured using the ^{31}P-MRS technique [7]. As vitamin D is primarily transferred to the fetus in the third trimester, premature infants are at high risk of vitamin D insufficiency and deficiency. Studies from the UK and Ireland have shown that at least two thirds of premature infants are likely to have vitamin D deficiency at birth [8,9] In addition, current neonatal nutritional strategies for early preterm infants may be insufficient to achieve recommended vitamin D intake and target serum 25(OH)D concentrations [8].

Serum vitamin D levels correlate with insulin sensitivity and vitamin D supplementation improves peripheral muscle insulin sensitivity, therefore it is important to consider vitamin D levels when investigating the association between preterm birth, insulin sensitivity and muscle function.

Few studies have explored the impact of preterm delivery on muscle metabolism and function in later life. We aimed to examine the association between gestational age and muscle function and metabolism using ^{31}P-MRS in late adolescence after adjustment for likely confounders including insulin sensitivity, fat mass, vitamin D status and physical activity levels.

2. Materials and Methods

2.1. Participants and Visit Schedule

This study was conducted in adolescents who were recruited from the Newcastle preterm birth growth study (PTBGS) cohort [10]. Participants were preterm infants (gestation range 24–34 weeks and mean birthweight ~1.2 kg) originally enrolled into one of two randomised neonatal nutrition trials [11,12]. Participants were excluded from the original studies if they had major neonatal morbidities such as severe neurological disease, chronic lung disease at discharge or were on regular daily medication. Of the 247 children in the PTBGS cohort, details were obtained for 235 using health care records, following confirmation from the general practitioner that children were alive and otherwise well. Families were contacted by letter, with one further follow up letter sent if no reply was received. The parents of 62 adolescents/adolescents themselves responded, of whom 60 attended for a half-day study visit at the Newcastle Magnetic Resonance Centre, Newcastle University Campus for Ageing and Vitality, UK. Study visits were conducted following an overnight (minimum 8-h) fast. Participants had the option of declining any of the study components. The protocol for the study has previously been published [10].

2.2. Anthropometry including Body Composition Determination

Participants underwent standard anthropometry (height, weight, waist circumference) by an appropriately trained clinician/researcher (RT). Each measurement was taken three times and averaged. Body mass index (BMI) was calculated (weight in kg divided by height in metres squared). Total body fat mass (FM) was measured by Air-Displacement Plethysmography (BOD POD™ system, COSMED, Concord California, USA) [13]. Tight-fitting swimsuits and a swim-cap were worn in the BODPOD to minimise clothing/hair volume interference with the measurement. Thoracic gas volume was not directly measured; instead a standardised, software-generated estimate was used to minimise the length of time in the BODPOD [14]. Standard deviation z-scores were calculated for birthweight, height, weight and BMI using reference data [15,16]. Self-assessed pubertal (Tanner) stage was recorded [17].

2.3. Biochemistry including Assessments of Insulin Sensitivity and Vitamin D Status

Oral glucose tolerance testing [18] was carried out and both Homeostatic model assessment (HOMA) modelling [19] and Matsuda Indexing [20] were used to assess IS based on T_{0min} and T_{120min} serum values. HOMA is a marker of hepatic IS and requires only a baseline glucose and insulin concentration. The Matsuda index is a measure of both hepatic and peripheral IS and is calculated following a glucose load. Vitamin D concentrations were measured because of the potential association with fat mass and oxidative muscle function [21,22]. Serum was stored frozen prior to assay for 25-OH Vitamin D quantitation using an ABSciex 5500 tandem mass spectrometer (Warrington, UK) and the Chromsystems (Munich, Germany) 25OHD kit for LC-MS/MS (intra- and inter-assay CV 3.7% and 4.8%, respectively) at Manchester University. Triglycerides were measured using a colorimetric method (Roche Diagnostics GmbH, Mannheim, Germany) with inter assay CV's of 0.9–2.0%.

2.4. Assessment of Physical Activity Levels

Study participants wore a lightweight, uniaxial accelerometer (ActiGraph™ Pensacola, Florida, USA) over 3 days following a study visit, which was pre-programmed to begin and stop recording activity prior to being issued to participants. They measured acceleration of different intensities in one (vertical) plane during sequential, pre-defined, short epochs (10 s). During wearing, any displacement of the hip (i.e., pelvis tilt or changing body position) during activity causes vertical displacement of the accelerometer which is recorded as counts per minute (cpm) [23]. Analysis of the activity data were performed using the Actilife program (version 5, MTI, Pensacola, Florida, USA) under the supervision of Dr Laura Basterfield (Human Nutrition Research Centre, Newcastle University). Using pre-defined, calorimetrically referenced cut-offs, the data recorded over three consecutive days was classified into sedentary ($\leq$100 cpm), light (101–2295 cpm), moderate (2296–4011 cpm) or vigorous ($\geq$4012 cpm) physical activity (MVPA) [24].

2.5. Magnetic Resonance Spectroscopy

A 3-Tesla Achieva MRI scanner (Philips) was used with a 14 cm ^{31}P surface coil placed over the calf muscles (Figure 1B) to acquire phosphorus spectra [25]. ^{31}P spectra were recorded over 3 min to assess resting mitochondrial function, then participants performed plantar flexion against resistance (at 35% MVC loading, see Supplementary Materials) at 0.5 Hz for 3 min. Participants then rested and MR phosphorous spectra were recorded every 10 s. ^{31}P spectra were analysed using the AMARES algorithm in jMRUI and prior knowledge [26]. From this, quantification of PCr, inorganic phosphate (Pi) and pH was obtained (Figure 1A). A single exponential fit was used to estimate half-time to recovery within the muscle (Figure 1D), represented by recovery of equilibrium of PCr ($\tau_{1/2}$PCr) and ADP ($\tau_{1/2}$ADP).

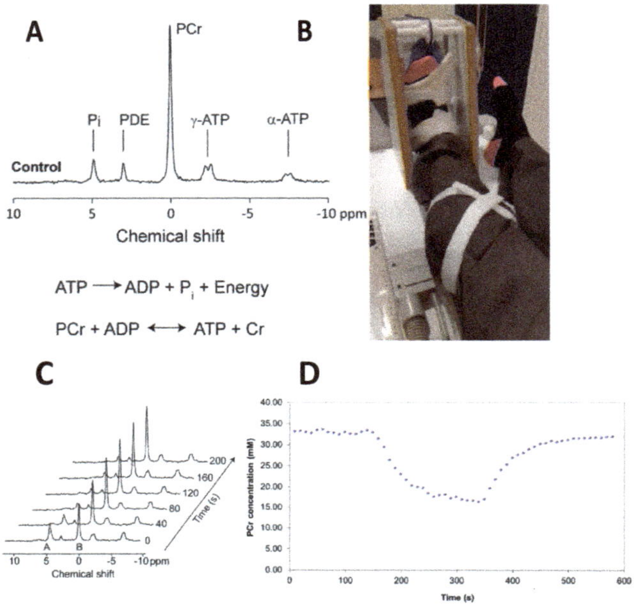

Figure 1. (**A**) The phosphorus spectrum of the human gastrocnemius/soleus muscle at rest, showing the resonances due to inorganic phosphate (Pi), phosphodiesters (PDE), phosphocreatine (PCr) and the α and γ phosphorus nuclei of ATP. The area under each peak indicates the concentration of that substance. (**B**) The apparatus used for the plantar flexion exercise showing the pedal, and the radiofrequency coil used to acquire signals from phosphorus-containing high energy compounds from the back of the leg during exercise and recovery. The pedal is attached to a weight within the scanner bore to provide a fixed resistance of 35% of the maximum voluntary contraction of the subject. (**C**) A dynamic series of phosphorus spectra acquired after the plantar flexion exercise has ceased, showing the changes in the inorganic phosphate peak and the phosphocreatine peak, which recovers to equilibrium. (**D**) Extracting the area under the curve of the phosphocreatine peak for each time point as concentration, showing the initial concentration at rest, depletion during the exercise and recovery by oxidative phosphorylation after exercise has ceased. The $\tau_{1/2}$PCr is calculated by fitting a monoexponential curve to the recovery. In this case, the $\tau_{1/2}$PCr was 33.2 s.

2.6. Statistics

The precise sample sized was linked to the number of respondents but according to effect size data from the cohort at earlier assessments where fat mass index was related to insulin sensitivity ($R^2 = 0.12$), 60 patients were sufficient to detect a within-cohort difference with 80% power at the 5% significance level. However, the analyses in this paper included more powerful linear regression methods, using mainly continuous data suggesting that the numbers involved in this study were adequate. Stata™ (v11/13 StataCorp, College Station, TX, USA) was used for all statistical analyses. Spearman correlation analysis was used to examine potential associations between paired variables. Mann–Whitney U or 't' tests indicated that the follow-up sample was broadly representative of the original cohort for key variables including gestational age, birthweight and birth weight SDS. No active selection process was used when contacting families (i.e., no discriminators based on previous cohort results) with all respondents included in the study. We are not, therefore, aware of any recruitment bias. Multiple linear regression modelling was used to examine interactions between variables using $\tau_{1/2}$PCr as the dependent variable. Key variables that could impact on muscle function were considered when comparing gestational age to muscle metabolism. Sex, birthweight, activity level, FMI, IS and vitamin D concentration were all analysed separately in univariate models, then a manual forwards stepwise approach used to inform the final variables for inclusion into the multivariable regression model. Non-significant terms were removed until the minimum number of significant variables remained. Age at follow-up was not included as it was felt that including both pubertal stage and age in a model may lead to collinearity (Rho = 0.62, $p < 0.001$). Indices of insulin sensitivity were logarithmically transformed as residuals deviated from homogeneity. Statistical significance was set at 5%.

3. Results

3.1. Baseline Characteristics and Recruitment Flowchart

60 adolescents (15.6 years old, range 12.1–18.8) attended a study visit, although not all agreed to each component (Table 1). Participants were representative of the original Newcastle PTBGS cohort and there was no difference between those consenting to each component and the overall cohort in terms of age at study, gender, gestation at birth, birthweight or body fat content recorded at previous visit.

Table 1. Subject characteristics at birth and time of follow-up and auxology, body composition and biochemistry at study visit. BMI: body mass index, SD: standard deviation.

Variable	Mean (SD) or Median (Range)
Sex (Male: Female)	25 (42%): 35 (58%)
Birth weight (kg), n = 60	1.37 (0.25)
Birthweight z-score, n = 60	−0.72 (−3.81, 1.37)
Gestation at birth (weeks), n = 60	31.0 (1.9)
Age (years), n = 60	15.6 (12.1–18.8)
Weight z-score, n = 60	0.02 (1.21)
Height z-score, n = 60	−0.19 (0.90)
BMI z-score, n = 60	0.16 (1.21)
Pubertal status by Tanner staging (1–5), n = 60	Stage 1—8% Stage 2—3% Stage 3—27% Stage 4—40% Stage 5—22%
25(OH)D (nmol/L), n = 46	59.3 (21.9–102.6)
Systolic blood pressure (mm Hg), n = 60	116.1 (13.0)
Diastolic blood pressure (mm Hg), n = 60	73.1 (7.24)
Mean blood pressure (mm Hg), n = 60	83.5 (7.5)
Cholesterol (mmol/L), n = 46	4.1 (3.2–6.5)
Triglyceride (mmol/L), n = 46	0.7 (0.4–2.6)
Total body fat mass from BodPod (kg/m^2), n = 58	3.4 (0.4–15.1)
Total body fat-free mass from BodPod (kg/m^2), n = 58	15.9 (13.2–20.1)
Waist circumference (cm), n = 60	71.7 (57.0–108.7)

3.2. Anthropometry

The height and weight of participants is shown in Table 1. Most (89%) were in mid to late puberty (Tanner stage 3–5) at time of assessment. Body composition data were consistent with UK age and sex-matched reference data. Median FMI for males was 1.93 (9th–25th centile) and LMI 16.55 (50th centile) and females FMI 5.45 (25th–50th centile) and LMI 15.70 (50th–75th centile). Markers of adiposity were also analysed with respect to the measured muscle kinetics and no significant correlation identified.

3.3. Insulin Sensitivity

Measures of IS using HOMA and Matsuda index are shown in Table 2.

Table 2. Exercise and muscle function parameters assessed by accelerometery, oral glucose tolerance test and magnetic resonance spectroscopy. HOMA: Homeostatic model assessment, PCr: phosphocreatine.

Variable	Mean (SD) or Median (IQR)	Male	Female	*p*-Value for Male v Female
Moderate to vigorous physical activity (mins/day) n = 44	45.0 (22.8)	52.1 (21.5)	39.7 (22.7)	0.06
Sedentary activity (mins/day), n = 44	500.0 (84.2)	483.1 (93.2)	512.9 (76.0)	0.02
Light activity (mins/day), n = 44	143.3 (47.5)	154.7 (44.9)	134.7 (48.5)	0.02
Insulin sensitivity assessed by Matsuda index, n = 50	4.9 (3.0–7.1)	5.6 (3.5–8.7)	4.0 (2.9–5.2)	0.13
Insulin sensitivity assessed by HOMA (%), n = 46	79.7 (65.9–114.1)	98.1 (66.9–118.4)	78.3 (62.6–111.0)	0.32
PCr recovery time, $\tau_{1/2}$PCr (s), n = 50	33.8 (7.3)	31.5 (7.9)	34.2 (8.8)	0.28

Body composition and greater fat mass, waist circumference, and higher BMI z-score were all associated with lower IS, but there was no correlation between gestational age or birthweight z-score and IS (Table 3). Spearman correlation analysis of recorded minimum pH during standardised exercise showed no correlation between minimum pH and IS measured by Matsuda (Rho:0.07, $p = 0.75$). Serum triglyceride levels were also analysed with respect to measured muscle kinetics and no significant correlation identified.

Table 3. Spearman's correlation analysis for. (**A**) measures of physical activity, assessed by accelerometry. (**B**) insulin sensitivity (* $p < 0.05$, ** $p < 0.01$). BMI: body mass index, FMI: fat mass index, MVPA: moderate-vigorous physical activity.

(A)

Variable	MVPA (Mean Mins)	Sedentary Activity (Mean Mins)	Light Activity (Mean Mins)
Gestational age	−0.26	0.02	0.04
FMI (Bodpod)	−0.18	0.03	−0.21
Current BMI z-score	0.00	0.11	−0.14
Waist circumference (cm)	−0.15	0.12	−0.25
Matsuda Index	0.03	0.05	0.32 *

(B)

Variable	Matsuda Index	HOMA %S
Gestational age	−0.05	−0.06
Birthweight z-score	−0.03	−0.16
FMI (Bodpod)	−0.41 **	−0.39 **
Waist circumference (cm)	−0.30 *	−0.34 *
BMI z-score	−0.41 **	−0.39 **

3.4. Accelerometery

Valid accelerometery results (>6 h/day wear-time) were obtained in 44/60 participants. Mean daily time spent in MVPA in the overall cohort was 45 min, 25% less than the nationally recommended 60 min per day [27,28]. Average step count was also less than the recommended 10,000 daily steps [29]. Males were more active than females (Table 2) with a significantly higher proportion of their time spent in light activity ($p = 0.02$) and a lower proportion in sedentary mode ($p = 0.02$), but there was no significant difference in the time spent in MVPA. There were no strong correlations between activity levels and gestational age or markers of adiposity. Time spent in light activity was significantly associated with the Matsuda Index of IS (Table 3). There was no correlation between accelerometer-measured activity levels and muscle metabolism, and no measurable effect of sex (Table 4).

Table 4. Univariable regression analysis for adjusted PCr recovery ($\tau_{1/2}$PCr), showing the unadjusted values for the variables that were considered for inclusion in the multivariable model. FMI: fat mass index, * indicate variables that were included in final model, + indicates log transformation.

Independent Variable	Co-eff	95% CI	*p*-Value
Gestational age at birth (days)	−0.21	−0.39, −0.03	0.03 *
Serum Vitamin D +	−0.11	−0.21, −0.01	0.03 *
Fat mass index (measured by BodPod)	−1.07	−4.36, 2.21	0.52
Mean step-count/day	1.70	−3.86, 7.26	0.54
Matsuda index of insulin sensitivity+	3.01	−1.32, 7.35	0.17
Birthweight z-score	1.15	−1.46, 3.75	0.38
Female sex	2.61	−2.23, 7.45	0.28

3.5. *Vitamin D (25-OHD) Concentrations*

The median serum Vitamin D concentration was 59.3 nmol/L (range 21.9–102.6 nmol/L; Table 1) and was deficient/insufficient in 12/46 (26%) participants. Levels were significantly higher in visits occurring between March-September compared to October-February ($p = 0.001$). Spearman correlation analysis showed a negative association between vitamin D levels and BMI (Rho: −0.31, $p = 0.046$) but not fat mass (Rho: −0.27, $p = 0.07$) or waist circumference (Rho: −0.28, $p = 0.06$). Vitamin D was positively associated with enhanced IS when measured by Matsuda index (Rho: 0.41, $p = 0.005$) and HOMA (Rho: 0.34, $p = 0.02$). The greater the vitamin D level, the shorter the half-time to recovery of equilibrium of PCr (co-eff-0.11, $p = 0.03$).

3.6. *Magnetic Resonance Spectroscopy*

Magnetic resonance spectroscopy was performed in 50 participants. Spearman rank correlation analysis and univariate linear regression modelling were used to determine independent factors associated with oxidative muscle function (measured by $\tau_{1/2}$PCr). Gestational age was negatively associated with $\tau_{1/2}$PCr, i.e., the greater the gestational age at birth, the shorter the half-time to recovery (Table 4). Birthweight z-score was not associated with MRS kinetics.

3.7. *Stepwise Linear Regression with $\tau_{1/2}$PCr as the Outcome Variable*

Multivariable linear regression modelling was undertaken, with $\tau_{1/2}$PCr as the outcome variable. Because IS and activity levels were associated with vitamin D levels, these parameters were tested for inclusion in the initial model. As anticipated, IS was related to puberty stage: Matsuda Index was significantly higher in those who were pre-pubertal (Tanner stage 1) compared to those who were Tanner stage 2–5; 8.83 v 5.16 (coefficient 1.21 (0.14, 2.25), $p = 0.03$). Pubertal staging was therefore considered in the stepwise model. Variables tested for inclusion within the final model are in Table 4. In the final regression model (data from 36 participants with MRS data and vitamin D levels recorded) gestational age at birth remained the most significant predictive factor of oxidative muscle function; those born more premature had longer phosphocreatine recovery times (co-efficient −0.26, $p = 0.005$). Higher vitamin D levels were also associated with faster recovery times (co-efficient—5.86, $p = 0.045$, p-value for overall model = 0.004, adjusted $R^2 = 0.24$. Testing for heteroskedasticity showed that the final terms (vitamin D and gestational age) were independent. Inclusion of Tanner Staging was not significant by likelihood ratio testing of this model with/without Tanner Staging included.

4. Discussion

We have shown that gestational age at birth is predictive of skeletal muscle oxidative function in later life as measured by $\tau_{1/2}$PCr. This demonstrates the life-long adverse metabolic consequences of preterm birth. We detected the anticipated associations between puberty stage, BMI, fat mass and activity levels with IS but, unlike gestational age, none of these variables predicted skeletal muscle oxidative function. We found that lower vitamin D concentrations were associated with worse skeletal muscle oxidative function as has been described previously [20].

There are few similar studies. Work by Bertocci showed that infants who were born preterm have a smaller PCr signal than their term born counterparts, using a similar MRS technique to that used here [30]. They speculated that preterm infants may have limited phosphate reserves such that when challenged by even a small increase in activity they deplete their reserves very quickly and take a long time to recover. However, this mechanism would not explain persistence of this effect in later life. Using other methods to measure oxidative capacity (aerobic fitness score), Rogers and colleagues demonstrated that at age 17, adolescents born preterm have reduced oxidative capacity and are more likely to become fatigued [31].

We believe that the association that we have identified is biologically plausible because post-mortem specimens from the skeletal muscle of infants born preterm show a predominance of type 2 (low-oxidative) muscle fibres which have a relatively low density of mitochondria [32–34]. In these studies, which looked at muscle groups such as the diaphragm and intercostal muscles, data suggest that typical development towards term age involved an increase in the density of type 1 (high oxidative) fibres. Some preterm infants may therefore experience an arrest or permanent alteration in the density of type 1 fibres associated with lower mitochondrial density that may then result in a prolonged PCr recovery in later life. Habitual activity levels might be associated with the oxidative capacity of the mitochondria if it was modifiable by muscle training, but we found no evidence of a correlation between an objective measurement of daily activity and ^{31}P-MRS spectroscopy. However, absence of such an association may reflect the fact that the test standardised to MVC is designed to deplete the PCr stores substantially to measure oxidative function during recovery of PCr, and thus is perhaps more extreme than the more usual low-level of aerobic exercise.

We noted a strong association between vitamin D concentrations and muscle kinetics which is important as it is potentially modifiable [21]. The relationship between lower serum vitamin D levels and longer $\tau_{1/2}$PCr recovery time was independent of the relationship between $\tau_{1/2}$PCr and gestational age at birth in our cohort. Vitamin D concentrations tend to be lower in obese individuals and have been shown to be lower at birth in babies born preterm [35]. In other populations there is also a well-documented association between lower vitamin D levels and markers of reduced IS [36–39]. Other data show that vitamin D replacement improves IS [40,41]. Both FM and IS were therefore considered for inclusion in the multivariable linear regression but were not significant variables in the final model.

Vitamin D has a wide range of effects in tissues and cells, but there are no definitive data to show that it has a direct effect on muscle at the myocyte membrane. It is possible that it may act at the mitochondrial genomic level upregulating either the cellular mechanisms needed to improve oxidative function, or more directly by influencing ATP synthesis [42]. Further studies could explore the potential for Vitamin D supplementation to improve muscle function in this group with a particular focus on patients with vitamin D levels at the lower end of the spectrum observed in this study.

Obtaining valid accelerometery data in the adolescent population is challenging and only 44/60 completed >6 h wear-time. The directly measured activity data from this cohort was similar to another cohort in our region which also noted that boys were more physically active than girls [24,43,44]. Another striking feature from our data was that light activity is most strongly associated with measures of IS. While there was no direct association between $\tau_{1/2}$PCr and any of the activity measures, increasing light activity may have an indirect effect on muscle oxidative function via either its positive association with IS or via mechanisms that link IS with vitamin D. The association of body habitus with IS across the cohort longitudinally [45] is in agreement with other published data describing the increasing influence of body habitus on IS with increasing chronological age [46].

The association between light physical activity and improved glucose disposal reflects the relationship between exercise and IS in muscle that has been observed in a range of different settings. Light activity appears to have the most impact as observed in animal models [47], older humans [48] and individuals at high risk of metabolic syndrome [49], and promotion of this may be more acceptable in adolescents than attempts to increase more vigorous forms of activity.

Limitations

This study has important limitations. The cohort is modest in size, however the group studied appeared to be representative of the initial cohort with respect to key characteristics. Our sample size was fixed by virtue of the size of the initial cohort and then the number of willing respondents, but the study was sufficiently powered to detect a change in $\tau_{1/2}$PCr of 10%. It is of note that the overall $\tau_{1/2}$PCr values are not indicative of major defects in oxidative function, as might be found in mitochondrial dysfunction, and indeed are similar to a group of healthy young adults also tested under the same protocol [50]. The differences may be relevant, however, in terms of an individual's ability to participate competitively in sporting activities and so should not be trivialised. Whilst the association between gestational age and muscle metabolism in premature infants is not dependent on term controls, future studies need to assess muscle function in the full spectrum of gestational age. We also cannot rule out the fact that the study may have been underpowered for the non-significant outcomes and similarly the sample size was too small to stratify by gender.

Assessing pubertal status in studies involving adolescents can be challenging although a recent meta-analysis concluded that there is moderate or substantial agreement between patient and clinician assessments [17]. The value of a clinician's assessment of pubertal stage needs to be balanced against the likelihood of a n associated reduction in participant numbers. Importantly, self-assessed pubertal stage was related to IS and the relevance of pubertal status in this study is primarily because of measured variables such as fat-mass and fat-free mass. Reassessment of metabolic outcomes including muscle function in early adulthood is important.

5. Conclusions

We noted a relationship between gestational age and muscle oxidative capacity determined using ^{31}P-MRS in adolescent children born preterm. This may be programmed by differential development of muscle fibre type as a result of preterm birth. The relationship between gestational age and muscle function in later life requires further investigation in a larger study but in the interim we recommend optimising vitamin D status and encouraging preterm-born children and adolescents to engage in regular light activity.

Supplementary Materials: The following supporting information can be downloaded at: https://www.mdpi.com/article/10.3390/nu14235045/s1, Methods S1. Reference [51] is cited in the supplementary materials.

Author Contributions: N.D.E., T.D.C., K.G.H., M.I.T. and R.T. designed the project. R.T., C.L.W. and K.G.H. undertook data collection/analysis. M.S.P. provided statistical expertise. N.D.E., R.T., C.L.W. and T.D.C. prepared the initial draft of the manuscript. All authors have read and agreed to the published version of the manuscript.

Funding: Nutricia UK provided funding for the initial controlled trials in infancy. Support for subsequent follow-up studies was provided by Novo Nordisk, Nutricia UK and the Special Trustees Newcastle Healthcare Charity. CW is funded by the Medical Research Council/MDUK (MR/N020588/1).

Institutional Review Board Statement: The study was conducted in accordance with the Declaration of Helsinki, and approved by the Sunderland 9 February 2011 from Sunderland Regional Ethics Committee (study number 10/H0904/67, 09/02/2011).

Informed Consent Statement: Informed consent was obtained from all subjects involved in the study.

Data Availability Statement: Data are available on request.

Acknowledgments: We would like to acknowledge the assistance of: Tim Hodgson, Louise Ward and Dorothy Wallace, Senior Research Radiographers at the Newcastle Magnetic Resonance Centre, the nursing staff at the Newcastle Clinical Research Facility, Jacqueline Berry from the University of Manchester for the vitamin D analysis, Christopher Boot, Consultant Clinical Scientist at Newcastle Laboratories and Laura Basterfield.

Conflicts of Interest: The authors have no conflict of interest to declare. Embleton declares research funding from Prolacta Biosciences US and Danone Early life Nutrition, and lecture honoraria from Nestle Nutrition Institute.

References

1. Parkinson, J.R.C.; Hyde, M.J.; Gale, C.; Santhakumaran, S.; Modi, N. Preterm Birth and the Metabolic Syndrome in Adult Life: A Systematic Review and Meta-analysis. *Pediatrics* **2013**, *131*, e1240–e1263. [CrossRef] [PubMed]
2. Thomas, E.L.; Parkinson, J.R.; Hyde, M.J.; Yap, I.K.; Holmes, E.; Doré, C.J.; Bell, J.D.; Modi, N. Aberrant Adiposity and Ectopic Lipid Deposition Characterize the Adult Phenotype of the Preterm Infant. *Pediatr. Res.* **2011**, *70*, 507–512. [CrossRef] [PubMed]
3. Kelley, D.E. Skeletal muscle fat oxidation: Timing and flexibility are everything. *J. Clin. Investig.* **2005**, *115*, 1699–1702. [CrossRef]
4. Kaseva, N.; Wehkalampi, K.; Strang-Karlsson, S.; Salonen, M.; Pesonen, A.K.; Räikkönen, K.; Tammelin, T.; Hovi, P.; Lahti, J.; Heinonen, K.; et al. Lower Conditioning Leisure-Time Physical Activity in Young Adults Born Preterm at Very Low Birth Weight. *PLoS ONE* **2012**, *7*, e32430. [CrossRef]
5. Lim, E.L.; Hollingsworth, K.G.; Smith, F.E.; Thelwall, P.E.; Taylor, R. Inhibition of lipolysis in Type 2 diabetes normalizes glucose disposal without change in muscle glycogen synthesis rates. *Clin. Sci.* **2011**, *121*, 169–177. [CrossRef] [PubMed]
6. Trenell, M.I.; Hollingsworth, K.G.; Lim, E.L.; Taylor, R. Increased Daily Walking Improves Lipid Oxidation Without Changes in Mitochondrial Function in Type 2 Diabetes. *Diabetes Care* **2008**, *31*, 1644–1649. [CrossRef] [PubMed]
7. Sinha, A.; Hollingsworth, K.G.; Ball, S.; Cheetham, T. Improving the Vitamin D Status of Vitamin D Deficient Adults Is Associated With Improved Mitochondrial Oxidative Function in Skeletal Muscle. *J. Clin. Endocrinol. Metab.* **2013**, *98*, E509–E513. [CrossRef] [PubMed]
8. Monangi, N.; Slaughter, J.L.; Dawodu, A.; Smith, C.; Akinbi, H.T. Vitamin D status of early preterm infants and the effects of vitamin D intake during hospital stay. *Arch. Dis. Child.-Fetal Neonatal Ed.* **2014**, *99*, F166–F168. [CrossRef]
9. McCarthy, R.A.; McKenna, M.J.; Oyefeso, O.; Uduma, O.; Murray, B.F.; Brady, J.J.; Kilbane, M.T.; Murphy, J.F.; Twomey, A.; O'Donnell, C.P.; et al. Vitamin D nutritional status in preterm infants and response to supplementation. *Br. J. Nutr.* **2013**, *110*, 156–163. [CrossRef]
10. Wood, C.L.; Tinnion, R.J.; Korada, S.M.; Cheetham, T.D.; Relton, C.L.; Cooke, R.J.; Pearce, M.S.; Hollingsworth, K.G.; Trenell, M.I.; Embleton, N.D. Growth and metabolic outcome in adolescents born preterm (GROWMORE): Follow-up protocol for the Newcastle Preterm Birth Growth study (PTBGS). *BMC Pediatr.* **2013**, *13*, 213. [CrossRef]
11. Cooke, R.J.; McCormick, K.; Griffin, I.J.; Embleton, N.; Faulkner, K.; Wells, J.C.; Rawlings, D.C. Feeding preterm infants after hospital discharge: Effect of diet on body composition. *Pediatr. Res.* **1999**, *46*, 461–464. [CrossRef] [PubMed]
12. Embleton, N.D.; Cooke, R.J. Protein requirements in preterm infants: Effect of different levels of protein intake on growth and body composition. *Pediatr. Res.* **2005**, *58*, 855–860. [CrossRef] [PubMed]
13. Fields, D.A.; Goran, M.I.; McCrory, M.A. Body-composition assessment via air-displacement plethysmography in adults and children: A review. *Am. J. Clin. Nutr.* **2002**, *75*, 453–467. [CrossRef] [PubMed]
14. Fields, D.A.; Hull, H.R.; Cheline, A.J.; Yao, M.; Higgins, P.B. Child-Specific Thoracic Gas Volume Prediction Equations for Air-Displacement Plethysmography. *Obes. Res.* **2004**, *12*, 1797–1804. [CrossRef]
15. Cole, T.J.; Freeman, J.V.; Preece, M.A. British 1990 growth reference centiles for weight, height, body mass index and head circumference fitted by maximum penalized likelihood. *Stat. Med.* **1998**, *17*, 407–429. Available online: http://www.ncbi.nlm.nih.gov/pubmed/9496720 (accessed on 11 July 2016). [CrossRef]
16. Vidmar, S.; Carlin, J.; Hesketh, K.; Cole, T. Standardizing anthropometric measures in children and adolescents with new functions for egen. *Stata J.* **2004**, *4*, 50–55. [CrossRef]
17. Campisi, S.C.; Marchand, J.D.; Siddiqui, F.J.; Islam, M.; Bhutta, Z.A.; Palmert, M.R. Can we rely on adolescents to self-assess puberty stage? A systematic review and meta-analysis. *J. Clin. Endocrinol. Metab.* **2020**, *105*, dgaa135. [CrossRef]
18. Colley, C.M.; Larner, J.R. The Use of Fortical in Glucose Tolerance Tests. *Ann. Clin. Biochem. Int. J. Biochem. Lab. Med.* **1990**, *27*, 496–498. [CrossRef]
19. Wallace, T.M.; Levy, J.C.; Matthews, D.R. Use and abuse of HOMA modeling. *Diabetes Care* **2004**, *27*, 1487–1495. [CrossRef]

20. Matsuda, M.; DeFronzo, R.A. Insulin sensitivity indices obtained from oral glucose tolerance testing: Comparison with the euglycemic insulin clamp. *Diabetes Care* **1999**, *22*, 1462–1470. [CrossRef]
21. Hossain, M.J.; Levinson, A.; George, D.; Canas, J.; Kumar, S.; Balagopal, P.B. Vitamin D Status and Cardiovascular Risk in Obesity: Effect of Physical Activity in Nonvitamin D Supplemented Adolescents. *Metab. Syndr. Relat. Disord.* **2018**, *16*, 197–203. [CrossRef] [PubMed]
22. Rock, C.L.; Emond, J.A.; Flatt, S.W.; Heath, D.D.; Karanja, N.; Pakiz, B.; Sherwood, N.E.; Thomson, C.A. Weight loss is associated with increased serum 25-hydroxyvitamin D in overweight or obese women. *Obesity* **2012**, *20*, 2296–2301. [CrossRef]
23. Evenson, K.R.; Catellier, D.J.; Gill, K.; Ondrak, K.S.; McMurray, R.G. Calibration of two objective measures of physical activity for children. *J. Sports Sci.* **2008**, *26*, 1557–1565. [CrossRef] [PubMed]
24. Basterfield, L.; Pearce, M.S.; Adamson, A.J.; Frary, J.K.; Parkinson, K.N.; Wright, C.M.; Reilly, J.J.; Gateshead Millennium Study Core Team. Physical Activity, Sedentary Behavior, and Adiposity in English Children. *Am. J. Prev. Med.* **2012**, *42*, 445–451. [CrossRef]
25. Jones, D.E.J.; Hollingsworth, K.G.; Taylor, R.; Blamire, A.M.; Newton, J.L. Abnormalities in pH handling by peripheral muscle and potential regulation by the autonomic nervous system in chronic fatigue syndrome. *J. Intern. Med.* **2010**, *267*, 394–401. [CrossRef] [PubMed]
26. Vanhamme, L.; van Huffel, S.; van Hecke, P.; van Ormondt, D. Time-Domain Quantification of Series of Biomedical Magnetic Resonance Spectroscopy Signals. *J. Magn. Reson.* **1999**, *140*, 120–130. [CrossRef] [PubMed]
27. Strong, W.B.; Malina, R.M.; Blimkie, C.J.; Daniels, S.R.; Dishman, R.K.; Gutin, B.; Hergenroeder, A.C.; Must, A.; Nixon, P.A.; Pivarnik, J.M.; et al. Evidence Based Physical Activity for School-age Youth. *J. Pediatr.* **2005**, *146*, 732–737. [CrossRef]
28. Basterfield, L.; Adamson, A.J.; Parkinson, K.N.; Maute, U.; Li, P.X.; Reilly, J.J.; Gateshead Millennium Study Core Team. Surveillance of physical activity in the UK is flawed: Validation of the Health Survey for England Physical Activity Questionnaire. *Arch. Dis. Child.* **2008**, *93*, 1054–1058. [CrossRef] [PubMed]
29. Rosenkranz, R.R.; Duncan, M.J.; Caperchione, C.M.; Kolt, G.S.; Vandelanotte, C.; Maeder, A.J.; Savage, T.N.; Mummery, W.K. Validity of the Stages of Change in Steps instrument (SoC-Step) for achieving the physical activity goal of 10,000 steps per day. *BMC Public Health* **2015**, *15*, 1197. [CrossRef]
30. Bertocci, L.A.; Mize, C.E.; Uauy, R. Muscle phosphorus energy state in very-low-birth-weight infants: Effect of exercise. *Am. J. Physiol.* **1992**, *262 Pt 1*, E289–E294. [CrossRef]
31. Rogers, M.; Fay, T.B.; Whitfield, M.F.; Tomlinson, J.; Grunau, R.E. Aerobic Capacity, Strength, Flexibility, and Activity Level in Unimpaired Extremely Low Birth Weight (<=800 g) Survivors at 17 Years of Age Compared With Term-Born Control Subjects. *Pediatrics* **2005**, *116*, e58–e65. [CrossRef] [PubMed]
32. Keens, T.G.; Bryan, A.C.; Levison, H.; Ianuzzo, C.D. Developmental pattern of muscle fiber types in human ventilatory muscles. *J. Appl. Physiol.* **1978**, *44*, 909–913. [CrossRef] [PubMed]
33. Schloon, H.; Schlottmann, J.; Lenard, H.G.; Goebel, H.H. The development of skeletal muscles in premature infants. I. Fibre size and histochemical differentiation. *Eur. J. Pediatr.* **1979**, *131*, 49–60. [CrossRef] [PubMed]
34. Vogler, C.; Bove, K.E. Morphology of skeletal muscle in children. An assessment of normal growth and differentiation. *Arch. Pathol. Lab. Med.* **1985**, *109*, 238–242. [PubMed]
35. Burris, H.H.; Van Marter, L.J.; McElrath, T.F.; Tabatabai, P.; Litonjua, A.A.; Weiss, S.T.; Christou, H. Vitamin D status among preterm and full-term infants at birth. *Pediatr. Res.* **2014**, *75*, 75–80. [CrossRef]
36. Chiu, K.C.; Chu, A.; Go, V.L.W.; Saad, M.F. Hypovitaminosis D is associated with insulin resistance and β cell dysfunction. *Am. J. Clin. Nutr.* **2004**, *79*, 820–825. [CrossRef]
37. Forouhi, N.G.; Luan, J.; Cooper, A.; Boucher, B.J.; Wareham, N.J. Baseline Serum 25-Hydroxy Vitamin D Is Predictive of Future Glycemic Status and Insulin Resistance: The Medical Research Council Ely Prospective Study 1990-2000. *Diabetes* **2008**, *57*, 2619–2625. [CrossRef]
38. Liu, E.; Meigs, J.B.; Pittas, A.G.; McKeown, N.M.; Economos, C.D.; Booth, S.L.; Jacques, P.F. Plasma 25-Hydroxyvitamin D Is Associated with Markers of the Insulin Resistant Phenotype in Nondiabetic Adults. *J. Nutr.* **2009**, *139*, 329–334. [CrossRef]
39. Baz-Hecht, M.; Goldfine, A.B. The impact of vitamin D deficiency on diabetes and cardiovascular risk. *Curr. Opin. Endocrinol. Diabetes Obes.* **2010**, *17*, 113–119. [CrossRef]
40. Belenchia, A.M.; Tosh, A.K.; Hillman, L.S.; Peterson, C.A. Correcting vitamin D insufficiency improves insulin sensitivity in obese adolescents: A randomized controlled trial. *Am. J. Clin. Nutr.* **2013**, *97*, 774–781. [CrossRef]
41. Kelishadi, R.; Salek, S.; Salek, M.; Hashemipour, M.; Movahedian, M. Effects of vitamin D supplementation on insulin resistance and cardiometabolic risk factors in children with metabolic syndrome: A triple-masked controlled trial. *J. Pediatr. (Rio J.)* **2014**, *90*, 28–34. [CrossRef] [PubMed]
42. Psarra, A.-M.G.; Solakidi, S.; Sekeris, C.E. The mitochondrion as a primary site of action of steroid and thyroid hormones: Presence and action of steroid and thyroid hormone receptors in mitochondria of animal cells. *Mol. Cell Endocrinol.* **2006**, *246*, 21–33. [CrossRef] [PubMed]
43. Jiménez-Pavón, D.; Kelly, J.; Reilly, J.J. Associations between objectively measured habitual physical activity and adiposity in children and adolescents: Systematic review. *Int. J. Pediatr. Obes.* **2010**, *5*, 3–18. [CrossRef]
44. Basterfield, L.; Adamson, A.J.; Pearce, M.S.; Reilly, J.J. Stability of habitual physical activity and sedentary behavior monitoring by accelerometry in 6- to 8-year-olds. *J. Phys. Act Health* **2011**, *8*, 543–547. [CrossRef] [PubMed]

45. Embleton, N.D.; Korada, M.; Wood, C.L.; Pearce, M.S.; Swamy, R.; Cheetham, T.D. Catch-up growth and metabolic outcomes in adolescents born preterm. *Arch. Dis. Child.* **2016**, *101*, 1026–1031. [CrossRef] [PubMed]
46. Tinnion, R.; Gillone, J.; Cheetham, T.; Embleton, N. Preterm birth and subsequent insulin sensitivity: A systematic review. *Arch. Dis. Child.* **2014**, *99*, 362–368. [CrossRef] [PubMed]
47. Fonseca, F.; Amaral, F.; Lima, N.; Ornelas, E.; Simardi, L.; Maifrino, L.B.M. Effect of different exercise intensities on the pancreas of animals with metabolic syndrome. *Diabetes Metab. Syndr. Obes. Targets Ther.* **2015**, *8*, 115. [CrossRef] [PubMed]
48. Loprinzi, P.D.; Lee, H.; Cardinal, B.J. Evidence to Support Including Lifestyle Light-Intensity Recommendations in Physical Activity Guidelines for Older Adults. *Am. J. Health Promot.* **2015**, *29*, 277–284. [CrossRef]
49. Herzig, K.-H.; Ahola, R.; Leppäluoto, J.; Jokelainen, J.; Jämsä, T.; Keinänen-Kiukaanniemi, S. Light physical activity determined by a motion sensor decreases insulin resistance, improves lipid homeostasis and reduces visceral fat in high-risk subjects: PreDiabEx study RCT. *Int. J. Obes.* **2014**, *38*, 1089–1096. [CrossRef]
50. Sinha, A.; Hollingsworth, K.G.; Ball, S.; Cheetham, T. Impaired quality of life in growth hormone-deficient adults is independent of the altered skeletal muscle oxidative metabolism found in conditions with peripheral fatigue. *Clin. Endocrinol.* **2014**, *80*, 107–114. [CrossRef]
51. Iotti, S.; Lodi, R.; Frassineti, C.; Zaniol, P.; Barbiroli, B. In vivo assessment of mitochondrial functionality in human gastrocnemius muscle by 31P MRS. The role of pH in the evaluation of phosphocreatine and inorganic phosphate recoveries from exercise. *NMR Biomed.* **1993**, *6*, 248–253. [CrossRef] [PubMed]

nutrients

MDPI

Article

Supplementation of Mother's Own Milk with Preterm Donor Human Milk: Impact on Protein Intake and Growth in Very Low Birth Weight Infants—A Randomized Controlled Study

Giannoula Gialeli [1], Anastasia Kapetanaki [1], Ourania Panagopoulou [1], Panagiota Vourna [1], Athanasios Michos [2], Christina Kanaka-Gantenbein [2], George Liosis [1] and Tania Siahanidou [2,*]

[1] Neonatal Intensive Care Unit, "Elena Venizelou" General and Maternal Hospital, 11521 Athens, Greece
[2] First Department of Pediatrics, Medical School, National & Kapodistrian University of Athens, 11527 Athens, Greece
* Correspondence: siahan@med.uoa.gr; Tel.: +30-2132013-517

Abstract: This randomized study investigates whether feeding very low birth weight (VLBW) infants with mother's own milk (MOM) supplemented with either preterm (PDM) or term donor milk (TDM), when MOM is insufficient, has a positive impact on infants' protein intake and growth. A hundred and twenty VLBW infants were randomized into two groups. Group A (43 infants) received MOM supplemented with PDM, whereas Group B (77 infants) was fed with MOM supplemented with TDM, for the first three weeks of life (donor milk period). Breast milk fortifier was added when milk feeds exceeded 50 mL/Kg/day. After the donor milk period, both groups were fed with formula when MOM was not available or the milk bank was unable to provide TDM. Protein intake was higher in Group A than in Group B at initiation of milk fortification ($p = 0.006$), as well as during the 3-week donor milk period ($p = 0.023$) and throughout hospitalization ($p = 0.014$). Moreover, Group A presented higher Δz-score for body weight ($p = 0.019$) and head circumference ($p = 0.001$) from birth to the end of donor milk period, and higher mean body weight at discharge ($p = 0.047$) compared to Group B. In conclusion, when donor milk is required, PDM positively impacts protein intake and growth in VLBW infants (NCT05675397).

Keywords: preterm donor milk; mother's own milk; growth; VLBW infants; protein; fortification

1. Introduction

Human milk is the best nutritional option for infants, especially those born preterm [1–7]. Feeding with mother's own milk (MOM) is considered to be an important factor in increasing the survival and improving outcomes of very low birth weight (VLBW) infants (<1500 g) in the last two decades [8–11]. However, a considerable number of mothers delivering preterm struggle to provide adequate milk the first days after delivery to meet their infants' requirements. When MOM is not sufficient, pasteurized donor milk (DM) is the best alternative according to current recommendations [7,12–14].

Nowadays, many maternity hospitals have organized milk banks in order to cater the needs of premature infants. Donor milk is primarily derived from mothers of term-born infants for the first six months of lactation [15]. This term milk presents significant differences compared to preterm human milk which has higher protein concentration and more caloric energy [16]. According to Bauer et al., protein content in extremely preterm human milk versus term human milk differs by 0.73 g/dl and provides almost 10 kcal/dl more energy [17].

According to ESPGHAN guidelines, VLBW infants have high needs of protein intake soon after birth [18]. For the first critical week of life, Stephens et al. have demonstrated that an increase in protein intake by 1 g/kg/day is associated with better neurodevelopmental outcome [19]. After this short period, preterm MOM needs fortification in order to meet the nutrient requirements of VLBW infants whose needs are dynamic and related to postnatal age, severity of illness, and need for catch-up growth [20–22]. In most neonatal intensive care units (NICUs), fortification is initiated when the fed milk volume reaches 50–100 mL/kg/day [23,24]. However, for VLBW infants, this delay may result in significant protein deficit during the first weeks of life. This is a primary concern in infants fed with term donor milk given the fact that protein amounts in human milk tend to decrease with postnatal age [25].

We hypothesized that feeding VLBW infants with preterm donor milk (PDM) in combination with MOM may positively influence the protein intake and, consequently, the infants' growth. The aim of the current study was to assess whether MOM supplementation with PDM has any beneficial effects on energy and protein intake and growth in VLBW infants.

2. Materials and Methods

2.1. Study Design and Participants

This is a randomized, controlled, double-blind study conducted in a level III NICU, at "Elena Venizelou" General and Maternal Hospital in Athens, Greece. VLBW infants with birth weight <1500 g and born to mothers who had agreed to feed their babies with donor milk for the first three weeks of life (donor milk period) if their own milk quantity was insufficient were enrolled in the study from April 2017 to August 2021. Infants were excluded if they had congenital anomalies, chromosomal disorders or metabolic diseases. Also, any infant fed with formula at any point during the donor milk period was not eligible to participate in the study.

The Ethics Committee of "Elena Venizelou" General and Maternal Hospital approved the investigation and each infant's parent provided written informed consent before participating in the study.

2.2. Eligible Donor Mothers

Mothers who gave birth at <35 weeks of gestation could become donors of preterm milk (PDM) until they reach 34^{+6} weeks of corrected gestational age and only during their first four weeks of lactation. Also, the Milk Bank of "Elena Venizelou" hospital provided term donor milk (TDM) from eligible mothers who expressed breast milk for a period up to six months post-delivery. All eligible donor mothers were serologically screened for infectious diseases including hepatitis B and C, Human Immunodeficiency virus, Cytomegalovirus, and Syphilis [26]

2.3. Collection and Storage of Donor Human Milk

DM was collected in a special container and was processed by the "Elena Venizelou" Milk Bank using the Holder Pasteurization method (human milk was heated to 62.5 °C for 30 min) and quickly cooled down to 25 °C within 10 min in an ice water bath; it was then stored in a refrigerator at a temperature of 0–4 °C for one to two days or frozen at −20 °C for three to six months. Single donor expressed human milk was collected and pasteurized separately.

2.4. Feeding Protocol and Analysis of Human Milk

Following enrollment, infants were randomly assigned using a sequentially numbered sealed opaque envelope system with a ratio 1:2 to be fed with MOM supplemented, if required, either with PDM (Group A) or with TDM (Group B). If MOM was completely unavailable, the infant was fed with pasteurized PDM or TDM following randomization. Neither the attending physicians nor the nurses were aware of the type of donor milk. Only the principal investigator (not involved in the care of enrolled infants) knew the type of donor milk provided.

Pasteurized PDM or TDM, as supplementary to MOM or for exclusive feeding, was provided to the study population for a three-week period after birth (defined as donor milk period) during which time the milk was analyzed regularly for protein and calorie content. After the donor milk period and until discharge, increasing demands were met with formula supplementation if MOM was not available or the milk bank was unable to provide TDM.

Parenteral nutrition was started immediately after birth for all infants. Feeding of unfortified MOM or pasteurized DM from the hospital's milk bank was initiated within the first three days of life. Powder breast milk fortifier (BMF) was added to human milk when milk intake reached 50–100 mL/kg/day. In all cases, a standard fortification with BMF (Nutricia Human Milk Fortifier) was applied (two sachets BMF per 100 mL of milk) according to the manufacturer's instructions. Each sachet of fortifier (2.2 g) provided 0.6 g of protein in the form of extensively hydrolyzed bovine whey protein and 8 kcal of energy. The fortifier was introduced at half dose (1 sachet per 100 mL) for two to three days and then increased to full dose (2 sachets per 100 mL).

Since sampling and pooling of milk samples after a full breast expression at each feed across a 24-hour period is considered the "gold standard" for human milk collection [16,27], MOM was collected throughout the last 24 h. Frozen DM (PDM or TDM) was thawed before it was administered to neonates within 24 h. A random representative sample of the human milk pool (MOM or DM) was analyzed, before fortification, once a week using a MIRIS Human Milk Analyzer (HMA™, Miris AB, Uppsala, Sweden). The Miris HMA is based on semi-solid mid-infrared (MIR) transmission spectroscopy. A calibration check was performed prior to analysis using the calibration solution provided by the supplier. For the analyzer, a 2 mL sample of milk was required, which was heated at 40 °C in a thermostatic bath before undergoing analysis. In this study, Miris HMA was used to record the amount of protein and caloric energy content of milk samples.

2.5. Data Collection

The following parameters were recorded in all infants during hospitalization:

- CRIB II score (Clinical Risk Index for Babies), a validated measure of initial mortality risk and illness severity within the first hour of admission [28].
- Anthropometric characteristics (body weight and length, head circumference) at birth, at the end of donor milk period and at discharge. The anthropometric characteristics were recorded as both absolute values and z-scores; z-scores were documented according to the revised Fenton growth charts using the PediTools [29]. Small for gestational age (SGA) status was defined as birthweight z-score less than −2 SD from the mean. The difference (Δz-score) of z-score for body weight, body length and head circumference from birth to the end of donor milk period, as well as from birth to discharge, was calculated.
- Total protein and energy intake through parenteral nutrition, MOM, DM and fortification.
- Neonatal/Infant Morbidity. In particular:
    - Culture-positive sepsis (clinical signs of infection plus positive blood, urine or cerebrospinal fluid culture).
    - Necrotizing Enterocolitis (NEC) if fulfilling criteria compatible with Bell's stage 2 or higher.
    - Bronchopulmonary dysplasia (BPD) defined as need for supplemental oxygen for more than 28 days.
    - Retinopathy of prematurity (ROP)—if fulfilling criteria compatible with Stage 3 according to international classification of retinopathy of prematurity (2005) [30].
    - Intraventricular hemorrhage (IVH)—any degree.
    - Patent ductus arteriosus (PDA) (presence of clinical signs plus ductal left to right shunt in echocardiography).

2.6. Statistical Analysis

Quantitative variables were expressed as mean values (standard deviation; SD) or as median (interquartile range; IQR), while qualitative variables were expressed as absolute and relative frequencies. For comparison of proportions, chi-square and Fisher's exact tests were used. Independent samples Student's t-tests or Mann-Whitney U tests were used, as appropriate, for comparisons between Group A and Group B. Repeated measurements analysis of variance (ANOVA) was applied to evaluate changes in total protein intake between groups over the donor milk period. In order to evaluate the change in pasteurized donor milk quantity received by the study population over the donor milk period, linear mixed regression was applied and regression coefficients (β) with standard errors (SE) were computed. Sensitivity analysis was also run after excluding infants born to mothers with multiple pregnancies. All reported p values are two-tailed. Statistical significance was set at $p < 0.05$ and analyses were conducted using the SPSS statistical software (version 22.0).

3. Results

A hundred and thirty-eight VLBW infants were enrolled in the study. Of them, 18 infants were excluded after randomization due to transportation, death before discharge or parental decision to withdraw the consent for their child participation. Finally, 120 infants allocated to Group A (n = 43) or Group B (n = 77) were studied (Figure 1).

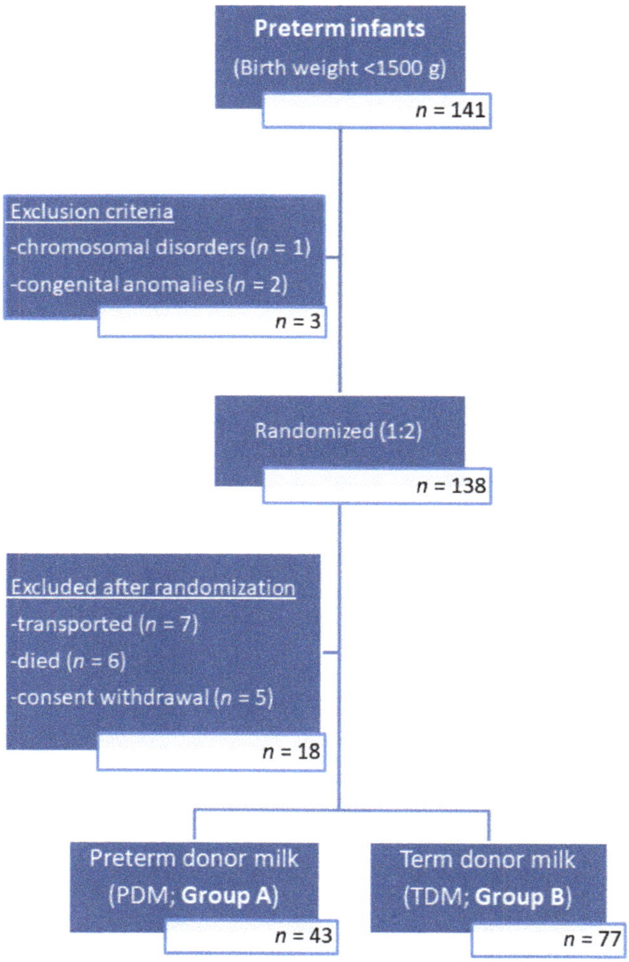

Figure 1. Flow chart of the study population.

Maternal age, gestational age, multiple pregnancies, infants' gender, anthropometric characteristics at birth, SGA status, CRIB II score and length of hospitalization did not differ significantly between Group A and Group B (Table 1).

Table 1. Demographic and clinical parameters of the study population.

	Total Population (N = 120)	**Group A (N = 43)**	**Group B (N = 77)**	***p*-Value**
	Mean (SD)	***Mean (SD)***	***Mean (SD)***	
Mother's age (years)	33.8 (5.1)	32.7 (5.0)	34.4 (5.0)	0.233 +
Gestational age (weeks)	29.7 (2.5)	29.7 (2.4)	29.7 (2.5)	0.959 +
	N (%)	*N (%)*	*N (%)*	
Pregnancy				
Single	88 (73.3)	30 (69.8)	52 (67.5)	0.484 ‡
Multiple	32 (26.7)	13 (30.2)	25 (32.5)	
Gender				
Females	47 (39.2)	14 (32.6)	33 (42.9)	0.268 ‡
Males	73 (60.8)	29 (67.4)	44 (57.1)	
SGA	10 (8.3)	3 (7.0)	7 (9.1)	0.489 ‡
	Mean (SD)	*Mean (SD)*	*Mean (SD)*	
Birth Weight (g)	1169.8 (234.1)	1182.9 (257.6)	1162.5 (221.3)	0.649 +
Birth Weight z-score	−0.48 (0.98)	−0.48 (0.93)	−0.48 (1.01)	0.987 +
Body length at birth (cm)	38.0 (3.3)	38.2 (3.1)	37.8 (3.3)	0.562 +
Body length z-score	−0.20 (1.14)	−0.13 (1.21)	−0.24 (1.11)	0.598 +
Head circumference at birth (cm)	26.6 (2.0)	26.5 (2.1)	26.7 (1.9)	0.720 +
Head circumference z-score at birth	−0.24 (1.26)	−0.38 (1.25)	−0.16 (1.26)	0.362 +
CRIB II score	6.9 (3.1)	6.8 (3.1)	6.9 (3.2)	0.878 +
	Median (IQR)	*Median (IQR)*	*Median (IQR)*	
Length of hospitalization (days)	56.5 (45.0–69.5)	58.0 (47.0–68.0)	55.0 (42.0–72.0)	0.465 ++

Group A: VLBW infants fed with MOM supplemented, if needed, with preterm donor milk (PDM); Group B: VLBW infants fed with MOM supplemented, if needed, with term donor milk (TDM); + Student's *t*-test; ++ Mann-Whitney test, ‡ Pearson's chi-square test.

PDM and TDM for feeding were derived from 26 and 43 donor mothers, respectively. As expected, gestational age was significantly lower in mothers who provided PDM compared to mothers who provided TDM ($p < 0.001$). No difference was recorded in maternal age ($p = 0.130$), parity ($p = 0.100$) and multiple gestation ($p = 0.138$) between preterm and term donor mothers (Table 2).

Table 2. Characteristics of donor mothers.

	Total Population (N = 69)	**PDM Mothers (N = 26)**	**TDM Mothers (N = 43)**	***p*-Value**
Gestational age, weeks	34.7 (4.6)	29.8 (2.7)	38.0 (2.0)	<0.001 +
Maternal age, years	33.7 (3.7)	32.9 (4.0)	34.3 (3.4)	0.130 +
Parity, N (%)				
1st	42 (60.9)	20 (76.9)	22 (51.2)	
2nd	26 (37.7)	6 (23.1)	20 (46.5)	0.138 ‡
3rd	1 (1.4)	0 (0)	1 (2.3)	
Multiple gestation, N (%)	6 (8.7)	4 (15.4)	2 (4.6)	0.138 ‡

PDM, preterm donor milk; TDM, term donor milk; + Student's *t*-test; ‡ Pearson's chi-square test.

The proportion of pasteurized DM (PDM or TDM) diminished significantly over time ($\beta = -3.56$; SE = 0.47; $p < 0.001$). However, the degree of change did not differ significantly between the two groups ($\beta = -0.35$; SE = 0.98; $p = 0.719$). Moreover, following the donor milk period, no difference was recorded in the proportion of formula supplementation until discharge between groups [mean (SD): 27.9 (24.4)% in Group A vs. 21.7 (25.2)% in Group B; $p = 0.123$).

3.1. Protein and Calorie Intake

Mean protein intake during the donor milk period was significantly higher in Group A than in Group B ($p = 0.023$). When protein intake was assessed at each week separately, a significant difference between groups was observed at week 3 after birth ($p = 0.01$).

Protein intake was also significantly higher in Group A than in Group B at initiation of breast milk fortification ($p = 0.006$) and throughout hospitalization ($p = 0.014$) (Table 3).

Table 3. Protein intake (g/kg/day) of the study population.

	Total Population (N = 120)	Group A (N = 43)	Group B (N = 77)	*p*-Value
	Mean (SD)	Mean (SD)	Mean (SD)	
During hospitalization	3.03 (0.57)	3.20 (0.60)	2.93 (0.54)	**0.014 +**
Donor milk period				
1st week	3.35 (1.05)	3.53 (1.10)	3.25 (1.01)	
2nd week	3.53 (1.13)	3.67 (1.05)	3.45 (1.17)	**0.023 ++**
3rd week	3.36 (0.99)	3.67 (0.96)	3.19 (0.97)	
At initiation of human milk fortification	3.24 (0.84)	3.57 (0.82)	2.92 (0.85)	**0.006 +**

Group A: VLBW infants fed with MOM supplemented, if needed, with preterm donor milk (PDM); Group B: VLBW infants fed with MOM supplemented, if needed, with term donor milk (TDM); in bold: significant *p*-values, $p < 0.05$; + Student's *t*-test, ++ repeated measurements analysis of variance (ANOVA).

Calorie intake during the donor milk period [median (IQR): 115.4 (105.0–129.7) kcal/kg/day in Group A vs. 114.0 (101.3–133.8) kcal/Kg/day in Group B] and during the entire hospitalization [107.0 (96.0–116.5) kcal/kg/day in Group A vs. 102.3 (92.6–111.2) kcal/kg/day in Group B] did not differ significantly between the two groups ($p = 0.782$ and $p = 0.164$, respectively).

3.2. Growth

At the end of donor milk period, no difference was recorded between Group A and Group B in body weight z-score [−1.12 (0.87) vs. −1.28 (0.84); $p = 0.309$), body length z-score [−0.41 (1.00) vs. −0.48 (1.06); $p = 0.705$) or head circumference z-score [−0.13 (0.95) vs. −0.38 (1.14); $p = 0.215$). However, Δz-score in body weight and head circumference from birth to the end of donor milk period differed significantly between Group A [−0.63 (0.34) and 0.26 (0.72), respectively] and Group B [−0.81 (0.39); $p = 0.019$ and −0.22 (0.72); $p = 0.001$, respectively]. No difference was found in Δz-score for body length between groups [−0.28 (0.66) vs. −0.25 (0.56); $p = 0.720$) (Figure 2).

At discharge, body weight was significantly higher in Group A [mean (SD): 2560.7 (423.4) g] than in Group B [2411.8 (370.5) g; $p = 0.047$] (Figure S1). However, body weight z-score [−1.61 (1.02) in Group A vs. −1.70 (0.94) in Group B] and Δz-score from birth to discharge [−1.13 (0.68) in Group A vs. −1.23 (0.86) in Group B] did not differ significantly between groups ($p = 0.627$ and $p = 0.542$, respectively).

Body length z-score [−0.92 (1.39) vs. −0.97 (1.11); $p = 0.814$) and Δz-score from birth to discharge [−0.79 (1.02) vs. −0.73 (0.73); $p = 0.708$), as well as head circumference z-score [−0.46 (0.98) vs. −0.55 (0.97); $p = 0.643$) and Δz-score [−0.08 (1.24) vs. −0.39 (1.11); $p = 0.169$) did not differ significantly between the two groups.

In the sensitivity analysis, after excluding infants from multiple pregnancies, the results of the study did not change.

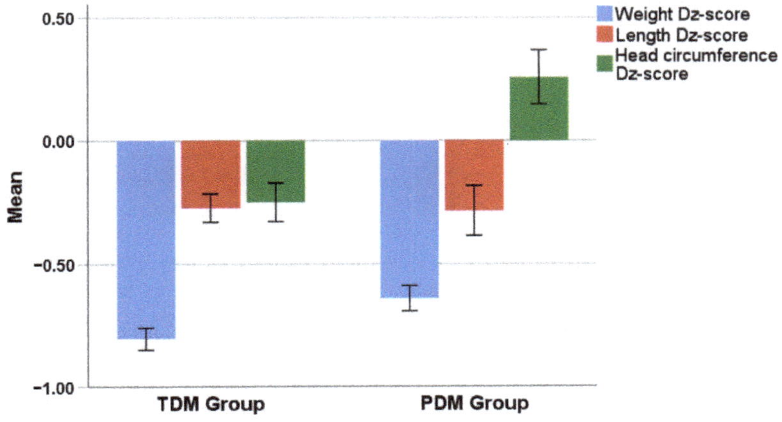

Figure 2. Δz-scores for body weight (p = 0.019), body length (p = 0.720) and head circumference (p = 0.001) from birth to the end of intervention (donor milk period) between preterm (PDM) and term donor milk (TDM) Group.

3.3. Clinical Characteristics and Morbidity during Hospitalization

No significant difference was found between groups in time to regain birth weight [median (IQR): 8.0 (7.0–13.0) days in Group A vs. 10.0 (8.0–14.0) days in Group B; p = 0.09] or in time to full enteral feeds of at least 150 mL/Kg/day [12.0 (9.0–18.0) days in Group A vs. 14.0 (10.0–21.0) days in Group B; p = 0.245].

Morbidity during hospitalization did not differ significantly between groups (Table 4).

Table 4. Morbidity of the study population during hospitalization.

	Total Population (N = 120)	Group A (N = 43)	Group B (N = 77)	*p*-Value
	N (%)	N (%)	N (%)	
Sepsis				
No	91 (75.8)	35 (81.4)	56 (72.7)	0.288 +
Yes	29 (24.2)	8 (18.6)	21 (27.3)	
Necrotizing enterocolitis				
No	118 (98.3)	42 (97.7)	76 (98.7)	1.000 ++
Yes	2 (1.7)	1 (2.3)	1 (1.3)	
Retinopathy of prematurity				
No	116 (96.7)	41 (95.3)	75 (97.4)	0.617 ++
Yes	4 (3.3)	2 (4.7)	2 (2.6)	
Bronchopulmonary dysplasia				
No	75 (62.5)	24 (55.8)	51 (66.2)	0.258 +
Yes	45 (37.5)	19 (44.2)	26 (33.8)	
Intraventricular hemorrhage				
No	116 (96.7)	42 (97.7)	74 (96.1)	1.000 ++
Yes	4 (3.3)	1 (2.3)	3 (3.9)	
Patent Ductus Arteriosus				
No	73 (84.9)	23 (85.2)	50 (84.7)	1.000 ++
Yes	13 (15.1)	4 (14.8)	9 (15.3)	

Group A: VLBW infants fed with MOM supplemented, if needed, with preterm donor milk (PDM); Group B: VLBW infants fed with MOM supplemented, if needed, with term donor milk (TDM); + Pearson's chi-square test; ++ Fisher's exact test.

4. Discussion

Optimal growth of VLBW infants is a primary goal in NICU but not easy to achieve. Growth failure was observed in 80% of VLBW infants in studies conducted under the Neonatal Research Network between 2008 and 2010 [31]. In 2013, among infants cared for in hospitals affiliated with the Vermont Oxford Network, 50.3% demonstrated growth failure at the time of hospital discharge [32]. Similarly, according to data obtained from the Korean Neonatal Network database from 2013 to 2014, the overall incidence of postnatal growth failure in VLBW infants was 45.5% [33]. Providing adequate nutrition is of paramount importance since growth failure has been associated with neurodevelopmental impairment. Especially protein intake has been strongly linked to the accomplishment of optimal growth and development in VLBW infants [34,35]. Stephens et al. have showed that an increase in protein intake by 1 g/kg per day during the first week of life was independently associated with more than an 8-point increase in Mental Developmental Index (MDI) at 18 months of age [19]. Growth failure occurs when nutrient intake is inadequate over a period of time. The exact timing and duration of this inadequacy has yet to be determined exactly in the preterm population. According to ESPGHAN guidelines [18] based on the protein needs and nitrogen utilization, the protein intake should be at least 3 g/kg/day for preterm infants up to a weight of approximately 1800 g. Unfortunately, in most studies the exact composition of human milk is unknown and clinicians estimate the nutrient content of each mother's milk according to specified references [16].

In this study, the composition of milk was accurately measured using a human milk analyzer (Miris HMA); the analyzer was used to capture the exact composition of MOM and DM at set time intervals. Miris HMA was not used as a tool for individualized fortification since breast milk samples in both groups were similarly fortified per manufacturer guidelines and regardless of measured protein concentration in order to fulfill the goals of the study. It is well known that the protein concentration of milk from mothers delivering preterm is initially higher than that from mothers delivering at term [36] but decreases after the first weeks of lactation [17]. This is the reason why, in this study, preterm donor milk was used only if expressed within the first four weeks after childbirth [37]. Maternal age, parity and multiple gestations that might have also impacted the breast milk nutrients composition [38,39] did not differ significantly between the two study groups.

The results of this study indicate that protein intake was greater in VLBW infants when MOM was supplemented with preterm rather than term donor milk. These infants fulfilled during the donor milk period the minimum protein requirements according to both ESPGHAN guidelines (3 g/kg/day) [18] and EMBA working group recommendation (3.5–4.5 g/kg/day) [24]. It is worth noting that on the day of initiation of human milk fortification, protein intake was significantly higher in Group A compared to Group B (3.57 g/kg/day vs. 2.92 g/kg/day, $p = 0.006$) which indicates the higher provision of protein by preterm donor milk *per se*. Although both groups achieved over 3 g/kg/day of protein intake during the first vulnerable week of life, as well as throughout the whole donor milk period, only Group A surpassed the amount of 3.5 g/kg/day which is in line with the most recent recommendations [24,40]. However, more studies are needed to determine the exact protein requirement for this population and whether it should be different in the extrauterine environment compared to the intrauterine one.

The above results demonstrate that feeding VLBW infants with PDM, when MOM is not sufficient, and starting fortification when the quantity of enteral feeds reaches 50–100 mL/kg/day, protein intake surpasses the amount of 3.5 g/kg/day as ESPGHAN (2022) recommends [40]. The precise time to commence fortifiers is not known. Few data exist whether early (<40 mL/kg/day) versus delayed (>75 mL/kg/day) initiation of fortification may be beneficial [41]. Current recommendations of ESPGHAN propose starting a fortifier when enteral intakes reach 40–100 mL/kg/day [40]. An individualized fortification strategy (i.e., adjustable or targeted) was also proposed [40].

Overall, there are great discrepancies in literature regarding the effect of early nutrition on anthropometric parameters of VLBW infants, especially when pasteurized donor milk is used. It is important to note in previous studies whether the results were documented before or after the practice of human milk fortification was initiated. Historically, before the era of human milk fortification, studies showed that infants fed with MOM supplemented with pasteurized DM exhibited growth retardation based on anthropometric measurements of body weight, length and head circumference over a period of time [42]. In contrast, studies conducted after the implementation of human milk fortification have shown that VLBW infants fed with MOM supplemented with donor milk have similar or even faster growth rates than the ones fed with MOM supplemented with preterm formula [43]. Ginovart et al. studied two groups of VLBW infants. The first group included 72 infants born prior to the initiation of human milk fortification and fed exclusively with formula. The second group included 114 infants born after the implementation of fortification of MOM and DM. The conclusion of that study was that formula may not be appropriate for initiation of feeding in preterm infants [44]. On the contrary, in a 2017 study by Madore et al. [45], very preterm infants fed MOM supplemented with donor milk had lower weight gain during the first month of life than those fed only MOM or MOM supplemented with preterm formula. Thus, further studies on this issue are needed.

In 2014, Dritsakou et al. [15] compared two groups of VLBW infants; one fed with MOM supplemented with term donor milk until discharge and the other fed exclusively with donor milk for the first three weeks of life followed by formula, if necessary, until discharge. Human milk was fortified in both groups. The first group showed greater head circumference and body length, whereas there was no difference in body weight between the two groups [15]. In the present study, donor milk is further categorized by mothers' length of gestation at birth (term versus preterm). No difference was found in infants' body length; however, Δz-score of body weight and head circumference from birth to the end of intervention differed significantly between groups. Moreover, body weight at discharge was by 6.2% higher in Group A than in Group B; this fact indicates that the nutrient composition of preterm versus term donor milk has a positive impact on infants' growth. It is also worth noting that Group A infants reached full enteral feeding two days earlier than Group B which is very important since it limits the use of indwelling catheters and the associated risk of infection [31].

The novelty in the design of this study was the comparison of PDM with TDM. To our knowledge, this is the first study that investigates the potential benefits of preterm donor milk on protein intake and growth in preterm infants. Only Fang et al. [46] evaluated recently, in 2021, whether preterm donor milk might have any beneficial effects in VLBW infants. However, in that study, preterm donor milk was compared to formula, not to term donor milk. Moreover, preterm donor milk was firstly expressed from mothers at 3.4 ± 2.2 weeks postpartum (when protein content naturally declines) whereas, in our study, preterm donor milk was expressed from delivery throughout the first four weeks postpartum.

Another strength of this study was the use of breast milk analyzer (Miris HMA) which allowed for the direct measurement of the exact protein concentration in MOM, PDM and TDM. In most studies, milk protein content is estimated using median calculated values in term donor milk [40,47] whereas in our study protein content was measured in each infant's feeds separately. This is one of the first studies in which the protein content of pasteurized preterm donor milk is determined. Landers et al. have also mentioned the reported preterm donor human milk composition from Australian mothers in order to provide evidence for the efficacy of feeding donor human milk to premature infants [48].

Limitations of this study were associated with the difficulty in recruiting mothers delivering preterm. As a result, preterm donor milk was in limited supply and thus the donor milk period was restricted to the first three weeks of life. The limited source of preterm donor milk has also impacted the number of infants enrolled in the study.

5. Conclusions

This study showed that feeding VLBW infants with MOM supplemented (when necessary) with pasteurized PDM has a positive impact on protein intake, as well as on body weight and head circumference at the end of the three-week intervention. Although the absolute value of body weight was also positively impacted at discharge, Δz-scores of anthropometric characteristics studied from birth to discharge did not differ significantly between groups. Whether, in our study population, the positive impact of PDM on growth during the initial vulnerable period of life might also have beneficial effects on neurodevelopment later in life remains to be further studied. Considering the unique nutritional needs of VLBW infants, milk banks should prioritize feeding them with milk expressed from mothers delivering prematurely when MOM is unavailable or insufficient. Efforts should be made to match, if possible, the prematurity level of donor milk to that of the infant.

To our knowledge, this is one of the first studies where PDM was used and analyzed for its nutritional content. Further research is required to establish the short- and long-term effects of feeding VLBW infants with PDM if required.

Supplementary Materials: The following supporting information can be downloaded at: https://www.mdpi.com/article/10.3390/nu15030566/s1, Figure S1: Body Weight at discharge in the two groups.

Author Contributions: Conceptualization, G.L.; methodology, G.L. and T.S.; software, G.G. and G.L.; validation, G.G. and C.K.-G.; formal analysis, G.G., T.S. and O.P.; investigation, G.G., A.K. and P.V.; resources, G.G., G.L., A.K., P.V. and O.P.; data curation, G.G., G.L. and A.M.; writing—original draft preparation, G.G., O.P., A.K. and P.V.; writing—review and editing, G.L., T.S., A.M. and C.K.-G.; visualization, G.L. and G.G.; supervision, G.L. and T.S.; project administration, T.S. All authors have read and agreed to the published version of the manuscript.

Funding: This research received no external funding.

Institutional Review Board Statement: The study was conducted in accordance with the Declaration of Helsinki, and approved by the Ethics Committee of Elena Venizelou General and Maternal Hospital (protocol code 6116/11-4-2017).

Informed Consent Statement: Informed consent was obtained from all subjects involved in the study.

Data Availability Statement: The data presented in this study are available on request from the corresponding author. The data are not publicly available due to privacy.

Acknowledgments: We would like to thank all participants and their families, as well as all of the clinical staff in the Neonatal Intensive Care Unit of "Elena Venizelou" General and Maternal Hospital.

Conflicts of Interest: The authors declare no conflict of interest.

Abbreviations

BMF, breast milk fortifier; BPD, bronchopulmonary dysplasia; CRIB, clinical risk index for babies, DM, donor milk; IVH, intraventricular hemorrhage; MOM, mother's own milk; NEC, necrotizing enterocolitis; NICUs, neonatal intensive care units; PDA, patent ductus arteriosus; PDM, preterm donor milk; ROP, retinopathy of prematurity; SGA, small for gestational age; TDM, term donor milk; VLBW, very low birth weight.

References

1. Morales, Y.; Schanler, R.J. Human milk and clinical outcomes in VLBW infants: How compelling is the evidence of benefit? *Semin. Perinatol.* **2007**, *31*, 83–88. [CrossRef]
2. Schanler, R.J.; Shulman, R.J.; Lau, C. Feeding strategies for premature infants: Beneficial outcomes of feeding fortified human milk versus preterm formula. *Pediatrics* **1999**, *103*, 1150–1157. [CrossRef]
3. Sen, S. Breast Milk and Breastfeeding: Benefits, Barriers, Maternal Predictors, and Opportunities for Innovation. *Clin. Ther.* **2022**, *44*, 170–171. [CrossRef] [PubMed]

4. Lyons, K.E.; Ryan, C.A.; Dempsey, E.M.; Ross, R.P.; Stanton, C. Breast Milk, a Source of Beneficial Microbes and Associated Benefits for Infant Health. *Nutrients* **2020**, *12*, 1039. [CrossRef] [PubMed]
5. Arnold, L.D.; Larson, E. Immunologic benefits of breast milk in relation to human milk banking. *Am. J. Infect. Control* **1993**, *21*, 235–242. [CrossRef]
6. Magnus, P.D. Benefits of breast milk. *Pediatrics* **1980**, *65*, 192–193. [CrossRef] [PubMed]
7. Eidelman, A.I. Breastfeeding and the use of human milk: An analysis of the American Academy of Pediatrics 2012 Breastfeeding Policy Statement. *Breastfeed Med.* **2012**, *7*, 323–324. [CrossRef] [PubMed]
8. Helenius, K.; Sjörs, G.; Shah, P.S.; Modi, N.; Reichman, B.; Morisaki, N.; Kusuda, S.; Lui, K.; Darlow, B.A.; Bassler, D.; et al. International Network for Evaluating Outcomes (iNeo) of Neonates. Survival in Very Preterm Infants: An International Comparison of 10 National Neonatal Networks. *Pediatrics* **2017**, *140*, e20171264. [CrossRef]
9. Lincetto, O.; Banerjee, A. World Prematurity Day: Improving survival and quality of life for millions of babies born preterm around the world. *Am. J. Physiol. Lung Cell Mol. Physiol.* **2020**, *319*, 871–874. [CrossRef] [PubMed]
10. McClure, E.M.; Goldenberg, R.L. Preterm neonatal survival: What is the role of prognostic models? *BJOG* **2022**, *129*, 539. [CrossRef]
11. van Beek, P.E.; Groenendaal, F.; Broeders, L.; Dijk, P.H.; Dijkman, K.P.; van den Dungen, F.A.M.; van Heijst, A.F.J.; van Hillegersberg, J.L.; Kornelisse, R.F.; Onland, W.; et al. Survival and causes of death in extremely preterm infants in the Netherlands. *Arch. Dis. Child Fetal Neonatal Ed.* **2021**, *106*, 251–257. [CrossRef] [PubMed]
12. ESPGHAN Committee on Nutrition; Arslanoglu, S.; Corpeleijn, W.; Moro, G.; Braegger, C.; Campoy, C.; Colomb, V.; Decsi, T.; Domellöf, M.; Fewtrell, M.; et al. Donor human milk for preterm infants: Current evidence and research directions. *J. Pediatr. Gastroenterol. Nutr.* **2013**, *57*, 535–542. [CrossRef] [PubMed]
13. Moro, G.E.; Arslanoglu, S.; Bertino, E.; Corvaglia, L.; Montirosso, R.; Picaud, J.C.; Polberger, S.; Schanler, R.J.; Steel, C.; van Goudoever, J.; et al. American Academy of Pediatrics; European Society for Pediatric Gastroenterology, Hepatology, and Nutrition. XII. Human Milk in Feeding Premature Infants: Consensus Statement. *J. Pediatr. Gastroenterol. Nutr* **2015**, *61*, 16–19. [CrossRef] [PubMed]
14. Committee on Nutrition, Section on Breastfeeding, Committee on Fetus and Newborn. Donor Human Milk for the High-Risk Infant: Preparation, Safety, and Usage Options in the United States. *Pediatrics* **2017**, *139*, 20163440. [CrossRef] [PubMed]
15. Dritsakou, K.; Liosis, G.; Valsami, G.; Polychronopoulos, E.; Skouroliakou, M. Improved outcomes of feeding low birth weight infants with predominantly raw human milk versus donor banked milk and formula. *J. Matern. Fetal Neonatal Med.* **2016**, *29*, 1131–1138. [CrossRef] [PubMed]
16. Ballard, O.; Morrow, A.L. Human milk composition: Nutrients and bioactive factors. *Pediatr. Clin. N. Am.* **2013**, *60*, 49–74. [CrossRef]
17. Bauer, J.; Gerss, J. Longitudinal analysis of macronutrients and minerals in human milk produced by mothers of preterm infants. *Clin. Nutr.* **2011**, *30*, 215–220. [CrossRef]
18. Agostoni, C.; Buonocore, G.; Carnielli, V.P.; De Curtis, M.; Darmaun, D.; Decsi, T.; Domellöf, M.; Embleton, N.D.; Fusch, C.; Genzel-Boroviczeny, O.; et al. ESPGHAN Committee on Nutrition. Enteral nutrient supply for preterm infants: Commentary from the European Society of Paediatric Gastroenterology, Hepatology and Nutrition Committee on Nutrition. *J. Pediatr. Gastroenterol. Nutr.* **2010**, *50*, 85–91. [CrossRef]
19. Stephens, B.E.; Walden, R.V.; Gargus, R.A.; Tucker, R.; McKinley, L.; Mance, M.; Nye, J.; Vohr, B.R. First-week protein and energy intakes are associated with 18-month developmental outcomes in extremely low birth weight infants. *Pediatrics* **2009**, *123*, 1337–1343. [CrossRef]
20. Rigo, J.; Hascoët, J.M.; Billeaud, C.; Picaud, J.C.; Mosca, F.; Rubio, A.; Saliba, E.; Radkë, M.; Simeoni, U.; Guillois, B.; et al. Growth and Nutritional Biomarkers of Preterm Infants Fed a New Powdered Human Milk Fortifier: A Randomized Trial. *J. Pediatr. Gastroenterol. Nutr.* **2017**, *65*, e83–e93. [CrossRef]
21. Atkinson, S.A. Special nutritional needs of infants for prevention of and recovery from bronchopulmonary dysplasia. *J. Nutr.* **2001**, *131*, 942–946. [CrossRef] [PubMed]
22. Anderson, D.M. Feeding the ill or preterm infant. *Neonatal Netw.* **2002**, *21*, 7–14. [CrossRef] [PubMed]
23. Huston, R.; Lee, M.; Rider, E.; Stawarz, M.; Hedstrom, D.; Pence, M.; Chan, V.; Chambers, J.; Rogers, S.; Sager, N.; et al. Early fortification of enteral feedings for infants <1250 grams birth weight receiving a human milk diet including human milk based fortifier. *J. Neonatal Perinat. Med.* **2020**, *13*, 215–221. [CrossRef] [PubMed]
24. Arslanoglu, S.; Boquien, C.Y.; King, C.; Lamireau, D.; Tonetto, P.; Barnett, D.; Bertino, E.; Gaya, A.; Gebauer, C.; Grovslien, A.; et al. Fortification of Human Milk for Preterm Infants: Update and Recommendations of the European Milk Bank Association (EMBA) Working Group on Human Milk Fortification. *Front. Pediatr.* **2019**, *22*, 7–76. [CrossRef] [PubMed]
25. Khaira, S.; Pert, A.; Farrell, E.; Sibley, C.; Harvey-Wilkes, K.; Nielsen, H.C.; Volpe, M.V. Expressed Breast Milk Analysis: Role of Individualized Protein Fortification to Avoid Protein Deficit After Preterm Birth and Improve Infant Outcomes. *Front. Pediatr.* **2022**, *9*, 652038. [CrossRef]
26. Italian Association of Human Milk Banks Associazione Italiana Banche del Latte Umano Donato. Guidelines for the establishment and operation of a donor human milk bank. *J. Matern. Fetal Neonatal Med.* **2010**, *23*, 1–20. [CrossRef]
27. Leghi, G.E.; Middleton, P.F.; Netting, M.J.; Wlodek, M.E.; Geddes, D.T.; Muhlhausler, B.S. A Systematic Review of Collection and Analysis of Human Milk for Macronutrient Composition. *J. Nutr.* **2020**, *1*, 1652–1670. [CrossRef]

28. Parry, G.; Tucker, J.; Tarnow-Mordi, W.; UK Neonatal Staffing Study Collaborative Group. CRIB II: An update of the clinical risk index for babies score. *Lancet* **2003**, *361*, 1789–1791. [CrossRef]
29. Chou, J.H.; Roumiantsev, S.; Singh, R. PediTools Electronic Growth Chart Calculators: Applications in Clinical Care, Research, and Quality Improvement. *J. Med. Internet Res.* **2020**, *22*, 16204. [CrossRef]
30. International Committee for the Classification of Retinopathy of Prematurity. The International Classification of Retinopathy of Prematurity revisited. *Arch. Ophthalmol.* **2005**, *123*, 991–999. [CrossRef]
31. Hay, W.W.; Ziegler, E.E. Growth failure among preterm infants due to insufficient protein is not innocuous and must be prevented. *J. Perinatol.* **2016**, *36*, 500–502. [CrossRef] [PubMed]
32. Horbar, J.D.; Ehrenkranz, R.A.; Badger, G.J.; Edwards, E.M.; Morrow, K.A.; Soll, R.F.; Buzas, J.S.; Bertino, E.; Gagliardi, L.; Bellù, R. Weight Growth Velocity and Postnatal Growth Failure in Infants 501 to 1500 Grams: 2000–2013. *Pediatrics.* **2015**, *136*, 84–92. [CrossRef] [PubMed]
33. Lee, S.M.; Kim, N.; Namgung, R.; Park, M.; Park, K.; Jeon, J. Prediction of Postnatal Growth Failure among Very Low Birth Weight Infants. *Sci. Rep.* **2018**, *27*, 3729. [CrossRef] [PubMed]
34. Brown, L.D.; Hay, W.W., Jr. The nutritional dilemma for preterm infants: How to promote neurocognitive development and linear growth, but reduce the risk of obesity. *J. Pediatr.* **2013**, *163*, 1543–1545. [CrossRef]
35. Hay, W.W., Jr.; Brown, L.D.; Denne, S.C. Energy requirements, protein-energy metabolism and balance, and carbohydrates in preterm infants. *World Rev. Nutr. Diet.* **2014**, *110*, 64–81. [CrossRef]
36. Mills, L.; Coulter, L.; Savage, E.; Modi, N. Macronutrient content of donor milk from a regional human milk bank: Variation with donor mother-infant characteristics. *Br. J. Nutr.* **2019**, *28*, 1155–1167. [CrossRef]
37. Lemons, J.A.; Moye, L.; Hall, D.; Simmons, M. Differences in the composition of preterm and term human milk during early lactation. *Pediatr. Res.* **1982**, *16*, 113–117. [CrossRef]
38. Dritsakou, K.; Liosis, G.; Valsami, G.; Polychronopoulos, E.; Skouroliakou, M. The impact of maternal- and neonatal-associated factors on human milk's macronutrients and energy. *J. Matern. Fetal Neonatal Med.* **2017**, *30*, 1302–1308. [CrossRef]
39. Borràs-Novell, C.; Herranz Barbero, A.; Balcells Esponera, C.; López-Abad, M.; Aldecoa Bilbao, V.; Izquierdo Renau, M.; Iglesias Platas, I. Influence of maternal and perinatal factors on macronutrient content of very preterm human milk during the first weeks after birth. *J. Perinatol.* **2023**, *43*, 52–59. [CrossRef]
40. Embleton, N.D.; Moltu, S.J.; Lapillonne, A.; van den Akker, C.H.P.; Carnielli, V.; Fusch, C.; Gerasimidis, K.; van Goudoever, J.B.; Haiden, N.; Iacobelli, S.; et al. Enteral Nutrition in Preterm Infants (2022): A Position Paper from the ESPGHAN Committee on Nutrition and invited experts. *J. Pediatr. Gastroenterol. Nutr.* **2022**, 00005176-990000000-00204. [CrossRef]
41. Alyahya, W.; Simpson, J.; Garcia, A.L.; Mactier, H.; Edwards, C.A. Early versus Delayed Fortification of Human Milk in Preterm Infants: A Systematic Review. *Neonatology* **2020**, *117*, 24–32. [CrossRef] [PubMed]
42. Castellano Yáñez, C.; Castillo Barrio, B.; Muñoz Labián, M.D.C.; Ortiz Movilla, R.; García Lara, N.R.; Royuela Vicente, A.; Marín Gabriel, M.A. Providing very preterm infants with donor human milk led to faster breastfeeding rates but worse biometric gains. *Acta Paediatr.* **2019**, *108*, 766–767. [CrossRef] [PubMed]
43. Hoban, R.; Schoeny, M.E.; Esquerra-Zwiers, A.; Kaenkumchorn, T.K.; Casini, G.; Tobin, G.; Siegel, A.H.; Patra, K.; Hamilton, M.; Wicks, J.; et al. Impact of Donor Milk on Short- and Long-Term Growth of Very Low Birth Weight Infants. *Nutrients* **2019**, *11*, 241. [CrossRef]
44. Ginovart, G.; Gich, I.; Gutiérrez, A.; Verd, S. A Fortified Donor Milk Policy is Associated with Improved In-Hospital Head Growth and Weight Gain in Very Low-Birth-Weight Infants. *Adv. Neonatal Care* **2017**, *17*, 250–257. [CrossRef]
45. Madore, L.S.; Bora, S.; Erdei, C.; Jumani, T.; Dengos, A.R.; Sen, S. Effects of Donor Breastmilk Feeding on Growth and Early Neurodevelopmental Outcomes in Preterm Infants: An Observational Study. *Clin. Ther.* **2017**, *39*, 1210–1220. [CrossRef] [PubMed]
46. Fang, L.; Zhang, M.; Wu, L.; Wang, R.; Lin, B.; Yao, J.; Chen, D. Is preterm donor milk better than preterm formula for very-low-birth-weight infants? *Food Nutr. Res.* **2021**, 65. [CrossRef] [PubMed]
47. Arslanoglu, S.; Moro, G.E.; Ziegler, E.E. Preterm infants fed fortified human milk receive less protein than they need. *J. Perinatol.* **2009**, *29*, 489–492. [CrossRef] [PubMed]
48. Landers, S.; Hartmann, B.T. Donor human milk banking and the emergence of milk sharing. *Pediatr. Clin. N. Am.* **2013**, *60*, 247–260. [CrossRef]

nutrients MDPI

Article

Effect of Targeted vs. Standard Fortification of Breast Milk on Growth and Development of Preterm Infants (≤32 Weeks): Results from an Interrupted Randomized Controlled Trial

Joanna Seliga-Siwecka [1], Justyna Fiałkowska [1] and Anna Chmielewska [2,*]

[1] Department of Neonatology and Neonatal Intensive Care, Medical University of Warsaw, 02–091 Warszawa, Poland
[2] Department of Clinical Sciences, Pediatrics, Umeå University, 901 87 Umeå, Sweden
* Correspondence: anna.chmielewska@umu.se; Tel.: +48-225966155

Abstract: Human milk is recommended for very low birth weight infants. Their nutritional needs are high, and the fortification of human milk is a standard procedure to optimize growth. Targeted fortification accounts for the variability in human milk composition. It has been a promising alternative to standard fixed-dose fortification, potentially improving short-term growth. In this trial, preterm infants (≤32 weeks of gestation) were randomized to receive human milk after standard fortification (HMF, Nutricia) or tailored fortification with modular components of proteins (Bebilon Bialko, Nutricia), carbohydrates (Polycal, Nutricia), and lipids (Calogen, Nutricia). The intervention started when preterms reached 80 mL/kg/day enteral feeds. Of the target number of 220 newborns, 39 were randomized. The trial was interrupted due to serious intolerance in five cases. There was no significant difference in velocity of weight gain during the supplementation period (primary outcome) in the tailored vs. standard fortification group: 27.01 ± 10.19 g/d vs. 25.84 ± 13.45 g/d, $p = 0.0776$. Length and head circumference were not significantly different between the groups. We found the feasibility of targeted fortification to be limited in neonatal intensive care unit practice. The trial was registered at clinicaltrials.gov NCT:03775785.

Keywords: breastmilk; fortification; preterm infant; targeted modification; neonatal intensive care unit; macronutrients; supplementation

1. Introduction

Preterm birth results in a high risk of mortality and is a cause of several morbidities, including extrauterine growth restriction [1–3]. Human milk (HM) is the optimal source of nutrition for premature infants [4]. Despite numerous proven benefits, the concentration of some nutrients in HM may be too low to meet the high nutritional needs of premature infants. To ensure optimal growth and development, human milk fortification (HMF) is recommended for all very low birth weight (VLBW, <1500 g birth weight) infants [4,5].

There are several modalities for fortifying HM. *Standard fortification* provides a fixed dose of a compound fortifier added to breastmilk based on the predefined composition of HM to achieve recommended nutritional values and is most widely used in the neonatal intensive care unit (NICU) [6,7]. However, measurements of protein, glucose, and lipids show interindividual and intraindividual variations; hence, other approaches have been suggested [8]. In an *adjustable fortification* strategy, blood urea nitrogen concentrations serve as a surrogate for the response to protein supplementation, and protein fortification is adjusted accordingly. *Tailored/targeted human milk fortification* is achieved by adding only nutritional components (protein, carbohydrates, and fat) to HM based on the results of repeated breast milk composition bedside analyses [5].

While standard breastmilk fortification is the most feasible strategy in a NICU, it does not account for the substantial variability in HM composition between mothers and between milk samples from the same individual [9]. Not accounting for this variability may lead to inappropriate nutritional intake in one-third of all preterm infants [10]. The effects of targeted (individualized) HMF, encompassing adjustable and targeted breastmilk fortification, have recently been systematically reviewed by Fabrizio et al. [11]. The Cochrane review and meta-analysis concluded that individualized HMF improves the short-term velocity of weight, length, and head circumference [11]. However, the studies included in these analyses were not uniform. Researchers have chosen multiple fortification regimes, ranging from adding one to adding all three nutrients [12–14]. Furthermore, differences in unit staffing and workload between healthcare systems and macronutrient products make it difficult to draw a clear conclusion and implement the results worldwide.

To our knowledge, this is the first randomized controlled trial to evaluate whether targeted HMF can optimize growth in infants born at a gestational age < 32 weeks using all three macronutrients in an Eastern European setting. The study protocol was approved by the local ethics committee and was published [2]. The trial was registered at clinicaltrials.gov (NCT03775785).

1.1. Objectives

Research Hypothesis

Tailored fortification of enteral nutrition improves weight gain velocity in preterm infants born at ≤32 weeks of gestation.

1.2. Study Objectives

1.2.1. Primary Objective

The primary objective was to determine whether tailored compared to the standard fortification of enteral nutrition improved weight gain velocity in preterm infants born at ≤32 weeks of gestation.

1.2.2. Secondary Objectives

Key Secondary Objectives

The key secondary objective was to determine the following anthropometric parameters in preterm infants born at ≤32 weeks of gestation at discharge and 4 months:

- feeding tolerance,
- velocity of weight gain,
- length and head growth

2. Materials and Methods

2.1. Trial Design

The trial was designed as a randomized observer- and patient-blinded controlled multicenter superiority trial, with two parallel groups with a 1:1 allocation ratio.

2.2. Participants

2.2.1. Study Setting

The study was initially planned as a multicenter trial; however, two out of three centers failed to randomize patients due to staff shortages. Finally, the study was completed at the Neonatal and Intensive Care Department of the Medical University of Warsaw.

The study site was a level III teaching hospital with approximately 2500–3000 (100 ≤ 32 weeks of gestation) deliveries per year. The local protocol was based on the standard fortification of own mothers' milk (OMM) and donor human milk (DHM).

2.2.2. Eligibility Criteria

All parents of infants born at less than 32 weeks of gestation and admitted to the NICU were approached by one of the research team members within the first week of life (as full enteral feeding is usually reached at a minimum of 7 days of life). Recruitment was conducted between June 2019 and June 2022. After obtaining written consent for participation in the trial, the patient's medical record number was immediately registered on a secure web-based platform, and demographic data were recorded.

2.2.3. Inclusion Criteria

Patients eligible for the trial had to comply with the following criteria at randomization:

1. Gestational age at birth $\leq$ 32 weeks
2. Enteral feeding of at least 80 mL/kg/day
3. 50% donor or maternal milk-based enteral feeding
4. Parenteral/legal guardian consent

2.2.4. Exclusion Criteria

1. Formula feeding
2. Small for gestational age (birth weight < 3rd percentile)
3. Presence of congenital abnormalities, which increase the risk of necrotizing enterocolitis such as hypoplastic left heart syndrome, transposition of the great arteries, omphalocele, gastroschisis
4. Necrotizing enterocolitis (NEC)
5. Withdrawal of feeding > 7 days
6. Sepsis
7. Death

2.2.5. Obtaining Informed Consent

All parents of infants born at less than 32 weeks of gestation and admitted to the study site were approached by one of the research team members within the first seven days of life. They provided oral and written information about the study. Parents were allowed to participate in an informed discussion with the attending physician and study personnel. The research team members obtained written consent from parents willing to allow their children to participate in the trial. Information consent forms and information sheets were provided in Polish for all parents. Given the limited diversity of our population, we did not recruit newborns of foreign parents unless they spoke Polish on a level that allowed a full understanding of the study.

Regarding additional consent provisions for collecting and using participant data and biological specimens, we did not plan to collect samples for ancillary studies.

2.2.6. Sample Size

The sample size required to compare two means in a two-sided equality test was estimated based on results from a prior double-blind, randomized clinical trial, investigating the effect of TG vs. SF of breast milk on the changes of anthropometric parameters and body composition in preterm children [15,16]. It was determined that a mean difference of weight gain of 1.9 g/kg/day between groups would be clinically important and feasible during the intervention. The following assumptions were made for the calculation: type I error (α) 5%, power 80%, equal sample sizes in both groups, the mean weight gain in the standard fortification group 19.3 g/kg/day, and the mean weight gain in the target fortification group 21.2 g/kg/day. To account for the higher uncertainty in measured weight gain due to differences between the studied and the quoted trial population, the standard deviation value taken from the prior trial was increased by 50% to 3.75.

The estimated minimum size of each group was 68. Accounting for a presumed 20% attrition rate due to potential dropouts, deviations from the protocol and loss to follow-up, the minimum sample size required was estimated at 156 infants or 78 infants per treatment arm.

2.3. Interventions

2.3.1. Explanation for the Choice of Comparators

Standard fortification (SF) assumes that HM has a protein level of 1.5g/dL. HM, however, is highly variable in nutrient content, both between mothers and between samples from the same mother [10,11]. A recent study suggested that not considering this variability leads to inadequate intake in approximately 25–40% of VLBW infants due to low protein and energy content [12]. Nonetheless, it is the most widely used strategy for HMF, and thus, its choice as a comparator is logical.

2.3.2. Intervention Description

After reaching 80 mL/kg/day of enteral feeding, patients were randomized to receive SF (Bebilon HMF, Nutricia®) or targeted fortification (TF) (protein: Bebilon Suplement Bialka, Nutricia®; lipids: Calogen, Nutricia®; carbohydrates: Polycal Nutricia®) [17]. The macro-and micronutrient contents have been previously published [17]. Milk fortification was routinely performed twice a day (at 8 am and 8 pm) for the following 12-h nursing shift. For the study, TF was integrated into this schedule and performed by experienced research nurses (RNs) [17].

One of the researchers (JSS) performed milk analysis in the NICU research laboratory at Princess Anna Mazowiecka Hospital three times per week (Monday/Wednesday/Friday) at 10:00 am and after protocol amendment twice per week (Tuesday/Thursday) from batches collected from the two previous days. A 10 mL aliquot from each batch of native breast milk was used for macronutrient analysis (Miris ® HMA) per the protocol [17]. The remaining batch was fortified using a routine fortifier. Macronutrient analysis determined the amount of extra fat, protein, or carbohydrate needed in the batch to obtain the final target fortified breast milk (FBM).

The mean of three measurements per batch (3×2–3 mL) was used to calculate the required amount of extra fat, protein, and carbohydrate for the following three days of fortification using a predefined Excel spreadsheet (Microsoft Inc., Redmond, Washington, USA). Milk analysis was performed for both treatment arms; however, only the intervention group received TF.

The desired macronutrient concentration in breast milk was 4.4 g/100 mL of fat, 3 g/100 mL of protein, and 8.8 g/ 100 mL of carbohydrate to meet the European Society for Paediatric Gastroenterology, Hepatology, and Nutrition (ESPGHAN) guidelines (6.6 g/kg/d of fat, 4.5 g/kg/d of protein, and 13.2 g/kg/d of carbohydrate) assuming an intake of 150 mL/kg/d.

Target fortification was conducted in three steps:

1. Determination of macronutrient concentration in OMM/HDM.
2. SF: Human milk fortifier, HMF Nutricia®.
3. TF: Adding fat, protein, or carbohydrates to achieve the target levels of macronutrients.

In cases where the macronutrient component after SF exceeded the target value, only other deficient macronutrient components were adjusted.

The patients were fed every 3 h via a gastric tube by RNs. Starting at 33 weeks of post-conceptional age (PCA), non-nutritive sucking stimulation was initiated by occupational therapists. At approximately 34 weeks of PCA, infants transitioned to bottle feeding. When breastfeeding was established, patients received TF as one or two bottled feeds.

As a safety assessment to ensure that an appropriate amount of fortifier was added, the osmolality of unfortified and FBM samples was measured using a 3320 Micro-Osmometer (Advance Instruments, Norwood, MA, USA). Bedside nurses were informed whether the osmolality of fortified milk was within the acceptable target range (400–600 mOsmol/kg) before milk was administered during the next 12-h shift. Osmolality lower or higher than the defined target range was considered a sample preparation error of fortification, and the single-nutrient fortification was omitted. TF prescription was completed before noon. The attending physician approved this prescription. Subsequently, individual additives were provided by the nutrition services. Bedside nurses prepared batches of FBM, including additives for target fortification, and divided them into single feeding portions to be administered to infants [17].

The intervention continued until 37 weeks of PCA or hospital discharge. The parents, attending physicians, and outcome assessors were blinded to the interventions.

2.3.3. Criteria for Discontinuing or Modifying Allocated Interventions

Criteria for discontinuing allocated intervention included

- Sepsis
- NEC
- Withdrawal of parental/guardian consent
- Poor feeding tolerance, defined as increasing abdominal distension >2 cm between inter-observer measurement or regurgitations after feeding >3 feeds per day

2.3.4. Strategies to Improve Adherence to Interventions

The medical notes of the infants included in the study were visibly marked to promote adherence to the study protocol. A flowchart explaining the inclusion, exclusion, and discontinuation criteria is available for the patient's medical notes.

2.3.5. Relevant Concomitant Care Permitted or Prohibited during the Trial

The participants continued to receive standard neonatal care. Interventions aimed at improving weight gain, such as increased daily intake (>160–170 mL/kg/day) or increased dosing of vitamin D (>1000 IU/L), or prescription of milk formula, were forbidden.

2.4. Outcomes

2.4.1. Primary Outcome

Weight gain velocity was measured starting from the day infants regained their birth weight to 4 weeks and then weekly until discharge. Length and head circumference were measured weekly until the patient was discharged.

2.4.2. Secondary Outcomes

1. Growth (weight, length, and head circumference) was assessed at discharge and four months of corrected age.
2. Feeding tolerance under the whole fortification period.
3. Morbidity: Incidence of NEC, retinopathy of prematurity (ROP), bronchopulmonary dysplasia (BPD), intraventricular hemorrhage (IVH), periventricular leukomalacia (PVL), sepsis, and pneumonia. The definitions are as follows:

The outcomes are defined as

- Feeding tolerance was defined as hemorrhagic residuals or vomiting of bile until pathological causes were ruled out (intestinal obstruction or ileus) [18]. Gastric residuals and abdominal girth were not routinely assessed. Isolated green or yellow residuals were considered unimportant.
- NEC: Stage II or III. Stage II requires clinical manifestations of a distended abdomen and radiological verification (intramural or portal gases). Stage III requires findings like in Stage II and more severe clinical symptoms (shock, need for a respirator). In surgically verified cases, radiological verification is not required [19].
- ROP: Stages I to V, diagnosed by an ophthalmologist according to international criteria [20].
- BPD: Need for oxygen, continuous positive airway pressure (CPAP,) or mechanical ventilation at 36+0 weeks of gestational age [21].
- IVH as defined by Volpe [18].
- PVL as defined by Volpe [18].

- Early- and late-onset sepsis was defined as positive blood or cerebral fluid culture at less and more than 72 h of age, respectively [22].

The schedule of enrolment, interventions (including any run-ins and washouts), assessments, and visits for participants are presented in Table 1.

Table 1. Baseline characteristics of study groups.

Variable	Tailored (n = 18)			Standard (n = 21)		
	n (%)	Mean ± SD	Median (Q1; Q3)	n (%)	Mean ± SD	Median (Q1; Q3)
Gender, male	9 (50.0)	-	-	10 (47.6)	-	-
Gestational week	-	29.22 ± 2.02	29.50 (28.00; 31.00)	-	28.24 ± 2.62	29.00 (26.00; 31.00)
Birth weight, g	-	1361.11 ± 454.30	1315.00 (1047.50; 1685.00)	-	1250.95 ± 429.68	1200.00 (1000.00; 1620.00)
Birth length, cm	-	41.33 ± 5.69	43.00 (37.50; 45.00)	-	38.88 ± 6.14	39.00 (35.00; 45.00)
Head circumference, cm	-	25.89 ± 7.21	28.25 (25.00; 30.00)	-	25.40 ± 6.58	27.00 (24.00; 29.00)
Birth weight z-score	-	0.39 ± 1.17	0.58 (-0.74; 1.13)	-	0.62 ± 1.19	0.54 (−0.06; 1.21)
Birth length z-score	-	1.42 ± 1.63	1.79 (0.22; 2.67)	-	1.03 ± 1.72	1.21 (−0.03; 2.14)
Head circumference z-score	-	0.55 ± 1.39	0.68 (-0.34; 1.64)	-	0.68 ± 1.09	0.98 (−0.05; 1.70)
80 mL/kg/day of maternal or human donor milk, day	-	6.44 ± 4.67	6.00 (4.00; 6.75)	-	7.90 ± 5.91	6.00 (5.00; 9.00)
50% donor or maternal milk-based enteral feeding	18 (100.0)	-	-	21 (100.0)	-	-
Milk type/source–mother	17 (94.4)	-	-	21 (100.0)	-	-
Milk type/source–formula	1 (5.6)	-	-	1 (4.8)	-	-
Milk type/source–donor	13 (72.2)	-	-	13 (61.9)	-	-

2.5. Recruitment

We planned to continue until a minimum of 200 valid observations were collected from every arm. As part of the antenatal consultation, women with threatened preterm labor were scheduled for a short meeting with a member of the recruitment team. During this appointment, they were offered to participate in the trial. To increase participant enrolment, the medical staff carried out a second patient screen during admission to the NICU. The enrolment period was extended from 2019 to 2022 (with intermittent withdrawals secondary to equipment failure). Recruitment rates were monitored monthly. In return, women were offered additional breastfeeding support by a certified lactation consultant, as reported previously [17].

2.6. Assignment of Interventions: Allocation

2.6.1. Sequence Generation

The allocation sequence was computer generated. Block randomization was performed with stratification by the delivery mode. Patients were randomly assigned to standard or tailored enteral nutrition fortification groups in a 1:1 ratio. The block size was varied and concealed until the primary endpoint analysis.

2.6.2. Concealment Mechanism

A member of the recruitment team approached caregivers within the infant's first 7 days of life. They explained the study and obtained written consent for participation in the trial. Subsequently, the patient's medical record number was registered on a secure web-based platform, and demographic data were recorded. The platform assigned a study number, together with the allocated treatment.

2.6.3. Implementation

A member [a physician not involved in patient care] of the research team prescribed the allocated fortification in the patient's drug chart. Milk fortification was routinely conducted twice a day (at 8 am and 8 pm) for each following 12-h nursing shift. For the study, TF was integrated into this schedule and performed by experienced RNs [14]. The intervention was performed by an RN blinded to the treatment allocation. Patient data, along with the allocation results, were sent to the statistical team. The randomization list remained with the statistical team for the entire study duration.

2.7. *Assignment of Interventions: Blinding*

2.7.1. Who Was Blinded

Bedside nurses, treating physicians, and clinical psychologists were blinded to the treatment allocation. Milk fortification was performed on a milk bank by an experienced RN. The prepared milk portions were transported to the unit. The feeding portions from both treatment arms did not differ in color or structure.

2.7.2. Procedure for Unblinding if Needed

The unblinding procedures were previously published. If unblinding was necessary, the allocation was disclosed to the treating physician.

2.8. *Plans for Assessment and Collection of Outcomes*

Primary Outcome

Weight gain velocity was measured starting from the day infants regained their birth weight to 4 weeks, then weekly until discharge using the Seca 336 Baby Scale®. Length and head circumference were measured weekly until discharge using a Seca 336 baby measuring rod®.

2.9. *Plans to Promote Participant Retention and Complete Follow-Up*

All randomized infants who prematurely discontinued the study intervention were considered off-study drug/on-study. They followed the same participant timetable as the infants who continued the study treatment.

Once an infant was enrolled or randomized, the study site made every reasonable effort to follow the infant for the entire study period.

The participants could withdraw from the study for any reason at any time. The investigator could withdraw the participants from the study to protect their safety.

2.10. *Data Management*

All data collection was completed electronically. Data integrity was enforced through various mechanisms. Referential data rules, valid values, range checks, and consistency checks against data already stored in the database (i.e., longitudinal checks) were supported. Modifications to the data written in the database were documented through either a data change or inquiry system. Data entered into the database were retrieved for viewing through data entry applications. The type of activity an individual user may undertake is regulated by the privileges associated with their user identification code and password.

2.11. *Confidentiality*

Complete patient and study information was stored on a secure, password-protected web-based platform. Only the researchers involved in the study were provided with a personalized login and password to access the study information. The statistical team did not have access to sensitive data, such as date of birth, address, or contact details. All records containing the patient details and relevant medical histories were stored separately in a locked file cabinet.

There were no plans for the collection, laboratory evaluation, and storage of biological specimens for genetic or molecular analysis in this trial/future use. We did not plan to perform any genetic or molecular analysis in this trial.

2.12. *Statistical Methods for Primary and Secondary Outcomes*

Baseline characteristics are presented according to the treatment groups. Categorical variables were presented as the number of counts and proportion of the group. Continuous variables are described as mean and standard deviation or median with interquartile range. Continuous variables were tested against the normality of distribution using the Shapiro–Wilk test and verified with skewness and kurtosis. In the justified cases, a visual assessment was performed. The equality of variance between groups was tested using Levene's test. For continuous variables distributed normally with homogenous variances, the Student's *t*-test was used to verify the differences in means. For continuous variables that were not normally distributed, comparisons were performed using the Mann–Whitney U test. Comparisons of groups for categorical variables were performed using the Pearson Chi-square test or Fisher's exact test, as appropriate. In addition, the risk ratio and mean or median difference (MD) are presented, along with 95% confidence intervals (CIs). Comparisons in time were performed using the paired *t*-test or Wilcoxon test. All statistical calculations assumed *alpha* = 0.05 and were performed with R statistical software, version R-4.1.2.

3. Results

3.1. Demographics

Between 2019 and 2022, 392 infants born below 32 weeks of gestation were admitted to the NICU and screened for eligibility. Initially, 344 infants were excluded from the study for the following reasons: declined consent (n = 200), paused recruitment (n = 100), and failure to meet the inclusion criteria (n = 44). Fifty-five infants were initially randomized; however, 16 did not receive the allocated intervention. Thirty-nine singleton (n = 25) and twin (n = 7) births at a median age of 29 (range, 26–31) weeks and a mean birth weight of 1306 (±454.3) g were randomly assigned to SF (n = 21) or TF (n = 18) (Figure 1). Siblings from multiple pregnancies were randomly assigned to different treatment groups.

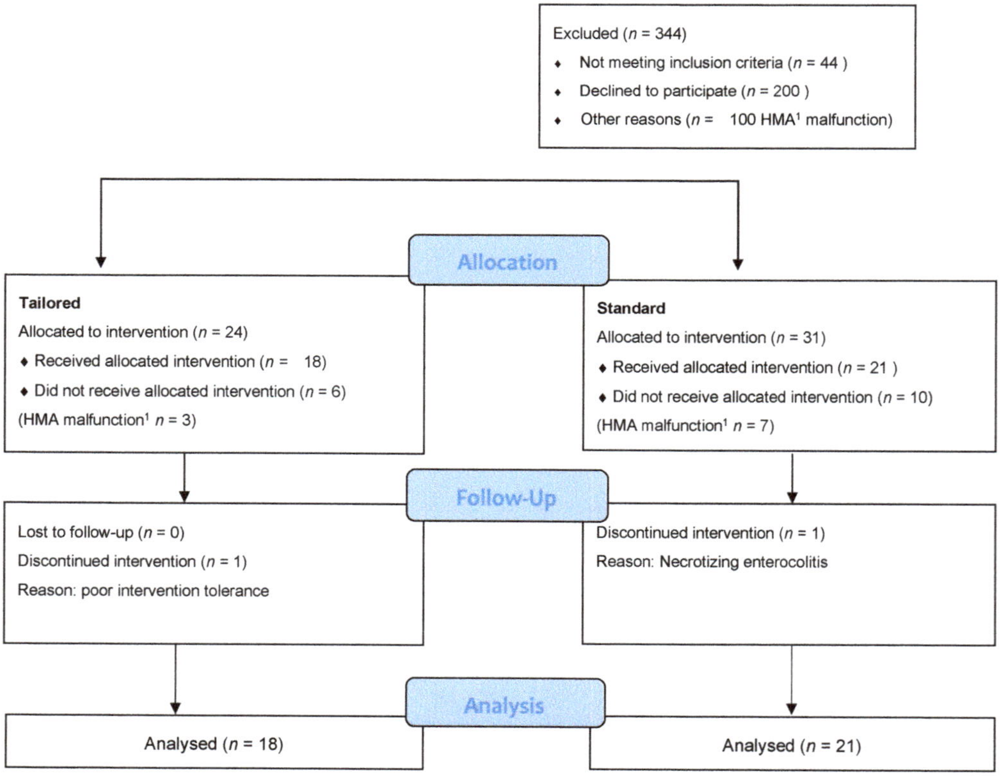

1. HMA- Human milk analyzer MIRIS®

Figure 1. Participant enrollment flowchart.

The baseline characteristics did not differ between the groups (Table 1).

3.2. Milk Composition

The average nutritional content of the breast milk was similar throughout the trial. There were no significant differences in baseline levels of macronutrients by the end of the first week of supplementation between the two groups: protein (2.0 ± 0.34 vs. 1.91 ± 0.22 g/100 mL, p = 0.328), glucose (7.60 vs. 7.40 g/100 mL, p = 0.219), lipids (3.48 ± 1.40 vs. 3.65 ± 1.20, p = 0.417), calories (71.06 ± 12.38 vs. 71.21 ± 12.04 kcal/100 mL, p = 0.972) (Table 2). Within each group, we noted differences in milk composition over the study period: protein concentration decreased significantly over the first four weeks [MD, 95% CI: −0.69 (−0.88, 0.50, p < 0.001 vs. −0.49 (−0.71, 0.27), p = 0.001], and the glucose concentration decreased over time in the standard group [MD, 95% CI: 0.49 (0.21, 0.77), p = 0.004] (Table 2).

Table 2. Milk composition during supplementation period.

Variable	Tailored	Standard	MD (95% CI)	*p*
Milk volume, mL				
Day 0	-	-	-	-
Week 1 (1/2)	241.60 ± 78.80	220.39 ± 65.79	21.21 (−30.10; 72.52)	0.406
Week 4 (2/2)	305.60 ± 106.79	264.00 ± 114.45	41.60 (−62.39; 145.59)	0.412
Last measurement	323.29 ± 114.93	313.60 ± 127.25	9.69 (−71.86; 91.25)	0.811
No. of HMF pieces				
Day 0	-	-	-	-
Week 1 (1/2)	8.94 ± 9.33	8.55 ± 7.94	0.38 (−5.55; 6.32)	0.896
Week 4 (2/2)	20.00 ± 7.48	17.20 ± 8.70	2.80 (−4.83; 10.43)	0.450
Last measurement	21.21 ± 7.43	16.50 ± 8.45	4.71 (−0.65; 10.06)	0.083
Protein, g/100 mL				
Day 0	2.02 ± 0.34	-	-	-
Week 1 (1/2)	2.00 ± 0.34	1.91 ± 0.22	0.09 (−0.10; 0.29)	0.328
Week 4 (2/2)	1.37 ± 0.24	1.32 ± 0.15	0.05 (−0.14; 0.24)	0.582
Last measurement	1.34 ± 0.26	1.38 ± 0.25	−0.04 (−0.21; 0.13)	0.640
Glucose, g/100 mL				
Day 0	7.50 (7.10; 7.80)	-	-	-
Week 1 (1/2)	7.60 (7.07; 7.80)	7.40 (7.05; 7.60)	0.20 (−0.10; 0.50)	0.219
Week 4 (2/2)	7.60 (7.53; 7.77)	7.90 (7.67; 8.00)	−0.30 (−0.50; 0.00)	**0.039**
Week 4 (2/2) (w/o one patient)	7.60 (7.60; 7.80)	7.90 (7.67; 8.00)	−0.30 (−0.40; 0.00)	0.069
Week 4 (2/2) (w/o one patient)	7.67 ± 0.18	7.86 ± 0.22	−0.19 (−0.39; 0.00)	0.051
Last measurement	7.70 (7.60; 7.80)	7.80 (7.60; 7.90)	−0.10 (-0.20; 0.10)	0.348
Fat, g/100 mL				
Day 0	3.36 ± 1.44	-	-	-
Week 1 (1/2)	3.48 ± 1.40	3.65 ± 1.20	8.00 (−17.00; 8.00)	0.417
Week 4 (2/2)	4.06 ± 1.56	3.82 ± 0.56	−0.10 (−0.80; 0.80)	0.940
Last measurement	4.19 ± 1.48	3.52 ± 1.05	0.68 (−0.17; 1.53)	0.113
Energy, kcal/100 mL				
Day 0	-	-	-	-
Week 1 (1/2)	71.06 ± 12.38	71.21 ± 12.04	−0.15 (-8.57; 8.27)	0.972
Week 4 (2/2)	73.50 ± 12.20	73.10 ± 4.93	0.40 (−8.35; 9.15)	0.925
Last measurement	75.35 ± 12.18	69.20 ± 10.06	6.15 (−1.27; 13.57)	0.101

HMF -human milk fortifier.

3.3. Nutritional Intake and Growth

Only one infant in each group received formula feeding. The rates of OMM and DHM feeding did not differ between the groups. The mean achieving 80 mL/kg/d of enteral feeding did not differ between the groups (SF 6.44 vs. TF 7.9, p = 0.21) (Table 1). All infants in both groups received 1 g of HMF Bebilon Nenatal Nutricia® per 25 mL of HM with a maximum dose of 6.6 g/kg. Forty-four percent (8 out of 18 newborns) required any type of nutrient throughout the study period. In the first week of the study, one infant required lipid supplementation only. Twenty-seven percent (5 out of 18) of patients required all three supplements for the entire study (Figure 2.)

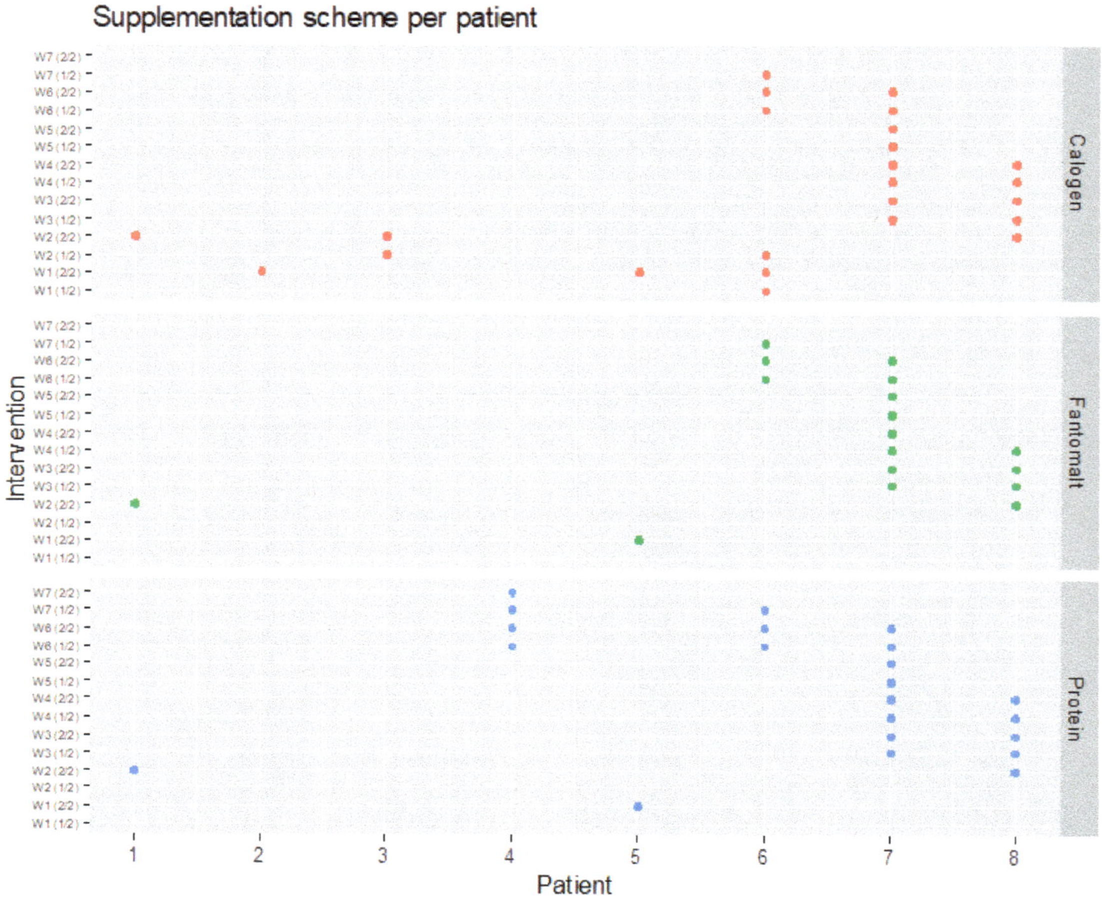

Figure 2. Supplementation per patient.

The average weight gain in g/d was higher in the tailored group compared to the standard group (27.01 ± 10.19 g/d vs. 25.84 ± 13.45 g/d, respectively); however, no significant difference was found ($p = 0.776$). No significant difference in weight gain in g/kg/d between the tailored and standard groups was found (15.76 ± 3.10 g/kg/d vs. 16.84 ± 10.04 g/kg/d, respectively, $p = 0.683$). Differences between groups at the level of statistical tendency were identified in the case of length and head circumference gain in cm/wk ($p = 0.056$ and $p = 0.074$, respectively) (Table 3).

There was significant total weight gain in the tailored and standard groups over the first 4 weeks of supplementation [MD = 632.11, 95% CI (359.94, 904.28), $p = 0.001$ and MD = 601.78, 95% CI (414.70, 788.86), $p < 0.001$, respectively]. The change in the weight z-score over the same period was not significant in either group ($p = 0.947$ and $p = 0.723$, respectively) (Table 3).

3.4. Secondary Outcomes

Secondary outcomes, such as IVH (stages 1–4), late-onset sepsis, BPD, ROP, and PVL, were similar between the targeted and standard fortification groups. Only one infant in the control group developed necrotizing enterocolitis and was not fed enterally for seven days (Table 4).

Table 3. Weight, length, and head circumference development for the first 4 weeks.

Variable	Week 1/at Birth	Week 4/Study End	MD (95% CI)	p
Week 1 to week 4, tailored group (n = 8)				
Weight, g	1379.56 ± 441.49	2011.67 ± 647.56	632.11 (359.94; 904.28)	**0.001**
Weight z-score	0.00 ± 1.14	0.02 ± 0.89	0.02 (−0.72; 0.76)	0.947
Week 1 to week 4, standard group (n = 8)				
Weight, g	1264.56 ± 365.98	1866.33 ± 570.42	601.78 (414.70; 788.86)	**<0.001**
Weight z-score	0.24 ± 1.15	0.29 ± 1.06	0.05 (−0.26; 0.36)	0.723
At birth to study end, tailored group (n = 18)				
Weight, g	1361.11 ± 454.30	2253.22 ± 838.63	892.11 (548.76; 1235.46)	**<0.001**
Length, cm	41.33 ± 5.69	48.50 ± 6.02	7.17 (4.81; 9.53)	**<0.001**
Head circumference, cm	25.89 ± 7.21	32.53 ± 3.06	6.64 (3.34; 9.93)	**0.001**
Weight z-score	0.39 ± 1.17	−0.38 ± 1.35	−0.78 (−1.05; −0.50)	**<0.001**
Length z-score	1.42 ± 1.63	1.30 ± 1.91	−0.12 (−0.88; 0.64)	0.749
Head circumference z-score	0.55 ± 1.39	0.74 ± 1.51	0.19 (−0.55; 0.93)	0.592
At birth to study end, standard group (n = 21)				
Weight, g	1250.95 ± 429.68	2041.48 ± 843.51	790.52 (465.30; 1115.75)	**<0.001**
Length, cm	39.42 ± 5.76	44.90 ± 7.10	5.48 (3.37; 7.58)	**<0.001**
Head circumference, cm	25.42 ± 6.75	30.70 ± 4.05	5.28 (1.71; 8.84)	**0.006**
Weight z-score	0.62 ± 1.19	−0.35 ± 1.21	−0.97 (−1.32; −0.61)	**<0.001**
Length z-score	1.21 ± 1.55	0.56 ± 1.80	−0.65 (−1.13; −0.18)	**0.009**
Head circumference z-score	0.66 ± 1.12	−0.05 ± 1.43	−0.72 (−1.15; −0.28)	**0.003**

Data presented as mean ± standard deviation. MD–mean (week 4/study end vs. week 1/at birth), CI–confidence interval. Measurements compared with Student's t-test for dependent groups.

Table 4. Secondary outcomes.

Variable	Tailored (n = 18)	Standard (n = 21)	p
Poor feeding tolerance	6 (33)	3 (14.3)	
Sepsis	0 (0.0)	0 (0.0)	-
Necrotizing enterocolitis	0 (0.0)	1 (4.8)	>0.999
Intraventricular haemorrhage 1	0 (0.0)	1 (4.8)	>0.999
Intraventricular haemorrhage 2	2 (11.1)	6 (28.6)	0.247
Intraventricular haemorrhage 3	0 (0.0)	2 (9.5)	0.490
Periventricular leukomalacia	0 (0.0)	0 (0.0)	-
Bronchopulmonary dysplasia	3 (17.7)	8 (38.1)	0.260
Retinopathy of premature	7 (38.9)	7 (33.3)	0.980
Death	0 (0.0)	0 (0.0)	-
Late onset sepsis	0 (0.0)	1 (4.8)	>0.999
Enteral feeding suspended for at least 7 days	1 (5.6)	1 (4.8)	>0.999
>50% formula feeding	2 (11.1)	1 (4.8)	0.586

Data presented as n (% of group). Groups compared with Fisher's exact test or Pearson's Chi-square test [1], as appropriate.

4. Discussion

4.1. Principal Findings

In this prematurely terminated randomized controlled trial, we did not find any statistically significant difference in the velocity of weight gain during the supplementation period in infants born before 32 weeks of gestation who received TF compared to those who received SF. Changes in length and head circumference did not differ between the groups.

We ceased recruitment due to five cases of intolerance to feeds in the TF group, such as significant abdominal distention (reported in two consecutive measurements), regurgitation, and posseting. These adverse events were reported to the local bioethical committee according to the study protocol, and the researchers decided to terminate the trial [17]. Recruitment was interrupted after 39 infants were randomized. Consequently, the power for detecting the difference in weight gain velocity between the groups (primary outcome) decreased from 1.9 g/kg/day to 3.2 g/kg/day. Additionally, TF was found to be labor-intensive and time-consuming for both mothers and medical personnel. This was the reason why mothers withdrew from the study. It is worth noting that most parents lived a long distance from the hospital; given the epidemiological time (COVID pandemic), these families were faced with the emotional burden of being away from their babies. Additional obligations, such as participating in a study, are an additional source of anxiety. We noted significant difficulties among the mothers in complying with the milk collection protocol. Another confounder in the study was that weekly fortification was not compensated for the dilutionary effect of omitting samples with high osmolarity (if osmolality exceeded the safety range after adding all necessary supplements, the fortification was omitted for the planned study period).

4.2. Comparison with Other Studies

Evidence confirming that TF using all three macronutrients improves growth in preterm infants is limited. To date, ten studies have been published on TF [12] [10,19–25]. Three of the six randomized controlled trials evaluated the use of all three macronutrients. A Cochrane review published in 2020 concluded that TF improves growth in the preterm population. However, it included seven studies, of which only two evaluated individualized target fortification as an intervention [11]. Pooled results from these trials (72 participants) showed that the mean weight gain velocity in the TF group was higher by 2.49 g/kg/day (0.44–4.54) compared to adjustable fortification. Since then, only one new study by Rochow et al. has been published, confirming previous findings. These studies were performed at a Canadian academic center involving a large multidisciplinary research team [13,26]. Furthermore, three members of the team performed the HM analysis, which we found impossible to replicate in busy clinical settings. Our findings were confirmed in an Australian study, where the authors concluded that TF was time-consuming and labor-intensive and did not lead to growth improvement [12]. In Europe, dieticians are not part of the clinical team, which significantly increases the workload of the rest of the staff when it comes to TF. Studies conducted in Asian and European settings evaluated the addition of only one macronutrient (in most cases, protein), and this was found to be clinically feasible and improved growth [14,24,27,28]. It is also worth noting that, in contrast to Rochow et al.'s study, the HMF used in our study did not contain lipids; thus, in cases of low-fat HM concentrations, higher amounts of supplementation were required. This probably led to higher osmolality results compared to the Canadian study and might be the reason for the observed low tolerance to tailored supplementation [25].

In the study mentioned above by Rochow et al., weight gain velocity during the first 21 days of intervention was higher in the TF group compared to the SF group (MD 1.9 g/kg/day, CI 0.9, 2.9) [10]. The fact that we could not show the difference in the weight gain velocity is probably due to a lack of power. With the 39 included patients, we only had the power to detect differences as large as 3.2 g/kg/day. Regarding feasibility, the difference may be accounted for by economic differences between the countries where the study sites were located. In Canada, the GDP is more than twice as high as than in Poland [29].

4.3. Strengths and Limitations

A randomized controlled trial design is the methodology of choice for studying the effects of an intervention. Moreover, blinding of the parents, NICU staff, and outcome accessors minimized bias related to allocation, intervention, and outcome assessment. Transparency is an additional strength of our study; we registered the study on a public research platform and published the complete protocol in a peer-reviewed journal [17].

Evidence on the effect of TF on outcomes other than weight gain velocity is lacking; thus, we aimed to study whether neurodevelopmental scores will improve in the TF group at 12 and 24 months of corrected age. However, due to the early cessation of the study, we could not show the difference between the groups as calculated during planning.

The most important limitation of the current study was that it ceased before recruiting the target number of participants. Another limitation is that we did not measure body composition according to the protocol (funds were not obtained). Consequently, despite the effort and funds invested in designing and commencing the trial, we could not obtain results that would add to the existing evidence in the field.

However, it is important to emphasize that we identified several potential obstacles to introducing individualized fortification in clinical practice in the NICU. First, frequent measurements of milk composition (twice per week) significantly increased the workload. The potential solution might be to perform the measurement less often, for example, once a week instead of twice a week. Rochow et al. showed that measurements twice weekly led to a mean macronutrient intake within a range of ±5% of the targeted levels [13].

4.4. Further Research

An ongoing randomized controlled trial designed by Belfort et al. will study the effect of individualized fortification on growth, body composition, and development [30]. There are important differences between this study, Rochow et al.'s 2021 study, and the current trial [4,25]. The intervention will begin with achieving an enteral intake of 140 mL/kg, compared to 80 mL/kg. Another difference is that protein and fat, but not carbohydrates, will be added to HM in the experimental arm. Surprisingly, the target protein concentration was set at 1 g/100 mL (compared with 3 g/mL in our trial, which aligns with the ESPGHAN guidelines) [4]. Milk analysis will be performed daily. It is of value for research purposes, but based on available evidence, it is not necessary to achieve desirable macronutrient intakes [31]. The sample size (N = 130) will allow the authors to detect a moderate effect of the intervention on growth. Still, it is probably too small to detect subtle differences in developmental scores.

To date, only single-center studies have been conducted. Future research should focus on generalizability and various clinical scenarios, as feeding protocols differ between units and fortifiers differ between brands. The potential role of tailored enteral nutrition should be confirmed in multicenter international trials.

5. Conclusions

Targeted milk modification is a strategy that may allow for the optimization of growth in premature infants; however, feasibility and poor tolerance of feeds may be important obstacles in introducing this strategy to NICU clinical practice. Further research should focus on outcomes, such as body composition and development, and emphasize practical aspects.

Author Contributions: Conceptualization, J.S.-S. and A.C.; methodology, J.S.-S. and A.C.; investigation, J.S.-S. and J.F. writing—original draft preparation, J.S.-S. and A.C. writing—review and editing, J.S.-S.; visualization, funding acquisition, J.S.-S. and A.C. All authors have read and agreed to the published version of the manuscript.

Funding: This research and APC were funded by The Nutricia Foundation Poland, grant number RG-4/2018.

Institutional Review Board Statement: The study was conducted in accordance with the Declaration of Helsinki and approved by the Bioethics Committee of the Medical University of Warsaw (protocol code KB/89/2018, date of approval: 21 May 2018).

Informed Consent Statement: Informed consent was obtained from all subjects involved in the study.

Data Availability Statement: Data are available upon reasonable request from the corresponding author.

Conflicts of Interest: The authors declare no conflict of interest. The funders had no role in the study design; collection, analyses, or interpretation of data; writing of the manuscript; or decision to publish the results.

References

1. Hu, F.; Tang, Q.; Wang, Y.; Wu, J.; Ruan, H.; Lu, L.; Tao, Y.; Cai, W. Analysis of Nutrition Support in Very Low-Birth-Weight Infants with Extrauterine Growth Restriction. *Nutr. Clin. Pract.* **2018**, *34*, 436–443. [CrossRef]
2. Ehrenkranz, R.A.; Younes, N.; Lemons, J.A.; Fanaroff, A.A.; Donovan, E.F.; Wright, L.L.; Katsikiotis, V.; Tyson, J.E.; Oh, W.; Shankaran, S.; et al. Longitudinal Growth of Hospitalized Very Low Birth Weight Infants. *Pediatrics* **1999**, *104*, 280–289. [CrossRef] [PubMed]
3. Clark, R.H.; Thomas, P.; Peabody, J. Extrauterine Growth Restriction Remains a Serious Problem in Prematurely Born Neonates. *Pediatrics* **2003**, *111*, 986–990. [CrossRef] [PubMed]
4. Agostoni, C.; Buonocore, G.; Carnielli, V.P.; De Curtis, M.; Darmaun, D.; Decsi, T.; Domellöf, M.; Embleton, N.D.; Fusch, C.; Genzel-Boroviczeny, O.; et al. Enteral Nutrient Supply for Preterm Infants: Commentary from the European Society of Paediatric Gastroenterology, Hepatology and Nutrition Committee on Nutrition. *J. Pediatr. Gastroenterol. Nutr.* **2010**, *50*, 85–91. [CrossRef] [PubMed]
5. Arslanoglu, S.; Boquien, C.-Y.; King, C.; Lamireau, D.; Tonetto, P.; Barnett, D.; Bertino, E.; Gaya, A.; Gebauer, C.; Grovslien, A.; et al. Fortification of Human Milk for Preterm Infants: Update and Recommendations of the European Milk Bank Association (EMBA) Working Group on Human Milk Fortification. *Front. Pediatr.* **2019**, *7*, 76. [CrossRef]
6. Reali, A.; Greco, F.; Fanaro, S.; Atzei, A.; Puddu, M.; Moi, M.; Fanos, V. Fortification of maternal milk for very low birth weight (VLBW) pre-term neonates. *Early Hum. Dev.* **2010**, *86* (Suppl. 1), 33–36. [CrossRef]
7. Di Natale, C.; Coclite, E.; Di Ventura, L.; Di Fabio, S. Fortification of maternal milk for preterm infants. *J. Matern.Fetal Neonatal Med.* **2011**, *24* (Suppl. 1), 41–43. [CrossRef]
8. Arslanoglu, S.; Moro, G.E.; Ziegler, E.E.; the WAPM Working Group on Nutrition. Optimization of human milk fortification for preterm infants: New concepts and recommendations. *J. Périnat. Med.* **2010**, *38*, 233–238. [CrossRef]
9. Wojcik, K.Y.; Rechtman, D.J.; Lee, M.L.; Montoya, A.; Medo, E.T. Macronutrient Analysis of a Nationwide Sample of Donor Breast Milk. *J. Am. Diet. Assoc.* **2009**, *109*, 137–140. [CrossRef] [PubMed]
10. Rochow, N.; Fusch, G.; Choi, A.; Chessell, L.; Elliott, L.; McDonald, K.; Kuiper, E.; Purcha, M.; Turner, S.; Chan, E.; et al. Target Fortification of Breast Milk with Fat, Protein, and Carbohydrates for Preterm Infants. *J. Pediatr.* **2013**, *163*, 1001–1007. [CrossRef]
11. Fabrizio, V.; Trzaski, J.M.; Brownell, E.A.; Esposito, P.; Lainwala, S.; Lussier, M.M.; Hagadorn, J.I. Individualized versus standard diet fortification for growth and development in preterm infants receiving human milk. *Cochrane Database Syst. Rev.* **2020**, *11*, CD013465.
12. McLeod, G.; Sherriff, J.; Hartmann, P.E.; Nathan, E.; Geddes, D.; Simmer, K. Comparing different methods of human breast milk fortification using measured v. assumed macronutrient composition to target reference growth: A randomised controlled trial. *Br. J. Nutr.* **2016**, *115*, 431–439. [CrossRef]
13. Fusch, G.; Mitra, S.; Rochow, N.; Fusch, C. Target fortification of breast milk: Levels of fat, protein or lactose are not related. *Acta Paediatr.* **2014**, *104*, 38–42. [CrossRef] [PubMed]
14. Arslanoglu, S.; Moro, G.E.; Ziegler, E.E. Adjustable fortification of human milk fed to preterm infants: Does it make a difference? *J. Perinatol.* **2006**, *26*, 614–621. [CrossRef] [PubMed]
15. Rochow, N.; Raja, P.; Liu, K.; Fenton, T.; Landau-Crangle, E.; Göttler, S.; Jahn, A.; Lee, S.; Seigel, S.; Campbell, D.; et al. Physiological adjustment to postnatal growth trajectories in healthy preterm infants. *Pediatr. Res.* **2016**, *79*, 870–879. [CrossRef]
16. Landau-Crangle, E.; Rochow, N.; Fenton, T.R.; Liu, K.; Ali, A.; So, H.Y.; Fusch, G.; Marrin, M.L.; Fusch, C. Individualized Postnatal Growth Trajectories for Preterm Infants. *J. Parenter. Enter. Nutr.* **2018**, *42*, 1084–1092. [CrossRef]
17. Seliga-Siwecka, J.; Chmielewska, A.; Jasinska, K. Effect of targeted vs. standard fortification of breast milk on growth and development of preterm infants (≤32 weeks): Study protocol for a randomized controlled trial. *Trials* **2020**, *21*, 946. [CrossRef]
18. Volpe, J.J. Neonatal Intraventricular Hemorrhage. *N. Engl. J. Med.* **1981**, *304*, 886–891. [CrossRef]
19. Polberger, S.; Räihä, N.C.R.; Juvonen, P.; Moro, G.E.; Minoli, I.; Warm, A. Individualized Protein Fortification of Human Milk for Preterm Infants: Comparison of Ultrafiltrated Human Milk Protein and a Bovine Whey Fortifier. *J. Pediatr. Gastroenterol. Nutr.* **1999**, *29*, 332–338. [CrossRef]
20. Şimşek, G.K.; Dizdar, E.A.; Arayıcı, S.; Canpolat, F.E.; Sarı, F.N.; Uraş, N.; Oguz, S.S. Comparison of the Effect of Three Different Fortification Methods on Growth of Very Low Birth Weight Infants. *Breastfeed. Med.* **2019**, *14*, 63–68. [CrossRef]
21. Maas, C.; Mathes, M.; Bleeker, C.; Vek, J.; Bernhard, W.; Wiechers, C.; Peter, A.; Poets, C.F.; Franz, A.R. Effect of Increased Enteral Protein Intake on Growth in Human Milk-Fed Preterm Infants: A Randomized Clinical Trial. *JAMA Pediatr.* **2017**, *171*, 16–22. [CrossRef] [PubMed]
22. De Halleux, V.; Rigo, J. Variability in human milk composition: Benefit of individualized fortification in very-low-birth-weight infants. *Am. J. Clin. Nutr.* **2013**, *98*, 529S–535S. [CrossRef] [PubMed]
23. Morlacchi, L.; Mallardi, D.; Giannì, M.L.; Roggero, P.; Amato, O.; Piemontese, P.; Consonni, D.; Mosca, F. Is targeted fortification of human breast milk an optimal nutrition strategy for preterm infants? An interventional study. *J. Transl. Med.* **2016**, *14*, 195. [CrossRef] [PubMed]
24. Bulut, O.; Coban, A.; Uzunhan, O.; Ince, Z. Effects of Targeted Versus Adjustable Protein Fortification of Breast Milk on Early Growth in Very Low-Birth-Weight Preterm Infants: A Randomized Clinical Trial. *Nutr. Clin. Pract.* **2019**, *35*, 335–343. [CrossRef]

25. Rochow, N.; Fusch, G.; Ali, A.; Bhatia, A.; So, H.Y.; Iskander, R.; Chessell, L.; el Helou, S.; Fusch, C. Individualized target fortification of breast milk with protein, carbohydrates, and fat for preterm infants: A double-blind randomized controlled trial. *Clin. Nutr.* **2021**, *40*, 54–63. [CrossRef] [PubMed]
26. Fusch, S.; Fusch, G.; Yousuf, E.I.; Rochow, M.; So, H.Y.; Fusch, C.; Rochow, N. Individualized Target Fortification of Breast Milk: Optimizing Macronutrient Content Using Different Fortifiers and Approaches. *Front. Nutr.* **2021**, *8*, 652641. [CrossRef]
27. Quan, M.; Wang, D.; Gou, L.; Sun, Z.; Ma, J.; Zhang, L.; Wang, C.; Schibler, K.; Li, Z. Individualized Human Milk Fortification to Improve the Growth of Hospitalized Preterm Infants. *Nutr. Clin. Pract.* **2019**, *35*, 680–688. [CrossRef]
28. Agakidou, E.; Karagiozoglou-Lampoudi, T.; Parlapani, E.; Fletouris, D.J.; Sarafidis, K.; Tzimouli, V.; Diamanti, E.; Agakidis, C. Modifications of Own Mothers' Milk Fortification Protocol Affect Early Plasma IGF-I and Ghrelin Levels in Preterm Infants. A Randomized Clinical Trial. *Nutrients* **2019**, *11*, 3056. [CrossRef]
29. Trading Economics. Available online: https://tradingeconomics.com/poland/gdp (accessed on 21 December 2022).
30. Belfort, M.B.; Woodward, L.J.; Cherkerzian, S.; Pepin, H.; Ellard, D.; Steele, T.; Fusch, C.; Grant, P.E.; Inder, T.E. Targeting human milk fortification to improve very preterm infant growth and brain development: Study protocol for Nourish, a single-center randomized, controlled clinical trial. *BMC Pediatr.* **2021**, *21*, 167. [CrossRef]
31. Fusch, G.; Rochow, N.; Choi, A.; Fusch, S.; Poeschl, S.; Ubah, A.O.; Lee, S.-Y.; Raja, P.; Fusch, C. Rapid measurement of macronutrients in breast milk: How reliable are infrared milk analyzers? *Clin. Nutr.* **2015**, *34*, 465–476. [CrossRef]

nutrients

MDPI

Article

Early-Life Slow Enteral Feeding Progression Pattern Is Associated with Longitudinal Head-Size Growth Faltering and Neurodevelopmental Impairment Outcomes in Extremely Preterm Infants

Yung-Chieh Lin [1,2], Chi-Hsiang Chu [3,4], Yen-Ju Chen [1,2], Ray-Bing Chen [4] and Chao-Ching Huang [1,5,*]

1 Department of Pediatrics, National Cheng Kung University Hospital, College of Medicine, National Cheng Kung University, Tainan 704302, Taiwan
2 Graduate Institute of Clinical Medicine, College of Medicine, National Cheng-Kung University, Tainan 701401, Taiwan
3 Department of Statistics, Tunghai University, Taichung 407224, Taiwan
4 Department of Statistics, Institute of Data Science, National Cheng Kung University, Tainan 701401, Taiwan
5 Department of Pediatrics, College of Medicine, Taipei Medical University, Taipei 110301, Taiwan
* Correspondence: huangped@mail.ncku.edu.tw; Tel.: +886-62353535-5273

Abstract: Objective: To determine whether feeding progression patterns in the first eight postnatal weeks, depicted by clustering analysis of daily enteral feeding volume, are associated with longitudinal head-circumference (HC) growth and neurodevelopmental outcomes in extremely preterm (EP) infants. Methods: 200 infants who were admitted at gestational ages 23–27 weeks between 2011 and 2018; survived to discharge; and underwent longitudinal HC growth measurements at birth, term-equivalent age (TEA), corrected age (CA) 6-month, 12-month, and 24-month; and neurodevelopmental assessment using the Bayley Scales of Infant Development at CA 24 months were included for analysis. Results: kmlShape analysis identified two distinct enteral feeding progression patterns: fast progression in 131 (66%) infants and slow progression in 69 (34%) infants. Compared to the fast progression group, the slow progression group showed significantly lower daily enteral volumes after day 13, was older in postnatal age reaching full feeding, had a higher rate of Delta z scores of HC (zHC) < -1 ($p < 0.001$) between birth and TEA, and displayed lower longitudinal zHC from TEA to CA 24 months. The slow progression group also showed higher rates of microcephaly [42% vs. 16%, $p < 0.001$; adjusted odd ratio (aOR): 3.269, $p = 0.001$] and neurodevelopmental impairment (NDI) (38% vs. 19%, $p = 0.007$; aOR: 2.095, $p = 0.035$) at CA 24 months. For NDI, the model including feeding progression patterns showed a lower Akaike information criterion score and a better goodness of fit than the model that did not include feeding patterns. Conclusion: Characterizing feeding progression pattern may help identify EP infants at high-risk of head-size growth faltering and NDI at early childhood.

Keywords: enteral feeding progression patterns; clustering analysis; growth faltering; head circumference; neurodevelopmental impairment; extremely preterm infants

1. Introduction

Extremely preterm (EP) infants with gestational age <28 weeks are at high risk of adverse growth and neurodevelopmental outcomes at follow-up [1–3]. Poor or inadequate nutritional support is associated with long-term neurodevelopmental problems [4,5]. In early postnatal weeks, the advancement of enteral feeding in EP infants can not only be affected by gastrointestinal morbidities but also be associated with non- gastrointestinal risks, such as respiratory failure requiring mechanical ventilation [6,7]. Therefore, the enteral feeding progression pattern may be associated with the well-being and neurodevelopmental outcomes of EP infants [6,8].

Monitoring the growth trajectories of head circumference (HC) starting from birth to discharge and periodically into early childhood is critical for neurodevelopmental outcomes in EP infants [9–11]. Head-size growth is more related to cognitive outcomes than bodyweight (BW) because head size is more relevant to brain volume and cortical maturation before 24 months of age [12–14]. Poor postnatal head-size growth has been associated with impaired neurodevelopmental outcome in EP infants [10,15–17]. Whether the slow-feeding progression pattern is associated with inadequate longitudinal HC growth and neurodevelopmental impairment (NDI) outcome at early childhood remains unknown.

kmlShape clustering analysis, a data partitioning method, allows the grouping of individuals whose trajectories have similar forms but with shifted positions in time [18]. This study compared the feeding progression patterns in the first 56 days after birth in EP infants using kmlShape analysis, and explored the associations of different feeding progression patterns with HC changes between birth and term-equivalent age (TEA) and from TEA to corrected age (CA) 6, 12, and 24 months, as well as neurodevelopmental outcomes at CA 24 months. We hypothesized that the early-life slow-feeding progression pattern is associated with longitudinal HC growth faltering and NDI outcomes in early childhood.

2. Materials and Methods

2.1. Study Settings and Design

Among the 298 EP infants who were born and admitted with gestational age at 23–27 weeks, 226 infants survived to discharge from a tertiary university hospital from January 2011 to December 2018. 213 (94%) infants received prospective longitudinal growth follow-up assessments at TEA and CA 6, 12, and 24 months. After excluding 13 children with congenital abnormalities, genetic syndromes, or perinatal or post-discharge brain injuries, 200 children were included in the analysis (Figure S1). This study was approved by the institutional review board of the University Hospital (approval code: ER-98-135; date: 28 June 2022). Informed consent was obtained from the parents of each infant.

2.2. Nutritional Care Policy

Preterm infants were cared for using the similar protocol of enteral feeding and parenteral nutrition soon after birth [6,19]. HC was measured weekly, and BW was measured daily. Soon after birth, infants were administrated with 3 g/kg/day of electrolyte-free amino acids via peripheral or central intravenous routes. Once the central intravenous route was established, lipid administration was initiated at 1 g/kg/day and gradually increased to 3–4 g/kg/day. When the baby's condition was stabilized, a tailor-made composited parenteral nutrition was prescribed. A trophic feeding volume of 10–20 mL/kg/day was started as soon as possible after birth, and maintained for 1 to 3 days or more, depending on the clinical status [20–22].

The daily total protein intake was controlled at 3.5–4.0 g/kg/day, and the daily total lipid intakes maintained at 3–4 g/kg/day. The glucose infusion was set at 7 g/kg/day initially and then 13–17 g/kg/day according to glucose tolerance [21,22]. Total fluid was targeted at 60–80 mL/kg in the first 24 h of life and increased with improving urine outputs. After the diuretic phase after birth, the daily fluid intake was maintained at 130 to 150 mL/kg/day with caloric density of 80–100 Kcal/kg/day.

Increase in the feeding volume by increments of 10–20 mL/kg/day was prescribed and evaluated daily. When the enteral feeding volume reached 100 mL/kg/day, feeding with fortified human milk (0.74 Kcal/mL) was initiated and intravenous lipid administration discontinued. Full enteral feeding was defined as the enteral feeding volume reaching 120 mL/kg/day [6,23–25] and intravenous parenteral fluids discontinued along with removal of intravenous catheters. Full enteral volume was set at 120 mL/kg/day, which is commonly used for preterm infants with balanced fluid maintenance without additional intravenous fluid support. Further milk volume advancement might be required for higher caloric requirement and growth [6,19].

The postnatal ages at initial feeding and full enteral feeding (120 mL/kg/day) were recorded. The daily enteral feeding volume in the first 8 postnatal weeks was calculated as mL/kg/day. The daily parenteral nutritional intake (mL/kg/day), the daily total nutritional fluid intake (mL/kg/day), and the daily total caloric intake (mL/kg/day) were also calculated.

After discharge, infants were regularly followed up with for health surveillance and growth and developmental supervision up to CA 24 months. Fortification of milk or the use of the post-discharge formula was shifted to the regular infant formula or unfortified human milk when the growth trajectories reached the adequate percentile [22,26].

2.3. Covariates

Small for gestational age (SGA) was defined as birth BW of less than the 10th percentile for GA. Neonatal morbidities were recorded, including respiratory distress syndrome (RDS) requiring surfactant therapy, hypotension requiring vasopressors, hemodynamically significant patent ductus arteriosus (hs-PDA) requiring surgery, postnatal steroid use, sepsis, intraventricular hemorrhage (IVH), cystic periventricular leukomalacia (cPVL), postnatal steroid, bacteremia, necrotizing enterocolitis (NEC), and non-NEC events requiring surgery [6]. Non-NEC events requiring surgery included meconium ileus, spontaneous intestine perforation, volvulus, and intestine adhesions [6].

2.4. Outcomes

The longitudinal growth of BW and HC was calculated from birth to TEA, and from TEA to CA 6, 12, and 24 months. BW and HC at TEA were recorded at the postmenstrual age of 37–42 weeks. A non-stretch tape was used and placed precisely at the broadest part of the forehead above the eyebrow, above the ears, and at the most prominent part of the occipital part of the head (https://www.cdc.gov/zika/pdfs/microcephaly_measuring.pdf, accessed on 28 February 2023). Each measurement represented a single measurement by experienced nurses. Re-measurement was required when obvious deviation from the standard growth trajectory curve was noted. The anthropometric z-scores for BW (zBW) and HC (zHC) at birth and TEA, respectively, were derived from Fenton's postnatal growth charts [27]. A delta z score (the zBW or zHC at TEA minus the zBW or zHC at birth) of -1 or less indicated growth delay in BW or HC during hospital stay [26,28–30]. The zBW and zHC at each follow-up visit were based on the standards provided by the World Health Organization [31]. Microcephaly was defined as a head circumference of < 10th percentile for the age.

Neurodevelopmental outcomes at CA 24 months were assessed using the Bayley Scales of Infant Development third edition (BSID-III) [32,33]. Child psychologists who performed neurodevelopmental assessments were blinded to the early-life feeding status. The severity of cerebral palsy was measured using the Gross Motor Function Classification System (GMFCS) as mild (level 1), moderate (level 2 or 3), or severe (level 4 or 5). NDI was defined as the presence of one or more of the following: cognitive composite score or motor composite score < 85 by BSID-III, moderate or severe cerebral palsy (GMFCS level $\geq$2), profound visual impairment, or profound hearing loss [32].

2.5. Statistical Analysis

The feeding patterns were analyzed using the "kmlShape" package in R to cluster meaningful groups [6,18]. Demographics and risks were compared using chi-square or Fisher's exact tests for categorical variables and the independent *t*-test or Mann–Whitney U test for continuous variables. Repeated-measures analysis of variance was used to compare the longitudinal anthropometric data between groups. For multiple comparisons at each time point, Bonferroni adjustment as a post hoc test was used to explore pairwise differences. A generalized estimating equation (GEE) was used to analyze the association between repeated measurements and factors. The dependence of longitudinal anthropometric variables on the risks, chosen a priori, and feeding pattern was first assessed using univariate analysis. Using logistic regression and adjusting for the risk factors selected from the candidate factors in the univariate analysis, the association between feeding patterns and NDI outcomes was analyzed. After univariate analysis, all candidate factors were included in the multivariable analysis and chosen by a stepwise procedure using the Akaike information criterion (AIC). AIC was used to identify better performance from the candidate models. The likelihood ratio test was also used to determine the goodness of fit of the two competing statistical models. Results were considered statistically significant if the p-value was less than 0.05.

3. Results

3.1. Risks Associated with Slow Progression Feeding Pattern

Of the 200 EP infants included for analysis, the mean gestational age was 25.6 ± 1.3 weeks, and the mean birth body weight was 839 ± 199 g. Based on the daily enteral feeding data from the first 56 postnatal days, the kmlShape analysis identified two distinct feeding progression patterns: a fast progression pattern in 131 (66%) infants (Figure S2A) and a slow progression pattern in 69 (34%) infants (Figure S2B). The slow progression pattern group was older in the postnatal ages at initial feeding and reaching full feeding and showed a significantly lower daily enteral feeding volume by postnatal day 13 ($p < 0.05$), and the differences increased up to day 56 (all $p < 0.05$) compared to the fast progression pattern group (Figure 1A).

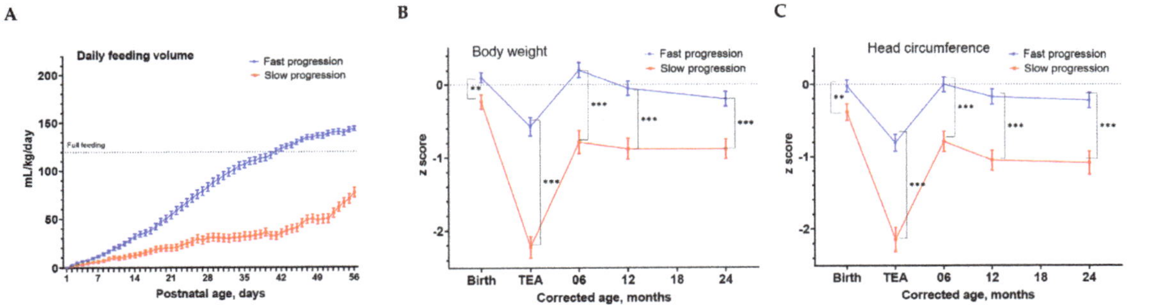

Figure 1. (**A**) Differences in the daily enteral feeding volumes in the first 56 postnatal days between the fast progression feeding pattern group and the slow progression feeding pattern group in extremely preterm infants. The statistical significances were observed from postnatal day 13 to day 56. Full feeding was defined as 120 mL/kg/days. Data were presented as mean ± SEM. Bonferroni adjustment was used for the multiple comparisons between the two different feeding progression patterns at each time points. Differences in the longitudinal anthropometric z-scores of bodyweights (**B**) and head circumference (**C**) from birth, term equivalent age (TEA), 6 months, 12 months, and up to 24 months of corrected age between the fast progression and slow progression feeding pattern. The blue line represents the fast progression pattern and the red line represents the slow progression pattern. Data were presented as mean ± SEM. Statistical significances: **: $p < 0.01$ and ***: $p < 0.001$.

Compared to the fast progression pattern group, the slow progression pattern group had significantly lower gestational age and birth zBW and zHC, and had higher proportions of hypotension, hs-PDA requiring surgery, late-onset sepsis, cPVL, and non-NEC gastrointestinal events requiring surgery (Table 1).

The total nutritional fluid intakes were comparable between the two feeding progression groups except for a lower intake on days 26, 27, 32, and 41 (all $p < 0.05$) in the fast progression group (Figure 2A). The slow progression group required a longer duration on parenteral nutritional intakes from day 7 to day 56 compared to the fast progression group (Figure 2B). In contrast, the fast progression group had higher total daily caloric intakes from day 32 to day 56 (all $p < 0.05$) compared to the slow progression group (Figure 2C).

Table 1. Differences of demographics, prenatal and neonatal risks, and exposures between the fast progression and slow progression pattern groups in extremely preterm infants.

Feeding Trajectories Risks and Exposures	Fast Progression N = 131	Slow Progression N = 69	*p* Values
Demographics			
Male, n (%)	64 (49)	40 (58)	0.237
Gestational age, weeks, mean (SD)	25.9 (1.3)	25.2 (1.3)	<0.001
Birth bodyweight z score, mean (SD)	0.10 (0.82)	−0.24 (0.81)	0.006
Small for gestational age, n (%)	7 (5)	6 (9)	0.377
Birth head circumference z score, mean (SD)	−0.02 (0.96)	−0.39 (0.95)	0.011
Maternal education level (<college), n (%)	50 (38)	29 (42)	0.649
Prenatal period			
Antenatal steroid, n (%)	123 (94)	66 (96)	0.751
Multiple gestation, n (%)	39 (30)	21 (30)	1.000
Preeclampsia, n (%)	20 (15)	12 (17)	0.690
Gestational diabetes, n (%)	4 (3)	1 (1)	0.661
Neonatal period			
Respiratory/hemodynamics, n (%)	109 (83)	62 (90)	0.291
RDS requiring surfactant therapy, n (%)	64 (49)	36 (52)	0.766
Hypotension requiring vasopressors, n (%)	82 (63)	57 (83)	0.006
hs-PDA requiring surgery, n (%)	26 (20)	28 (41)	0.002
Postnatal steroid, n (%)	26 (20)	21 (30)	0.114
Infection events, n (%)	17 (13)	30 (43)	0.001
Early-onset sepsis, n (%)	5 (4)	5 (7)	0.318
Late-onset sepsis, n (%)	14 (11)	26 (38)	<0.001
Severe brain injury, n (%)	10 (8)	11 (16)	0.089
IVH (≥III), n (%)	8 (6)	6 (9)	0.563
cPVL, n (%)	4 (3)	9 (13)	0.012
GI morbidities, n (%)	13 (10)	25 (36)	<0.001
NEC ≥ stage II, n (%)	10 (8)	12 (17)	0.055
Non-NEC events requiring surgery, n (%)	4 (3)	16 (23)	<0.001
Feeding progression			
Postnatal age at initial feeding, days, mean (SD)	4.2 (3.9)	5.9 (5.3)	0.024
Postnatal age at reaching full feeding, days, mean (SD)	33 (9.5)	56 (20.6)	<0.001
Growth differences between TEA and birth			
Delta z score of bodyweight <−1, n (%)	60 (46)	59 (86)	<0.001
Delta z score of head circumference <−1, n (%)	55 (42)	50 (73)	<0.001

RDS: respiratory distress syndrome; PDA: hemodynamic significant patent ductus arteriosus; NEC: Necrotizing enterocolitis; IVH: intraventricular hemorrhage; cPVL: cystic periventricular leukomalacia; TEA: term equivalent age; EUGR: extrauterine growth restriction; Delta z scores: the differences in z scores of bodyweight or head circumference between TEA and birth.

3.2. *Slow Progression Feeding Pattern Negatively Associated with the Trend Changes of Longitudinal Head-Size Growth*

The slow progression group had significantly higher rates of delta z scores < -1 in BW (86% vs. 46%, $p < 0.001$) and in HC (73% vs. 42%, $p < 0.001$) between TEA and birth than the fast progression group (Table 1). The longitudinal anthropometric zBW and zHC show that the slow progression group was associated with significantly lower zBW (Figure 1B) and zHC (Figure 1C) at TEA, and also at CA 6, 12, and 24 months compared to the fast progression group. The zHC of the fast progression group was −0.7 at TEA but increased to 0 at CA 6, 12, and 24 months. In contrast, the zHC of the slow progression group was well below −2 at TEA and remained persistently at −1 from CA 6 to 24 months.

Univariate followed by multivariate analysis by GEE for the risks associated with the trend changes of zHC showed that lower gestational age, SGA, RDS requiring surfactant therapy, severe IVH, and slow-feeding progression pattern were significantly associated with negative coefficients with repeated zHC measurements from birth to CA 24 months (Table S1).

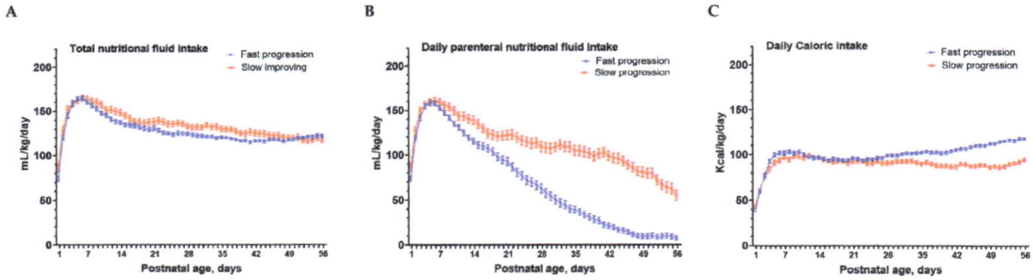

Figure 2. Differences of total nutritional fluid intake (mL/kg/day, (**A**)), the daily parenteral nutritional fluid intake (mL/kg/day, (**B**)), and total caloric intake (Kcal/kg/day, (**C**)) in the first 56 postnatal days between the fast progression and slow progression enteral feeding progression groups. Data were presented as mean ± SEM. Bonferroni adjustment was used for the multiple comparisons between the two feeding groups at each time point. Significant statistical differences were observed in the parenteral nutritional fluid intake from day 13 to day 56; the total nutritional fluid intake on days 26, 27, 32, and 41; the total caloric intake from day 32 to day 56.

3.3. *Microcephaly and Neurodevelopmental Impairment Outcomes at Corrected Age 24 Months after Slow-Feeding Progression Pattern*

We then compared the differences in the proportion of infants with microcephaly (HC < 10th percentile) and NDI outcomes at CA 24 months between the two early-life different feeding progression patterns. The slow progression group was associated with significantly higher rates of microcephaly [42% vs. 16%, $p < 0.001$; adjusted odd ratio (aOR): 3.269, $p = 0.001$] and NDI (38% vs. 19%, $p = 0.007$; aOR: 2.095, $p = 0.035$) than the fast progression group (Table 2).

Table 2. Differences in proportions of microcephaly and neurodevelopmental impairment outcomes at corrected age 24 months between the fast progression and slow progression feeding pattern groups in early life.

Early-Life Feeding Trajectories	Slow Progression	Fast Progression		* Adjusted Odds Ratio (aOR)		
Outcomes	**N = 69**	**N = 131**	***p* Values**	**aOR**	**95% CI**	***p* Values**
Head circumference < 10th percentile, n (%)	28 (42)	21 (16)	<0.001	3.269	1.634, 6.54	0.001
Neurodevelopmental impairment, n (%)	26 (38)	25 (19)	0.007	2.095	1.052, 4.171	0.035
Moderate to severe cerebral palsy, n (%)	8 (11.6)	6 (4.6)	0.082	2.507	0.799, 7.866	0.115
Cognitive impairment, n (%)	15 (22)	19 (15)	0.252	1.462	0.663, 3.223	0.347
Profound hearing/vision impairment, n (%)	7 (10.1)	6 (4.6)	0.142	1.923	0.597, 6.193	0.273

* Adjusted with gestational age and gender.

3.4. *The Model including Feeding Patterns Better Predicted Neurodevelopmental Outcomes*

Univariate and multivariate logistic regression analyses were performed to examine early-life medical risks and feeding progression patterns associated with NDI at CA 24 months (Table 3). The model that does not include feeding progression patterns (Model 1) identified three risk factors, namely male sex (aOR 2.316, 95% CI [1.136–4.720], $p = 0.021$), lower maternal education level (2.231, [1.124–4.431], $p = 0.022$), and severe brain injury (4.331, [1.641–11.616], $p = 0.004$), as being significantly associated with NDI. After adding feeding patterns to the multivariate model (Model 2), four risk factors, that is, male sex (2.224, [1.078–4.575], $p = 0.030$), lower maternal education level (2.200, [1.098–4.406], $p = 0.026$), severe brain injury (3.854, [1.408–10.550], $p = 0.009$), and slow progression feeding pattern (2.232, [1.114–4.473], $p = 0.024$), demonstrated significantly negative impacts on neurodevelopmental outcomes. The model including feeding progression patterns showed a lower AIC score and had a better model goodness of fit using the log likelihood ratio test ($p = 0.024$) than the model that did not include feeding progression patterns.

Table 3. Logistic regression analysis for early-life medical risks and feeding patterns associated with neurodevelopmental impairment outcomes at corrected age 24 months.

Logistic Regression Model		Univariate			Multivariate Model 1, Without Feeding Progression Patterns			Multivariate Model 2, With Feeding Progression Patterns		
	Ref.	OR	95% CI	p	aOR	95% CI	p	aOR	95% CI	p
Small for gestational age	None	0.512	0.110, 2.392	0.395	—	—	—	—	—	—
Gestational age 23–25 weeks	26–27	1.868	0.983, 3.551	0.056	—	—	0.225	—	—	0.634
Male	Female	2.859	1.444, 5.661	0.003	2.316	1.136, 4.720	0.021	2.224	1.078, 4.575	0.030
Low maternal education level	(≥college)	2.099	1.101, 3.999	0.024	2.231	1.124, 4.431	0.022	2.200	1.098, 4.406	0.026
Pulmonary/hemodynamics [a]	None	2.369	0.783, 7.171	0.127	—	—	—	—	—	—
Infection events [b]	None	1.157	0.554, 2.418	0.698	—	—	—	—	—	—
NEC ≥ stage II	None	1.421	0.544, 3.710	0.473	—	—	—	—	—	—
Severe brain injury [c]	None	4.786	1.88, 12.183	0.001	4.331	1.614, 11.616	0.004	3.854	1.408, 10.550	0.009
Slow progression feeding pattern	Fast	2.564	1.334, 4.928	0.005				2.232	1.114, 4.473	0.024
Model goodness of fit										
Akaike information criterion				NA		212.57				209.48
Log likelihood						204.57				199.48 *

[a] Any of RDS requiring surfactant therapy, hypotension requiring vasopressors, hs-PDA requiring surgery, or postnatal systemic steroid; [b] Any of early-onset sepsis or late-onset sepsis; [c] Any of severe IVH or cPVL; * Log likelihood test for model goodness of fit is applied for the comparison between model 1 and model 2 ($p = 0.024$). Low maternal education level: education level below college.

4. Discussion

Under the similar enteral feeding and nutritional support protocol, we investigated the impacts of two different early-life feeding progression patterns, established by the daily enteral feeding volume in the first 8 postnatal weeks, on the longitudinal head-size growth from birth to CA 24 months, and microcephaly and neurodevelopment outcomes at CA 24 months in EP infants. We found that the slow-feeding progression pattern occurred in one third of EP infants who could be distinguished from the fast progression feeding pattern as early as postnatal day 13. The slow progression group required a longer duration on parenteral nutritional intakes from day 7, while the two feeding progression groups had similar daily caloric intakes in the first postnatal weeks. Compared to the fast progression group, the slow progression group showed growth faltering in zHC not only from birth to TEA but also from TEA to CA 24 months. The slow progression group also had significantly higher rates of microcephaly and NDI at CA 24 months. The model that included early-life feeding patterns demonstrated more negative impacts on neurodevelopmental outcomes than the model without including feeding progression patterns. Taken together, these findings suggest that close monitoring of feeding progression patterns in the early postnatal weeks provides important information on the longitudinal head-size growth and neurodevelopmental outcomes in EP infants.

4.1. Characterizing the Patterns of Early-Life Feeding Progression

The goal to achieve normal growth and neurodevelopment for infants born extremely preterm is to provide adequate nutritional supports through daily feeding. However, the enteral feeding progression is largely affected by the degree of gut immaturity, and the occurrence of gastrointestinal and non-gastrointestinal medical morbidities of these infants in the NICU. On the enteral feeding progression, we found that two thirds of EP infants showing the fast progression pattern had better head-size growth and neurodevelopmental outcomes compared to the slow progression pattern group. Early full enteral feeding, which appears to be feasible in these clinically stable EP infants, has been associated with better short outcome in late-onset sepsis and reduced length of hospital stays [34–36]. However, in these stable infants, studies fail to establish a link between increased protein and energy intakes of recommended levels and neurodevelopmental outcome at follow-up, and the evidence between early protein supplement and reduced postnatal faltering growth is weak [37–41]. A large, randomized trial also demonstrated a faster volume increment of enteral feeding (daily increments of 30 mL/kg) compared to a slower increment (daily increments of 18 mL/kg) failed to improve survival without NDI at CA 24 months [42,43].

Yet, very limited studies have investigated the underlying causes and growth and neurodevelopmental outcomes of the EP infants who fail to follow the trajectory of feeding progression [6,44]. We found that enteral feeding progression was very difficult to achieve in one third of EP infants due to gut immaturity and the presence of medical morbidities. The infants who followed the slow progression pattern and required prolonged parenteral nutritional intakes could be identified by the first 2 weeks after birth. Despite the comparable daily total nutritional fluid intakes and caloric intakes between the slow progression and fast progression groups in the first 4 weeks after birth, the slow progression groups showed long-term head-size growth faltering, and higher rates of microcephaly and NDI at CA 24 months.

4.2. Early-Life Feeding Patterns, Extrauterine Head-Size Growth by TEA, and Longitudinal Head-Size Growth from TEA to CA 24 Months

Studies on the risks for extrauterine growth restriction have included the risks, morbidities, and nutritional feeding practices in the NICU [25,45–47]. Head-size growth in the first two years after birth is associated with neurodevelopmental outcome in very preterm infants [10,12,13,15–17,48]. We focused on the daily enteral feeding volumes in the first 8 postnatal weeks to depict early-life feeding progression patterns that might associate with the extrauterine head-size growth at TEA status as well as at follow-up. Studies suggest that infants with extrauterine growth restriction at discharge/TEA frequently show continued growth restriction at follow-up [49–51]. Head-size growth needs to be monitored with longitudinal growth curves for the best result in EP infants [10,52,53]. We found that the slow progression feeding group was not only associated with extrauterine growth restriction in HC between TEA and birth but also with persistent head-size growth faltering from TEA to CA 24 months. Gut microbiota is important for growth in young infants [54,55]. The specific gut microbiota that were involved with the faltering of head-size changes in the slow progression feeding group remain to be elucidated.

4.3. Close Relationship between Early-Life Feeding Patterns, Longitudinal Head-Size Growth and Neurodevelopmental Outcomes

The relationship between growth patterns and neurodevelopment outcomes in preterm infants has been investigated [10,48,56,57]. In-hospital growth velocity in BW and HC between birth and discharge/TEA shows significant effects on neurodevelopmental outcome [12,15,48]. However, whether extrauterine growth restriction at discharge is associated with neurodevelopmental outcomes remains controversial [28,58,59]. The longitudinal growth faltering in HC from birth to TEA and into early childhood may have a higher negative predictive value for NDI than cross-sectional ones or just at TEA [10,26,28,59]. We found that slow progression feeding patterns were associated with a high rate of NDI by persistently faltering in head-size growth curves from TEA to CA 24 months. These findings indicate the close relationship between early-life feeding progression patterns, longitudinal head-size growth, and NDI outcomes in EP infants.

4.4. Early-Life Slow Progression Feeding Pattern Depicted by Clustering Analysis as an Important Risk for Head-Size Growth Faltering and NDI

In addition to the well-known neonatal risks that have been associated with NDI, our study demonstrated the early-life adverse feeding patterns are also an important risk for NDI. Monitoring the daily enteral feeding volume in preterm infants is a part of routine care worldwide [42]. More than 90% of infants in our NICU were fully or partially fed with human milk up to TEA [19,60,61]. kmlShape analysis stratified the heterogenic trajectories within the study populations according to their shapes after examining their time series and longitudinal data [18,62]. kmlShape clustering analysis has been applied to examine time series and longitudinal data according to their shapes in order to capture the heterogenic trajectories within the study populations. Using kmlShape clustering analysis of respiratory patterns based on the daily type of ventilation support in the first 8 weeks after birth in preterm infants, one study had shown that early-life respiratory trajectories were associated with neurodevelopmental outcomes in extremely preterm infants [32]. For the first time, we established early-life feeding progression patterns by performing clustering analysis on data from daily enteral feeding, and further linked the feeding patterns with the head-size growth trajectory and NDI in EP infants.

4.5. Limitations

This prospective registration and follow-up cohort of EP infants has limitations inherent to observational studies from a single academic center. The generalizability of the results to other centers needs to be validated through further prospective multicenter studies. The macronutrients, energy, and protein intakes during hospitalization may be associated with a free fat mass/fat mass at discharge, a potential marker for growth and neurodevelopment outcomes in infants [63,64]. The evaluations of macronutrients, energy, and protein intakes during hospitalization and free fat mass or fat mass at TEA and follow-up were not available in this study. A single head circumference measurement at designated time points instead of considering the average of consecutive measurements and the lack of an interobserver agreement assessment of measurements could also be study limitations.

5. Conclusions

Early-life feeding progression pattern may serve as a risk factor for long-term head-size growth faltering and neurodevelopmental outcomes. EP infants who followed the slow progression feeding pattern were at high risk of longitudinal head-size growth faltering, microcephaly, and NDI at early childhood. Characterizing the adverse feeding progression pattern in the first two weeks after birth may help identify high-risk infants earlier for further nutritional interventions to improve outcomes.

Supplementary Materials: The following supporting information can be downloaded at: https://www.mdpi.com/article/10.3390/nu15051277/s1, Figure S1: A flowchart of the extremely preterm infants included for analysis; Figure S2: The kmlShape clustering analysis characterizes the feeding progression trajectories of extremely preterm infants; Table S1: The early-life medical risks and slowly feeding progression pattern that are associated with the trend changes of head circumference z scores from birth to 24 months of corrected age in extremely preterm infants: univariate and multivariate GEE analyses.

Author Contributions: Conceptualization, C.-C.H.; methodology, Y.-C.L.; validation, Y.-J.C. and R.-B.C.; formal analysis, C.-H.C. and R.-B.C.; investigation, Y.-C.L. and Y.-J.C.; resource, C.-C.H.; data curation, C.-H.C., R.-B.C., and C.-C.H.; writing—original draft preparation, Y.-C.L.; writing—review and editing, C.-C.H.; visualization, Y.-C.L.; supervision, C.-C.H.; project administration, C.-C.H.; funding acquisition, C.-C.H. All authors have read and agreed to the published version of the manuscript.

Funding: This study was supported by grants from the Taiwan Ministry of Science and Technology (MOST 111-2314-B-006 -012; MOST 110-2314-B-006-113; NSTC-111-2314-B006-001) and the grant of National Cheng Kung University Hospital (NCKUH-11101001; NCKUH-11201003).

Institutional Review Board Statement: The study was conducted according to the guidelines of the Declaration of Helsinki, and approved by the Institutional Review Board of National Cheng Kung University Hospital (approval code: ER-98-135, date: 28 June 2022).

Informed Consent Statement: Informed consent was obtained from the parents of each infant during hospitalization and at the follow-up visits.

Data Availability Statement: The corresponding author had full access to the dataset used and analyzed during the current study. The datasets used during the current study are available from the corresponding author upon reasonable request.

Acknowledgments: The authors thank the Taiwan Premature Baby Foundation and all team members in charge of the data collection and assessment of the children. None of these individuals were compensated for their contributions. Data described in the manuscript, code book, and analytic code will be made available upon request pending reasonable application and approval through the institute of the corresponding author.

Conflicts of Interest: The authors declare no conflict of interest.

References

1. Shankaran, S. Childhood neurodevelopmental outcome following extremely preterm birth. *Lancet Child Adolesc. Health* **2018**, *2*, 843–844. [CrossRef] [PubMed]
2. Younge, N.; Goldstein, R.F.; Bann, C.M.; Hintz, S.R.; Patel, R.M.; Smith, P.B.; Bell, E.F.; Rysavy, M.A.; Duncan, A.F.; Vohr, B.R.; et al. Survival and Neurodevelopmental Outcomes among Periviable Infants. *N. Engl. J. Med.* **2017**, *376*, 617–628. [CrossRef]
3. Duncan, A.F.; Bann, C.M.; Dempsey, A.; Peralta-Carcelen, M.; Hintz, S.; Eunice Kennedy Shriver National Institute of Child Health; Development Neonatal Research Network. Behavioral Deficits at 18–22 Months of Age Are Associated with Early Cerebellar Injury and Cognitive and Language Performance in Children Born Extremely Preterm. *J. Pediatr.* **2019**, *204*, 148–156.e4. [CrossRef] [PubMed]
4. Lithoxopoulou, M.; Rallis, D.; Christou, H.; Goutsiou, E.; Varaklioti, A.; Karagianni, P.; Tsakalidis, C.; Domeyer, P.; Kuriakeli, G.; Soubasi, V. Early caloric deprivation in preterm infants affects Bayley-III scales performance at 18–24 months of corrected age. *Res. Dev. Disabil.* **2019**, *91*, 103429. [CrossRef] [PubMed]
5. Coviello, C.; Keunen, K.; Kersbergen, K.J.; Groenendaal, F.; Leemans, A.; Peels, B.; Isgum, I.; Viergever, M.A.; de Vries, L.S.; Buonocore, G.; et al. Effects of early nutrition and growth on brain volumes, white matter microstructure, and neurodevelopmental outcome in preterm newborns. *Pediatr. Res.* **2018**, *83*, 102–110. [CrossRef]

6. Lin, Y.C.; Chu, C.H.; Chen, Y.J.; Chen, R.B.; Huang, C.C. Gestational Age-Related Associations between Early-Life Feeding Trajectories and Growth Outcomes at Term Equivalent Age in Very Preterm Infants. *Nutrients* **2022**, *14*, 1032. [CrossRef]
7. Kwok, T.C.; Dorling, J.; Gale, C. Early enteral feeding in preterm infants. *Semin. Perinatol.* **2019**, *43*, 151159. [CrossRef]
8. Walsh, V.; Brown, J.V.E.; Copperthwaite, B.R.; Oddie, S.J.; McGuire, W. Early full enteral feeding for preterm or low birth weight infants. *Cochrane Database Syst. Rev.* **2020**, *12*, Cd013542. [CrossRef]
9. Landau-Crangle, E.; Rochow, N.; Fenton, T.R.; Liu, K.; Ali, A.; So, H.Y.; Fusch, G.; Marrin, M.L.; Fusch, C. Individualized Postnatal Growth Trajectories for Preterm Infants. *JPEN J. Parenter. Enter. Nutr.* **2018**, *42*, 1084–1092. [CrossRef]
10. Raghuram, K.; Yang, J.; Church, P.T.; Cieslak, Z.; Synnes, A.; Mukerji, A.; Shah, P.S. Head Growth Trajectory and Neurodevelopmental Outcomes in Preterm Neonates. *Pediatrics* **2017**, *140*, e20170216. [CrossRef]
11. Guellec, I.; Marret, S.; Baud, O.; Cambonie, G.; Lapillonne, A.; Roze, J.C.; Fresson, J.; Flamant, C.; Charkaluk, M.L.; Arnaud, C.; et al. Intrauterine Growth Restriction, Head Size at Birth, and Outcome in Very Preterm Infants. *J. Pediatr.* **2015**, *167*, 975–981.e2. [CrossRef]
12. Cheong, J.L.Y.; Hunt, R.W.; Anderson, P.J.; Howard, K.; Thompson, D.K.; Wang, H.X.; Bear, M.J.; Inder, T.E.; Doyle, L.W. Head growth in preterm infants: Correlation with magnetic resonance imaging and neurodevelopmental outcome. *Pediatrics* **2008**, *121*, E1534–E1540. [CrossRef]
13. Tan, M.; Abernethy, L.; Cooke, R. Improving head growth in preterm infants—A randomised controlled trial II: MRI and developmental outcomes in the first year. *Arch. Dis. Child.-Fetal Neonatal Ed.* **2008**, *93*, F342–F346. [CrossRef] [PubMed]
14. Vinall, J.; Grunau, R.E.; Brant, R.; Chau, V.; Poskitt, K.J.; Synnes, A.R.; Miller, S.P. Slower Postnatal Growth Is Associated with Delayed Cerebral Cortical Maturation in Preterm Newborns. *Sci. Transl. Med.* **2013**, *5*, 168ra8. [CrossRef]
15. Ehrenkranz, R.A.; Dusick, A.M.; Vohr, B.R.; Wright, L.L.; Wrage, L.A.; Poole, W.K.; Neonatal, N.I.H.H.D. Growth in the neonatal intensive care unit influences neurodevelopmental and growth outcomes of extremely low birth weight infants. *Pediatrics* **2006**, *117*, 1253–1261. [CrossRef] [PubMed]
16. Ranke, M.B.; Krageloh-Mann, I.; Vollmer, B. Growth, head growth, and neurocognitive outcome in children born very preterm: Methodological aspects and selected results. *Dev. Med. Child. Neurol.* **2015**, *57*, 23–28. [CrossRef] [PubMed]
17. Lee, K.A.; Hayes, B.C. Head size and growth in the very preterm infant: A literature review. *Res. Rep. Neonatol.* **2015**, *5*, 1–6. [CrossRef]
18. Genolini, C.; Ecochard, R.; Benghezal, M.; Driss, T.; Andrieu, S.; Subtil, F. kmlShape: An Efficient Method to Cluster Longitudinal Data (Time-Series) According to Their Shapes. *PLoS ONE* **2016**, *11*, e0150738. [CrossRef]
19. Lin, Y.C.; Chen, Y.J.; Huang, C.C.; Shieh, C.C. Concentrated Preterm Formula as a Liquid Human Milk Fortifier at Initiation Stage in Extremely Low Birth Weight Preterm Infants: Short Term and 2-year Follow-up Outcomes. *Nutrients* **2020**, *12*, 2229. [CrossRef]
20. Terrin, G.; Di Chiara, M.; Sabatini, G.; Senterre, T.; De Curtis, M. Enteral Nutrition in Preterm Neonates. In *Textbook of Pediatric Gastroenterology, Hepatology and Nutrition: A Comprehensive Guide to Practice*; Guandalini, S., Dhawan, A., Eds.; Springer International Publishing: Cham, Switzerland, 2022; pp. 65–85.
21. Brune, K.D.; Donn, S.M. Enteral Feeding of the Preterm Infant. *NeoReviews* **2018**, *19*, e645–e653. [CrossRef]
22. Taiwan-Society-of-Neonatology. *Recommendation on Nutritional Care of Taiwan Preterm Infants*; Taiwan Society of Neonatology: Taiwan, 2015.
23. Salas, A.A.; Cuna, A.; Bhat, R.; McGwin, G., Jr.; Carlo, W.A.; Ambalavanan, N. A randomised trial of re-feeding gastric residuals in preterm infants. *Arch. Dis. Child. Fetal Neonatal Ed.* **2015**, *100*, F224–F228. [CrossRef]
24. Glackin, S.J.; O'Sullivan, A.; George, S.; Semberova, J.; Miletin, J. High flow nasal cannula versus NCPAP, duration to full oral feeds in preterm infants: A randomised controlled trial. *Arch. Dis Child. Fetal Neonatal Ed.* **2017**, *102*, F329–F332. [CrossRef]
25. Travers, C.P.; Wang, T.; Salas, A.A.; Schofield, E.; Dills, M.; Laney, D.; Yee, A.; Bhatia, A.; Winter, L.; Ambalavanan, N.; et al. Higher or Usual Volume Feedings in Very Preterm Infants: A Randomized Clinical Trial. *J. Pediatr.* **2020**, *224*, 66–71. [CrossRef] [PubMed]
26. Fenton, T.R.; Dai, S.; Lalari, V.; Alshaikh, B. Neonatal and Preterm Infant Growth Assessment. *Clin. Perinatol.* **2022**, *49*, 295–311. [CrossRef]
27. Fenton, T.R.; Nasser, R.; Eliasziw, M.; Kim, J.H.; Bilan, D.; Sauve, R. Validating the weight gain of preterm infants between the reference growth curve of the fetus and the term infant. *BMC Pediatr.* **2013**, *13*, 92. [CrossRef]
28. Fenton, T.R.; Cormack, B.; Goldberg, D.; Nasser, R.; Alshaikh, B.; Eliasziw, M.; Hay, W.W.; Hoyos, A.; Anderson, D.; Bloomfield, F.; et al. "Extrauterine growth restriction" and "postnatal growth failure" are misnomers for preterm infants. *J. Perinatol.* **2020**, *40*, 704–714. [CrossRef]
29. Kim, Y.J.; Shin, S.H.; Cho, H.; Shin, S.H.; Kim, S.H.; Song, I.G.; Kim, E.K.; Kim, H.S. Extrauterine growth restriction in extremely preterm infants based on the Intergrowth-21st Project Preterm Postnatal Follow-up Study growth charts and the Fenton growth charts. *Eur. J. Pediatr.* **2020**, *180*, 817–824. [CrossRef] [PubMed]
30. Pampanini, V.; Boiani, A.; De Marchis, C.; Giacomozzi, C.; Navas, R.; Agostino, R.; Dini, F.; Ghirri, P.; Cianfarani, S. Preterm infants with severe extrauterine growth retardation (EUGR) are at high risk of growth impairment during childhood. *Eur. J. Pediatr.* **2015**, *174*, 33–41. [CrossRef]
31. Kalliomaki, M.; Collado, M.C.; Salminen, S.; Isolauri, E. Early differences in fecal microbiota composition in children may predict overweight. *Am. J. Clin. Nutr.* **2008**, *87*, 534–538. [CrossRef] [PubMed]

32. Yu, W.H.; Chu, C.H.; Lin, Y.C.; Chen, R.B.; Iwata, O.; Huang, C.C. Early-life respiratory trajectories and neurodevelopmental outcomes in infants born very and extremely preterm: A retrospective study. *Dev. Med. Child. Neurol.* **2022**, *64*, 1246–1253. [CrossRef] [PubMed]
33. Chen, L.W.; Wang, S.T.; Wang, L.W.; Kao, Y.C.; Chu, C.L.; Wu, C.C.; Chiang, C.H.; Huang, C.C. Early Neurodevelopmental Trajectories for Autism Spectrum Disorder in Children Born Very Preterm. *Pediatrics* **2020**, *146*, e20200297. [CrossRef]
34. Alshaikh, B.; Dharel, D.; Yusuf, K.; Singhal, N. Early total enteral feeding in stable preterm infants: A systematic review and meta-analysis. *J. Matern. Fetal Neonatal Med.* **2021**, *34*, 1479–1486. [CrossRef]
35. Behnke, J.; Estreich, V.; Oehmke, F.; Zimmer, K.P.; Windhorst, A.; Ehrhardt, H. Compatibility of rapid enteral feeding advances and noninvasive ventilation in preterm infants-An observational study. *Pediatr. Pulmonol.* **2022**, *57*, 1117–1126. [CrossRef] [PubMed]
36. Thoene, M.; Anderson-Berry, A. Early Enteral Feeding in Preterm Infants: A Narrative Review of the Nutritional, Metabolic, and Developmental Benefits. *Nutrients* **2021**, *13*, 2289. [CrossRef] [PubMed]
37. Cester, E.A.; Bloomfield, F.H.; Taylor, J.; Smith, S.; Cormack, B.E. Do recommended protein intakes improve neurodevelopment in extremely preterm babies? *Arch. Dis. Child. Fetal Neonatal Ed.* **2015**, *100*, F243–F247. [CrossRef] [PubMed]
38. Strommen, K.; Blakstad, E.W.; Moltu, S.J.; Almaas, A.N.; Westerberg, A.C.; Amlien, I.K.; Ronnestad, A.E.; Nakstad, B.; Drevon, C.A.; Bjornerud, A.; et al. Enhanced nutrient supply to very low birth weight infants is associated with improved white matter maturation and head growth. *Neonatology* **2015**, *107*, 68–75. [CrossRef]
39. Balakrishnan, M.; Jennings, A.; Przystac, L.; Phornphutkul, C.; Tucker, R.; Vohr, B.; Stephens, B.E.; Bliss, J.M. Growth and Neurodevelopmental Outcomes of Early, High-Dose Parenteral Amino Acid Intake in Very Low Birth Weight Infants: A Randomized Controlled Trial. *JPEN J. Parenter. Enter. Nutr.* **2018**, *42*, 597–606. [CrossRef]
40. Lafeber, H.N.; van de Lagemaat, M.; Rotteveel, J.; van Weissenbruch, M. Timing of nutritional interventions in very-low-birth-weight infants: Optimal neurodevelopment compared with the onset of the metabolic syndrome. *Am. J. Clin. Nutr.* **2013**, *98*, 556S–560S. [CrossRef]
41. Yang, J.; Chang, S.S.; Poon, W.B. Relationship Between Amino Acid and Energy Intake and Long-Term Growth and Neurodevelopmental Outcomes in Very Low Birth Weight Infants. *JPEN J. Parenter. Enter. Nutr.* **2016**, *40*, 820–826. [CrossRef]
42. Dorling, J.; Abbott, J.; Berrington, J.; Bosiak, B.; Bowler, U.; Boyle, E.; Embleton, N.; Hewer, O.; Johnson, S.; Juszczak, E.; et al. Controlled Trial of Two Incremental Milk-Feeding Rates in Preterm Infants. *N. Engl. J. Med.* **2019**, *381*, 1434–1443. [CrossRef]
43. Tahir, W.; Monahan, M.; Dorling, J.; Hewer, O.; Bowler, U.; Linsell, L.; Partlett, C.; Berrington, J.E.; Boyle, E.; Embleton, N.; et al. Economic evaluation alongside the Speed of Increasing milk Feeds Trial (SIFT). *Arch. Dis. Child. Fetal Neonatal Ed.* **2020**, *105*, 587–592. [CrossRef]
44. Hartel, C.; Haase, B.; Browning-Carmo, K.; Gebauer, C.; Kattner, E.; Kribs, A.; Segerer, H.; Teig, N.; Wense, A.; Wieg, C.; et al. Does the enteral feeding advancement affect short-term outcomes in very low birth weight infants? *J. Pediatr. Gastroenterol. Nutr.* **2009**, *48*, 464–470. [CrossRef]
45. Fabrizio, V.; Shabanova, V.; Taylor, S.N. Factors in Early Feeding Practices That May Influence Growth and the Challenges that Arise in Growth Outcomes Research. *Nutrients* **2020**, *12*, 1939. [CrossRef] [PubMed]
46. Zozaya, C.; Avila-Alvarez, A.; Arruza, L.; Garcia-Munoz Rodrigo, F.; Fernandez-Perez, C.; Castro, A.; Cuesta, M.T.; Vacas, B.; Couce, M.L.; Vento Torres, M.; et al. The Effect of Morbidity and Sex on Postnatal Growth of Very Preterm Infants: A Multicenter Cohort Study. *Neonatology* **2019**, *115*, 348–354. [CrossRef] [PubMed]
47. Fischer, C.J.; Maucort-Boulch, D.; Essomo Megnier-Mbo, C.M.; Remontet, L.; Claris, O. Early parenteral lipids and growth velocity in extremely-low-birth-weight infants. *Clin. Nutr.* **2014**, *33*, 502–508. [CrossRef] [PubMed]
48. Belfort, M.B.; Rifas-Shiman, S.L.; Sullivan, T.; Collins, C.T.; McPhee, A.J.; Ryan, P.; Kleinman, K.P.; Gillman, M.W.; Gibson, R.A.; Makrides, M. Infant Growth Before and After Term: Effects on Neurodevelopment in Preterm Infants. *Pediatrics* **2011**, *128*, E899–E906. [CrossRef] [PubMed]
49. Peila, C.; Spada, E.; Giuliani, F.; Maiocco, G.; Raia, M.; Cresi, F.; Bertino, E.; Coscia, A. Extrauterine Growth Restriction: Definitions and Predictability of Outcomes in a Cohort of Very Low Birth Weight Infants or Preterm Neonates. *Nutrients* **2020**, *12*, 1224. [CrossRef]
50. Zhang, X.; Donnelly, B.; Thomas, J.; Sams, L.; O'Brien, K.; Taylor, S.N.; Jump, C.S. Growth in the High-Risk Newborn Infant Post-Discharge: Results from a Neonatal Intensive Care Unit Nutrition Follow-up Clinic. *Nutr. Clin. Pract.* **2020**, *35*, 738–744. [CrossRef]
51. Martínez-Jiménez, M.D.; Gómez-García, F.J.; Gil-Campos, M.; Pérez-Navero, J.L. Comorbidities in childhood associated with extrauterine growth restriction in preterm infants: A scoping review. *Eur. J. Pediatr.* **2020**, *179*, 1255–1265. [CrossRef]
52. Villar, J.; Giuliani, F.; Barros, F.; Roggero, P.; Coronado Zarco, I.A.; Rego, M.A.S.; Ochieng, R.; Gianni, M.L.; Rao, S.; Lambert, A.; et al. Monitoring the Postnatal Growth of Preterm Infants: A Paradigm Change. *Pediatrics* **2018**, *141*, e20172467. [CrossRef]
53. Young, A.; Andrews, E.T.; Ashton, J.J.; Pearson, F.; Beattie, R.M.; Johnson, M.J. Generating longitudinal growth charts from preterm infants fed to current recommendations. *Arch. Dis. Child. Fetal Neonatal Ed.* **2020**, *105*, 646–651. [CrossRef] [PubMed]
54. Healy, D.B.; Ryan, C.A.; Ross, R.P.; Stanton, C.; Dempsey, E.M. Clinical implications of preterm infant gut microbiome development. *Nat. Microbiol.* **2022**, *7*, 22–33. [CrossRef] [PubMed]

55. Uzan-Yulzari, A.; Turta, O.; Belogolovski, A.; Ziv, O.; Kunz, C.; Perschbacher, S.; Neuman, H.; Pasolli, E.; Oz, A.; Ben-Amram, H.; et al. Neonatal antibiotic exposure impairs child growth during the first six years of life by perturbing intestinal microbial colonization. *Nat. Commun.* **2021**, *12*, 443. [CrossRef] [PubMed]
56. Nash, A.; Dunn, M.; Asztalos, E.; Corey, M.; Mulvihill-Jory, B.; O'Connor, D.L. Pattern of growth of very low birth weight preterm infants, assessed using the WHO Growth Standards, is associated with neurodevelopment. *Appl. Physiol. Nutr. Metab.* **2011**, *36*, 562–569. [CrossRef]
57. Frondas-Chauty, A.; Simon, L.; Branger, B.; Gascoin, G.; Flamant, C.; Ancel, P.Y.; Darmaun, D.; Roze, J.C. Early growth and neurodevelopmental outcome in very preterm infants: Impact of gender. *Arch. Dis. Child. Fetal Neonatal Ed.* **2014**, *99*, F366–F372. [CrossRef] [PubMed]
58. Ruys, C.A.; Hollanders, J.J.; Broring, T.; van Schie, P.E.M.; van der Pal, S.M.; van de Lagemaat, M.; Lafeber, H.N.; Rotteveel, J.; Finken, M.J.J. Early-life growth of preterm infants and its impact on neurodevelopment. *Pediatr. Res.* **2019**, *85*, 283–292. [CrossRef]
59. De Rose, D.U.; Cota, F.; Gallini, F.; Bottoni, A.; Fabrizio, G.C.; Ricci, D.; Romeo, D.M.; Mercuri, E.; Vento, G.; Maggio, L. Extra-uterine growth restriction in preterm infants: Neurodevelopmental outcomes according to different definitions. *Eur. J. Paediatr. Neurol.* **2021**, *33*, 135–145. [CrossRef]
60. Chen, C.-H.; Chiu, H.-Y.; Lee, S.-C.; Chang, H.-Y.; Chang, J.-H.; Chen, Y.-J.; Kang, L.; Shen, S.-P.; Lin, Y.-C. Growth of Very Preterm Infants in a Low-Resourced Rural Setting after Affiliation with a Human Milk Bank. *Children* **2022**, *9*, 80. [CrossRef]
61. Lin, Y.-C.; Chang, W.-H.; Li, T.-C.; Iwata, O.; Chen, H.-L. Health Risk of Infants Exposed to Lead and Mercury Through Breastfeeding. *Expo. Health* **2022**, *15*, 255–267. [CrossRef]
62. MacBean, V.; Lunt, A.; Drysdale, S.B.; Yarzi, M.N.; Rafferty, G.F.; Greenough, A. Predicting healthcare outcomes in prematurely born infants using cluster analysis. *Pediatr. Pulmonol.* **2018**, *53*, 1067–1072. [CrossRef] [PubMed]
63. Bua, J.; Risso, F.M.; Bin, M.; Vallon, F.; Travan, L.; Paviotti, G. Association between body composition at term equivalent age and Bayley scores at 2 years in preterm infants. *J. Perinatol.* **2021**, *41*, 1852–1858. [CrossRef] [PubMed]
64. Ramel, S.E.; Haapala, J.; Super, J.; Boys, C.; Demerath, E.W. Nutrition, Illness and Body Composition in Very Low Birth Weight Preterm Infants: Implications for Nutritional Management and Neurocognitive Outcomes. *Nutrients* **2020**, *12*, 145. [CrossRef] [PubMed]

nutrients

MDPI

Article

Growth and Duration of Inflammation Determine Short- and Long-Term Outcome in Very-Low-Birth-Weight Infants Requiring Abdominal Surgery

Corinna Peter [1], Abdulmonem Abukhris [1], Julia Brendel [2], Carolin Böhne [1], Bettina Bohnhorst [1] and Sabine Pirr [1,*]

[1] Department of Paediatric Pneumology, Allergology and Neonatology, Hannover Medical School, Carl-Neuberg-Str. 1, 30625 Hannover, Germany
[2] Department of Paediatric Surgery, Hannover Medical School, Carl-Neuberg-Str. 1, 30625 Hannover, Germany
* Correspondence: pirr.sabine@mh-hannover.de; Tel.: +49-511-532-9121; Fax: +49-511-532-3895

Abstract: Necrotizing enterocolitis (NEC), spontaneous intestinal perforation (SIP) and meconium-related ileus (MI) requiring surgical intervention are associated with a high risk of severe short- and long-term complications in very-low-birth-weight (VLBW) infants including poor growth, cholestasis and neurodevelopmental impairment. This retrospective study aimed to identify risk factors for such complications in a cohort of 55 VLBW preterm infants requiring surgery with enterostomy creation due to NEC, SIP or MI. Long-term follow-up was available for 43 (78%) infants. Multiple regression analyses revealed that the duration of inflammation and longitudinal growth determined the risk of cholestasis and neurodevelopmental outcome at 2 years corrected age independent of the aetiology of the intestinal complication. Direct bilirubin increased by 4.9 μmol/L (95%CI 0.26–9.5), 1.4 μmol/L (95%CI 0.6–2.2) and 0.8 μmol/L (95%CI 0.22–1.13) with every day of elevated (Interleukin-6) IL-6, (C-reactive protein) CrP and parenteral nutrition. The mental development index at 2 years corrected age decreased by 3.8 (95%CI −7.3–−0.36), 0.4 (95%CI 0.07–0.80) and 0.3 (95%CI 0.08–0.57) with every day of elevated IL-6 and every 1 point decrease in weight percentile at discharge and 2 years. These data stress the importance of optimal timing for the initial surgery in order to prevent prolonged inflammation and an early reversal of the enterostomy in case of poor growth or insufficient enteral nutrition.

Keywords: childhood outcomes; cholestasis; enterostomy; intestinal complication; longitudinal growth restriction; neurodevelopmental delay; parenteral nutrition; preterm infants

1. Introduction

Neonatal abdominal disorders such as necrotizing enterocolitis (NEC), spontaneous intestinal perforation (SIP) and meconium-related ileus (MI) requiring surgical intervention are associated with a high mortality in very-low-birth-weight (VLBW) preterm neonates. Surviving infants face severe short- and long-term morbidities such as poor growth, cholestasis and neurodevelopmental impairment [1]. The latter was reported to affect up to 61% of surviving infants at a corrected age (CA) of 18 to 36 months [2]. The risk of cholestasis increases significantly with prolonged parenteral nutrition and any cause of systemic inflammation [3,4], which are both frequently present in infants suffering from surgical NEC, SIP or MI. In these infants, cholestasis is mostly transient and only rarely accompanied by liver failure [3]. However, it is associated with poor growth [5], which in turn is a predictor for an adverse neurodevelopmental outcome in preterm infants [6]. A better understanding of risk factors associated with short- and long-term morbidities of surgically treated NEC, SIP and MI is needed to guide treatment strategies for improved outcomes and to reliably counsel parents.

This study aimed to identify risk factors that help to assess the probability for adverse short- and long-term outcomes in VLBW infants suffering from surgical NEC, SIP or MI.

2. Methods

2.1. Study Design and Population

In a single-centre retrospective study, all in- or outborn preterm neonates treated at the neonatal intensive care unit (NICU) of Hannover Medical School between January 2006 and December 2018 were included when fulfilling the following criteria: birth weight < 1500 g (VLBW) and surgery with the creation of an enterostomy due to NEC, SIP or MI. NEC, SIP and MI were diagnosed at the presence of clinical criteria (including bowel distension, abdominal tenderness and/or discoloration, feeding intolerance, regurgitation, bilious or stool vomiting) by ultrasound and radiography as well as laboratory evaluation. The indication for surgery was given in case of fulminant progress and/or signs of intestinal perforation or suspected perforation. Clinical data of those infants were obtained from the hospital information system. Infants with major congenital malformations or syndromes were excluded from the analysis. Furthermore, infants who were either transferred to another hospital for further treatment or died within 14 days after surgery were omitted due to missing data on weight gain and nutrition after initial surgery as well as short-term morbidity.

Data collection included baseline patient characteristics, details on the primary surgery with enterostomy creation, any re-laparotomy if required and the reversal of the enterostomy, as well as enteral and parenteral nutrition prior to and after surgery, number of central-line-associated bloodstream infections (CLABSI) and blood transfusions. Furthermore, laboratory values to assess the occurrence of cholestasis (direct bilirubin) and the inflammatory response (C-reactive protein (CrP) and Interleukin-6 (IL-6)) after primary surgery were evaluated. The normal level for direct bilirubin is <5 μmol/L; therefore, cholestasis was defined as a direct bilirubin > 35 μmol/L [4] and infants were routinely monitored until discharge. CrP and IL-6 serum levels were routinely measured at an interval of 1 to 2 days until negative to guide antibiotic treatment. Only elevated levels in association with the initial surgery or surgeries in case of the necessity of multiple procedures were considered for the analysis. Values > 10 mg/L for CrP and >150 ng/L for IL-6 were considered elevated [7,8]. In order to analyse weight gain after the initial surgery, body weight measurements were collected on a weekly basis. Weekly weight gain was expressed as a percentage of weight change relative to the weight at the time of initial surgery. We did not adjust for any weight gain from oedema directly following surgery as this to some extent was expected in all infants included in our study. Finally, data on growth throughout the onward treatment as well as growth and neurodevelopmental outcomes at 2 years of CA were collected. Growth was assessed using weight, head circumference (HC) and corresponding percentiles according to Voigt et al. and Brandt preterm growth charts up to 42 weeks postmenstrual age and beyond, respectively [9,10]. Any changes in weight or HC percentiles over time were calculated against birth percentiles and expressed as delta percentile (delta percentile = current percentile–birth percentile).

2.2. Long-Term Outcome Measures

According to the German National Neonatal Follow-up Program, infants were routinely invited at 2 years CA for the assessment of growth and neurodevelopmental outcome by an experienced neonatologist or paediatric neurologist. All age-related outcomes were corrected for prematurity. For the evaluation of cognitive development, the German version of the Bayley Scales of Infant Development III (Bayley-III) was applied [11]. If Bayley was not feasible due to a lack of cooperation, language barrier or major disabilities, the Griffiths Mental Development Scales edition II was used [12]. Cognitive development was expressed as Bayley-III score or Griffiths development quotient, which are age standardized (MDI, mental development index, normal population mean 100, standard deviation 15). Moderate or severe neurodevelopmental delay was defined as a Bayley-III score or Griffiths development quotient < 85 [13]. Patients who were lost to follow-up were not considered.

2.3. Statistical Analysis

Data were evaluated in the pseudonymised form using Excel 2016® (Microsoft Corporation, Redmond, WA, USA) and GraphPad® (GraphPad Prism Version 9.3.1 for Windows, GraphPad Software, San Diego, CA, USA) and tested for Gaussian distribution using the Shapiro–Wilk normality test. Continuous variables were presented as median and range, and categorical variables as frequencies and percentages. For analyses, Mann–Whitney *U* tests, Chi^2 tests and Kruskal–Wallis tests for multiple comparisons were applied. Spearman's correlation coefficient was used to estimate the relationship between individual variables. To identify influencing factors on the 2-year outcome or cholestasis, multiple linear regression analyses were performed using the MDI or the maximum direct bilirubin as the dependent variable and building linear models taking clinical characteristics of the infants into account. As potential influencing factors, we included the gestational age, birth weight, maximum inflammation values and duration of inflammation data and number of CLABSIs in both models. In the cholestasis model, we additionally included duration of parenteral nutrition, out-born status and number of transfusions and surgeries, and in the 2-year outcome model intraventricular haemorrhage and delta weight percentile data for initial surgery, discharge and 2-year CA. In order to remove the insignificant variables, we applied a backward elimination process to iteratively remove the least important variables until only significant factors remained in the model. The significance level was set at 0.05.

3. Results

3.1. Patient Characteristics

Between January 2006 and December 2018, a total of 1251 VLBW preterm infants were treated on the NICU of Hannover Medical School. Of those, 63 patients (5.0%) developed NEC, with 45 infants requiring surgery. SIP was diagnosed in 53 infants (4.2%), and MI in 26 patients (2.1%), all of whom underwent surgery. All operated infants received an enterostomy. Sixty-nine of these surgically treated infants (55.6%) were excluded from further analyses due to an early transfer to another hospital, death or major malformations (one congenital disorder of glycosylation (CDG) syndrome; one Cornelia-de-Lange-syndrome; two complex cardiac defects). Figure 1 provides further details on patient recruitment.

Of the thirty-one infants who died within 14 days after the initial surgery, nineteen died in the course of a fulminant NEC, eleven suffered from SIP and one from MI. Ten of those infants died from septic complications caused by the SIP/MI, one infant suffered from a fungal sepsis and one infant died from respiratory complications (pulmonary emphysema). No further deaths occurred during in-house treatment. Of the fifty-five infants included in the analyses, sixteen were treated for NEC, thirty-two infants for SIP and seven infants received a surgical intervention for MI. None of the infants with MI were diagnosed with cystic fibrosis. Ten infants required the creation of more than one enterostomy in the same or a second surgical session (five infants received a jejuno- and an ileostomy, two an ileo- and a colostomy and three infants two ileostomies each). In the remaining forty-five infants a single enterostomy was created, with three infants received a jejunostomy, forty an ileostomy and two a colostomy. Information regarding the neurodevelopmental outcome at a CA of 2 years was available for 43 out of the 55 remaining infants (78.2%). Twelve infants were lost to follow-up.

NEC was diagnosed at a median postnatal age of 16.5 days (range 3 to 50 days). SIP and MI were diagnosed significantly earlier at a postnatal age of 9.0 days (range 2 to 40 days) ($p = 0.0071$). All out-born infants ($n = 20$) were transferred to the Hannover Medical School for the diagnosis of NEC ($n = 7$), SIP ($n = 11$) or MI ($n = 3$) prior to the initial surgery with a median age of 9 days (range 1–55 days). Baseline characteristics of all patients are presented in Table 1.

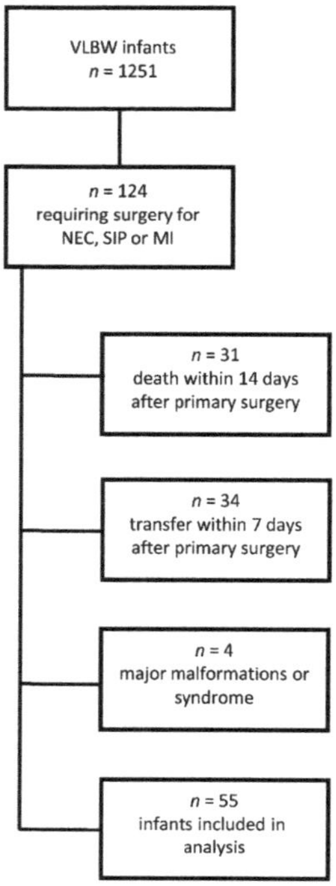

Figure 1. Flow chart of infant recruitment.

Table 1. Baseline characteristics of infants included in the analysis (n = 55).

Characteristic	Median (Range) or n (%)
Gestational age, weeks	25.3 (23.1–32.3)
Birth weight, grams	710 (315–1450)
Birth weight percentile	30 (1–92)
HC at birth, cm	23 (19–29)
HC percentile at birth	30 (1–80)
Sex, male	36 (65.5)
Out-born	21 (33.2)
Age at primary surgery, days	12 (2–50)
Age at reversal of enterostomy, days	75 (37–280)
Bronchopulmonary dysplasia, moderate or severe	8 (14.5)
Intraventricular haemorrhage > 2°	7 (12.7)

HC, head circumference.

No significant differences were found for gestational age, weight and head circumference at birth, rate of cholestasis and neurodevelopmental delay at 2 years CA between infants suffering from NEC, SIP or MI (Table 2).

3.2. Cholestasis

Cholestasis occurred in 20 patients (36.4%) and was diagnosed at a median age of 59 days (range 10–156) with a maximum direct bilirubin of 80 µmol/L (median, range 37–180 µmol/L). The characteristics and clinical parameters of infants with and without cholestasis and their statistical analyses are summarized in Table 3.

Table 2. Clinical characteristics and data availability of the infants included in the analyses stratified for aetiology of the intestinal complication, shown as median and range or *n* and %.

	NEC *n* = 16	SIP *n* = 32	MI *n* = 7	*p* Value [a]
Gestational age, weeks	25.8 (24.3–32.3)	25.0 (23.1–30.4)	26.0 (23.3–32.0)	0.26
Birth weight, grams	663 (380–1370)	713 (315–1450)	790 (645–1375)	0.69
Head circumference, cm	23.5 (19–29)	22.9 (20–28)	22 (22–28.5)	0.75
Cholestasis	9 (56.3)	10 (31.3)	1 (14.3)	0.11
Data on neurodevelopmental outcome available	12 (75.0)	26 (81.3)	5 (71.4)	0.80
Neurodevelopmental delay at 2 years CA	8 (66.7)	15 (57.7)	2 (40.0)	0.60

[a] Kruskal–Wallis test. CA, corrected age.

Table 3. Characteristics of infants (*n* = 55) with vs. without cholestasis, shown as median and range or *n* and %. Significant differences are marked in bold.

	Cholestasis *n* = 20	No Cholestasis *n* = 35	*p* Value
Gestational age, weeks	25.4 (23.1–31.7)	25.7 (23.3–32.3)	0.71 [a]
Birth weight, grams	760 (315–1370)	695 (575–1450)	0.77 [a]
Birth weight percentile	25 (1–92)	30 (5–90)	0.63 [a]
Sex, male	11 (55.0)	25 (71.4)	0.22 [b]
Out-born	12 (60.0)	9 (25.7)	**0.01** [b]
Aetiology of intestinal complication	NEC 9 (45.0) SIP 10 (50.0) MI 1 (5.0)	NEC 7 (20.0) SIP 22 (62.9) MI 6 (17.1)	0.47 [b]
CrP max, mg/L	145.5 (21–275)	75 (1.7–401)	**0.03** [a]
Duration of CrP elevation, days	19 (2–104)	6 (0–20)	**<0.0001** [a]
IL-6 max, ng/L	2040 (18–15,900)	153.5 (30–11,000)	0.07 [a]
Duration of IL-6 elevation, days	4 (0–10)	0 (0–7)	**0.0005** [a]
Enteral nutrition prior to initial surgery	18 (90.0)	31 (88.6)	0.87 [b]
Duration of parenteral nutrition after initial surgery, days	24 (3–96)	10 (4–59)	**0.001** [a]
Type of enteral nutrition after initial surgery, exclusive formula	11 (55.0)	22 (62.9)	0.57 [b]
Duration between creation and reversal of enterostomy, days	63.5 (33–251)	58 (18–121)	0.50 [a]
Short bowel syndrome prior to reversal of enterostomy [c]	4 (20.0)	2 (5.7)	0.10 [b]
Number of CLABSIs	1 (0–4)	0 (0–2)	**0.04** [a]
Number of blood transfusions	9 (5–36)	5 (1–16)	**0.0005** [a]
Number of laparotomies before reversal of enterostomy	2 (1–9)	1 (1–7)	**0.03** [a]
Age at initial surgery, days	15 (7–40)	10 (2–50)	0.09 [a]

[a] Mann–Whitney *U* test. [b] Chi^2 test. [c] Malabsorptive condition caused by the lack of functional small intestine due to a very proximal enterostomy and the subsequent continuous dependency on parenteral nutrition NEC, necrotizing enterocolitis; SIP, spontaneous intestinal perforation; MI, meconium-related ileus; CrP, C-reactive protein; IL-6, interleukin-6; CLABSIs, central-line-associated bloodstream infections.

Of note, outborn infants showed a significantly longer duration of CrP elevation after the initial surgery (median duration and range in days outborn 13 (0–104), inborn 7 (0–38), $p = 0.025$). Infants with cholestasis showed a significantly poorer weight gain starting 3 weeks after the initial surgery (Figure 2).

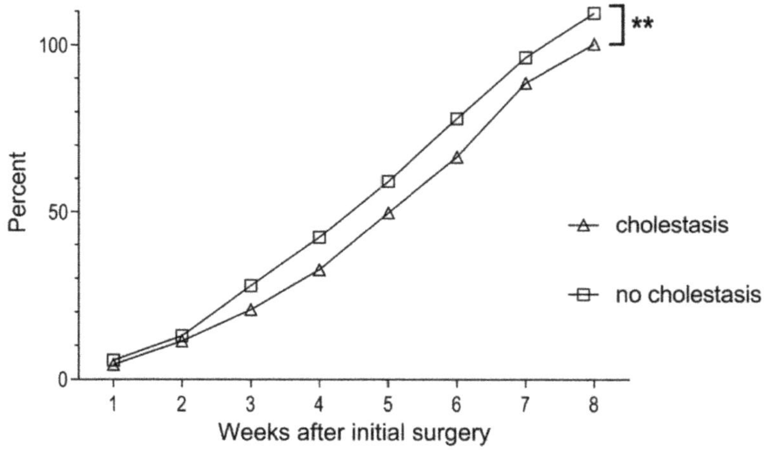

Figure 2. Median weight gain per week after initial surgery in percent of weight at surgery for infants with and without cholestasis. Paired *t*-test, ** $p = 0.0011$.

A multiple regression analysis including all 55 infants revealed that direct bilirubin values were determined by the duration of IL-6 and CrP elevation and of parenteral nutrition after the initial surgery. Every additional day of parenteral nutrition increased direct bilirubin by 0.8 µmol/L (95%CI 0.22–1.13, $p = 0.004$). Furthermore, direct bilirubin rose by 1.4 µmol/L (95%CI 0.6–2.2, $p = 0.001$) and 4.9 µmol/L (95%CI 0.26–9.5, $p = 0.039$) for every day with an elevated CrP and IL-6, respectively.

3.3. Outcome at 2 Years CA

In total, the follow-up data of 43 patients (78.2%) were available at a CA of 2 years. The outcome parameters of neurodevelopment and growth for these infants are summarized in Table 4.

Table 4. Outcome at 2 years CA ($n = 43$).

Outcome Parameter	Median (Range) or *n* (%)
Neurodevelopmental delay, moderate or severe	25 (58.1)
MDI	90 (50–120)
Body weight, grams	10,800 (8300–15,700)
Weight percentile	20 (1–83)
Delta weight percentile [a]	−6 (−70–+47)
HC, cm	46.8 (38.6–52)
HC percentile	4 (1–80)
Delta HC percentile [a]	−19 (−69–+50)

[a] Delta percentiles were calculated against birth measurements. MDI, mental development index; HC, head circumference.

Table 5 shows a comparison of the clinical parameters and characteristics of the initial hospital stay and growth parameters up to 2 years CA between infants with and without neurodevelopmental delay. Significant differences between both groups were found for weight development at the initial surgery and at 2 years CA, as well as for the duration but not the extent of IL-6 elevation after initial surgery as a marker for inflammation. A multiple regression analysis including all 43 infants revealed that poor growth during the initial hospital stay and up to 2 years CA as well as a longer duration of IL-6 elevation after the initial surgery significantly determined MDIs at 2 years CA. The MDI decreased by 0.4 (95%CI 0.07–0.80, $p = 0.021$) and 0.3 (95%CI 0.08–0.57, $p = 0.011$) for every 1 point decrease in weight percentile at discharge and 2 years CA, respectively. Furthermore, every day with an elevated IL-6 reduced the MDI at 2 years CA by 3.8 (95%CI −7.3–−0.36, $p = 0.032$).

Table 5. Clinical parameters and characteristics of infants ($n = 43$) with vs. without neurodevelopmental delay at 2 years CA, shown as median and range or n and %. Significant differences are marked in bold.

	Neurodevelopmental Delay $n = 25$	**No Neurodevelopmental Delay** $n = 18$	p **Value**
Gestational age, weeks	25.0 (23.1–32.3)	25.6 (23.3–32.0)	0.82 [b]
Aetiology of intestinal complication	NEC 8 (32.0) SIP 15 (60.0) MI 2 (8.0)	NEC 4 (22.2) SIP 11 (61.1) MI 3 (16.7)	0.60 [c]
Outborn	7 (28.0)	5 (27.8)	0.99 [c]
Sex (male)	19 (76.0)	11 (61.1)	0.29 [c]
Age at initial surgery, days	9 (2–50)	12 (2–37)	0.87 [b]
Number of transfusions	7 (1–36)	6.5 (1–32)	0.93 [b]
Number of CLABSIs	0 (0–3)	0.5 (0–4)	0.45 [b]
Number of laparotomies before reversal of enterostomy	2 (1–9)	1 (1–5)	0.24 [b]
Bronchopulmonary dysplasia, moderate or severe	5 (20.0)	1 (5.5)	0.18 [c]
Intraventricular haemorrhage > 2°	5 (20.0)	2 (11.1)	0.44 [c]
Maximum CrP, mg/L	114 (7–474)	121 (1.7–327)	0.96 [b]
Duration of CrP elevation, days	9.5 (0–104)	9.5 (0–38)	0.62 [b]
Maximum IL-6, ng/L	688.5 (18–15,900)	1889 (34–11,000)	0.99 [b]
Duration of IL-6 elevation, days	2 (0–10)	0 (0–5)	**0.048** [b]
	Growth percentiles at birth		
Weight, grams	690 (315–1450)	788 (510–1375)	0.38 [b]
Weight percentile	30 (1–90)	40 (9–90)	0.15 [b]
HC, cm	22.5 (19–28)	23.3 (21–28.5)	0.53 [b]
HC percentile	30 (1–80)	40 (15–70)	0.40 [b]
	Growth percentiles at initial surgery		
Weight percentile	15 (1–50)	20 (1–50)	0.70 [b]
Delta weight percentile [a]	−15 (−66–0)	−9 (−45–5)	**0.02** [b]
HC percentile	8 (1–40)	9 (1–40)	0.70 [b]
Delta HC percentile [a]	−23.5 (−69–0)	−15 (−55–0)	0.18 [b]
	Growth percentiles at discharge		
Weight percentile	4 (1–85)	3.5 (1–30)	0.96 [b]
Delta weight percentile [a]	−24 (−70–27)	−23.5 (−80–−8)	0.15 [b]
HC percentile	1 (1–98)	1 (1–50)	0.74 [b]
Delta HC percentile [a]	−20 (−70–28)	−23 (−69–10)	0.60 [b]

Table 5. *Cont.*

	Neurodevelopmental Delay $n = 25$	No Neurodevelopmental Delay $n = 18$	p Value
	Growth percentiles at 2 years CA		
Weight percentile	20 (1–60)	30 (1–83)	0.57 [b]
Delta weight percentile [a]	−18.5 (−70–45)	6.5 (−69–47)	**0.03** [b]
HC percentile	2 (1–80)	4 (1–26)	0.89 [b]
Delta HC percentile [a]	−16 (−69–50)	−27.5 (−66–0)	0.25 [b]

[a] Delta percentiles were calculated against birth measurements. [b] Mann–Whitney U test. [c] Chi^2 test. NEC, necrotizing enterocolitis; SIP, spontaneous intestinal perforation; MI, meconium-related ileus; CLABSIs, central-line-associated bloodstream infections; CrP, C-reactive protein; IL-6, interleukin-6; HC, head circumference; CA, corrected age.

4. Discussion

This study analysed a cohort of VLBW preterm infants requiring surgery with the creation of an enterostomy due to NEC, SIP or MI. The aim of the study was to identify risk factors for short- and long-term complications, in order to improve treatment strategies and counselling of parents. We found that in these particular patients, the duration of the inflammation and longitudinal growth determined the risk of cholestasis and neurodevelopmental outcome at 2 years CA independent of the aetiology of the intestinal complication.

The rate of cholestasis in preterm infants varied greatly with the degree of prematurity, birth weight and the presence of additional risk factors. Previous studies identified those infants at the greatest risk of developing a cholestasis with a birth weight below 750 g, those lacking enteral feeding and receiving prolonged parenteral nutrition and those with intestinal complications including NEC and SIP [4]. The risk of cholestasis continuously increases with the duration of parenteral nutrition [4]. Accordingly, in our cohort, infants with cholestasis presented with a longer duration of parenteral nutrition after the initial surgery. Furthermore, infants without cholestasis showed a better weight gain in the first weeks after the initial surgery. This might be due to the higher number of infants with sufficient enteral nutrition among those patients [14]. Consequently, infants suffering from insufficient enteral nutrition and developing cholestasis might benefit from an early reversal of the enterostomy in order to enable enteral nutrition, avoid prolonged parenteral nutrition and subsequent cholestasis and allow optimal growth [15]. Moreover, it has previously been reported that next to prolonged parenteral nutrition, cholestasis itself is associated with growth delay [5]. The risk of developing cholestasis is further aggravated by the presence of any cause of a systemic inflammatory response [4]. Our study confirmed these findings as infants with cholestasis showed a significantly higher incidence of CLABSIs, a greater need for re-laparotomies, higher maximum CrP values and a longer duration of CrP and IL-6 elevation after the initial surgery. However, regression analyses revealed that the risk of cholestasis was not determined by the number of re-laparotomies or the maximum elevation of CrP but by the duration of the systemic inflammation. Furthermore, infants with cholestasis were more likely to be outborn with the need for transfer for the initial surgical treatment. This might result in a significantly longer duration of inflammation, and therefore a higher rate of cholestasis in these infants. The duration of IL-6 elevation showed the strongest elevating effect on direct bilirubin levels. In this regard, the time between the indication for surgery and surgery itself should be kept as short as possible. In our cohort, gestational age and birth weight did not show a significant association with the risk of cholestasis as reported previously [4]. This is most likely due to the very restricted patient cohort included in our analyses. Furthermore, we did not find an association for the lack of enteral feeds prior to the initial surgery with the later risk of cholestasis. Veenstra et al. reported a decreased risk of later cholestasis if preterm infants received enteral nutrition within the first week of life [16]. However, in our cohort, all but six infants received enteral feeds prior to the initial surgery, two of whom later developed cholestasis. Finally, in our cohort, infants with cholestasis more frequently required a blood transfusion, a risk factor that has previously been reported by other authors [17]. However, it might merely be an indicator of the degree of illness in these infants as the regression analysis did not reveal a significant effect on direct bilirubin values.

Preterm infants have long been recognized as a population at high risk for neurodevelopmental impairment. Especially in the context of declining mortality rates, attention has increasingly turned to the measurement of long-term morbidities and associated risk factors [1]. Several factors have been identified as predictors of an adverse neurodevelopmental outcome including low gestational age and birth weight, sex, bronchopulmonary dysplasia, intraventricular haemorrhage and growth restriction [1,18]. Furthermore, the risk of severe neurodevelopmental delay is significantly increased in infants suffering from NEC, SIP or MI [19,20]. Therefore, 25 to 61% of surviving infants showed severe impairment at 18 to 36 months CA with the highest risks among extremely-low-birth-weight (ELBW) infants requiring surgical treatment. The numbers vary widely as the definitions used for neurodevelopmental delay and for NEC differ between studies [2]. In our cohort, the proportion of infants with moderate or severe neurodevelopmental delay at a CA of 2 years was at the upper range compared to other studies (58%) [2]. This could be explained by our restricted inclusion criteria (VLBW infants with NEC, SIP or MI who required surgical intervention). These criteria probably also masked the previously described association of gestational age and low birth weight with the neurodevelopmental outcome in our cohort [1,18]. Furthermore, we did not find significant correlations between severe intraventricular haemorrhage or bronchopulmonary dysplasia and neurodevelopmental delay most likely due to the low number of included patients. However, our analyses revealed a significant association between adverse neurodevelopmental outcome and extrauterine growth restriction not only during onward treatment but up to a CA of 2 years. Accordingly, De Rose et al. recently reported that longitudinal extrauterine growth restriction is a predictor for adverse neurodevelopmental outcome in preterm infants born before 30 weeks of gestation [6]. However, longitudinal growth does not differ between infants with NEC or SIP or compared to infants without these complications at a CA of 2 or 6 years [19,21].

Finally, in our study, the duration of IL-6 elevation as a biomarker for systemic inflammation was significantly associated with the neurodevelopmental outcome at a CA of 2 years. Several clinical and animal studies identified inflammation as an important contributor to adverse neurodevelopment [22–24]. The mechanisms of systemic inflammation-induced neuronal injury have not been fully elucidated, but systemic inflammation is known to disrupt the blood–brain barrier and incite a local inflammatory response in the brain [23,24]. Several previous studies have assessed the relationship between inflammation-related proteins in neonatal blood and subsequent neurodevelopmental outcomes [25–27]. They reported several significantly elevated cytokines and chemokines (i.e., IL-6) in cord blood and blood samples of the first weeks of life in preterm infants that later developed neurodevelopmental impairment [26,27]. An integrative review of 37 studies identified an elevation of IL-6, IL-1β, IL-8 and TNF-α during the first 3 weeks of life as potential, independent predictors of brain injury and neurodevelopmental impairment [28]. In our study, only measures of IL-6 and CrP were available for analyses as these were part of the routine work-up at expected inflammation/infection. Lee et al. found an association between CrP and plasma TNF-α levels during systemic inflammatory episodes induced by clinical infection or NEC with poor neurodevelopmental outcomes among preterm infants born before 30 weeks of gestation [25]. IL-6 was not included in their analyses. The ELGAN Study included repeated protein analyses during the first 4 weeks of life at weekly intervals and showed a stronger association when inflammation markers were elevated on more than one time point [26,27]. However, it remained unclear whether elevated inflammation markers on two or more time points reflected repeated episodes or a sustained elevation. To our knowledge, this is the first study demonstrating that it is not the extent but the duration of IL-6 elevation that determines the risk of neurodevelopmental impairment independent from the aetiology of the intestinal complication in a patient group at exceptionally high risk.

Not surprisingly, none of the infants with MI were diagnosed with cystic fibrosis, as the MI of the preterm infant must be distinguished from the meconium ileus of the term-born infant which often is associated with cystic fibrosis.

The limitations of this study are the retrospective approach restricting available data and the small number of included patients. This is due to the overall low incidence of NEC, SIP and MI in preterm infants and our single-centre approach. However, a multi-centre design carries the bias of treatment variabilities between centres and would have required a treatment alignment before the study. Furthermore, a relatively high number of infants had to be excluded from analysis due to early death or transfer after initial surgery. A further limitation is the use of different test tools for the evaluation of neurodevelopmental delay at 2 years CA, and the relatively short follow-up period, which is too short to gain true insight into the long-term prognosis as specific deficits in neurodevelopment might not emerge until later [19,20].

5. Conclusions

This study provides evidence of the high risk of cholestasis and neurodevelopmental delay in VLBW infants requiring surgery with the creation of an enterostomy for NEC, SIP or MI. As risk factors for cholestasis, we identified prolonged parenteral nutrition and sustained inflammation. The latter was also significantly associated with neurodevelopmental delay at a CA of 2 years next to longitudinal growth failure. For the first time, we demonstrated that it is not the extent but the duration of the elevation of the inflammation-associated proteins CrP and IL-6 that determines the risk of cholestasis and neurodevelopmental delay in this patient group regardless of the underlying disease, i.e., NEC, SIP or MI. These data stress the importance of optimal timing for the initial surgery once the indication is given in order to prevent prolonged inflammation as well as for an early reversal of the enterostomy in case of poor growth or insufficient enteral nutrition. Furthermore, they provide guidance for parent counselling at the time of initial diagnosis.

Author Contributions: Conceptualization, C.P., B.B. and S.P.; Methodology, C.P. and S.P.; Validation, C.P. and S.P.; Formal Analysis, C.P., A.A. and S.P.; Investigation, A.A. and C.B.; Resources, B.B.; Data Curation, A.A., C.B. and J.B.; Writing—Original Draft Preparation, C.P. and S.P.; Writing—Review and Editing, A.A., C.B., J.B. and B.B.; Visualization, S.P.; Supervision, B.B. All authors have read and agreed to the published version of the manuscript.

Funding: This research received no external funding.

Institutional Review Board Statement: Protocols were approved by the Institutional Review Board of the Hannover Medical School (no. 9855_BO_K_2021 on 25 June 2021) and were in accordance with the Helsinki Declaration of the World Medical Association.

Informed Consent Statement: Informed consent was obtained from all subjects involved in the study.

Data Availability Statement: The data presented in this study are available on reasonable request from the corresponding author. The data are not publicly available due to restrictions in the data access agreement by the institution's Ethical Board and Data Protection Board.

Conflicts of Interest: The authors declare no conflict of interest.

Abbreviations

CA: corrected age; CLABSI: central-line-associated bloodstream infection; CrP: C-reactive protein; HC: head circumference; IL-6: Interleukin-6; MDI: mental development index; MI: meconium-related ileus; NEC: necrotizing enterocolitis; NICU: neonatal intensive care unit; SIP: spontaneous intestinal perforation; VLBW: very-low-birth-weight.

References

1. Patel, R.M. Short- and Long-Term Outcomes for Extremely Preterm Infants. *Am. J. Perinatol.* **2016**, *33*, 318–328. [CrossRef] [PubMed]
2. Jones, I.H.; Hall, N.J. Contemporary Outcomes for Infants with Necrotizing Enterocolitis—A Systematic Review. *J. Pediatr.* **2020**, *220*, 86–92.e3. [CrossRef]
3. Choi, H.J.; Kim, I.; Lee, H.-J.; Oh, H.J.; Ahn, M.K.; Baek, W.I.; Kim, Y.E.; Oh, S.H.; Lee, B.S.; Namgoong, J.-M.; et al. Clinical characteristics of neonatal cholestasis in a tertiary hospital and the development of a novel prediction model for mortality. *Ebiomedicine* **2022**, *77*, 103890. [CrossRef] [PubMed]
4. Satrom, K.; Gourley, G. Cholestasis in Preterm Infants. *Clin. Perinatol.* **2016**, *43*, 355–373. [CrossRef] [PubMed]
5. Niccum, M.; Khan, M.N.; Middleton, J.P.; Vergales, B.D.; Syed, S. Cholestasis affects enteral tolerance and prospective weight gain in the NICU. *Clin. Nutr. ESPEN* **2019**, *30*, 119–125. [CrossRef] [PubMed]
6. De Rose, D.U.; Cota, F.; Gallini, F.; Bottoni, A.; Fabrizio, G.C.; Ricci, D.; Romeo, D.M.; Mercuri, E.; Vento, G.; Maggio, L. Extra-uterine growth restriction in preterm infants: Neurodevelopmental outcomes according to different definitions. *Eur. J. Paediatr. Neurol.* **2021**, *33*, 135–145. [CrossRef]
7. Goepfert, A.R.; Andrews, W.W.; Carlo, W.; Ramsey, P.S.; Cliver, S.P.; Goldenberg, R.L.; Hauth, J.C. Umbilical cord plasma interleukin-6 concentrations in preterm infants and risk of neonatal morbidity. *Am. J. Obstet. Gynecol.* **2004**, *191*, 1375–1381. [CrossRef]
8. Rallis, D.; Balomenou, F.; Kappatou, K.; Karantanou, K.; Tzoufi, M.; Giapros, V. C-reactive protein in infants with no evidence of early-onset sepsis. *J. Matern. Fetal. Neonatal Med.* **2021**, *35*, 5659–5664. [CrossRef]
9. Voigt, M.; Rochow, N.; Schneider, K.T.M.; Hagenah, H.-P.; Scholz, R.; Hesse, V.; Wittwer-Backofen, U.; Straube, S.; Olbertz, D. New Percentile Values for the Anthropometric Dimensions of Singleton Neonates: Analysis of Perinatal Survey Data of 2007–2011 from all 16 States of Germany. *Z. Geburtshilfe Neonatol.* **2014**, *218*, 210–217. [CrossRef]
10. Brandt, I. Growth dynamics of low-birth-weight infants with emphasis on the perinatal period. In *Human Growth: A Comprehensive Treatise*, 2nd ed.; Falkner, F., Tanner, J.M., Eds.; Plenum Press: New York, NY, USA, 1986; Volume 1, pp. 415–475. [CrossRef]
11. Bayley, N. *Bayley Scales of Infant and Toddler Development*, 3rd ed.; APA Psyc Tests; APA: Worcester, MA, USA, 2005. [CrossRef]
12. Griffiths, R.; Huntley, M. *Griffiths Mental Developmental Scales—Revised: Birth to 2 Years (GMDS 0-2)*; APA Psyc Tests; APA: Worcester, MA, USA, 1996. [CrossRef]
13. Johnson, S.; Moore, T.; Marlow, N. Using the Bayley-III to assess neurodevelopmental delay: Which cut-off should be used? *Pediatr. Res.* **2014**, *75*, 670–674. [CrossRef]
14. Radmacher, P.G.; Looney, S.W.; Rafail, S.T.; Adamkin, D.H. Prediction of Extrauterine Growth Retardation (EUGR) in VVLBW Infants. *J. Perinatol.* **2003**, *23*, 392–395. [CrossRef] [PubMed]
15. Wolf, L.; Gfroerer, S.; Fiegel, H.; Rolle, U. Complications of newborn enterostomies. *World J. Clin. Cases* **2018**, *6*, 1101–1110. [CrossRef] [PubMed]
16. Veenstra, M.; Danielson, L.; Brownie, E.; Saba, M.; Natarajan, G.; Klein, M. Enteral nutrition and total parenteral nutrition components in the course of total parenteral nutrition–associated cholestasis in neonatal necrotizing enterocolitis. *Surgery* **2014**, *156*, 578–583. [CrossRef] [PubMed]
17. Steinbach, M.; Clark, R.H.; Kelleher, A.S.; Flores, C.; White, R.; Chace, D.H.; Spitzer, A.R.; For the Pediatrix Amino-Acid Study Group. Demographic and nutritional factors associated with prolonged cholestatic jaundice in the premature infant. *J. Perinatol.* **2008**, *28*, 129–135. [CrossRef]
18. Salas, A.; Carlo, W.A.; Ambalavanan, N.; Nolen, T.L.; Stoll, B.J.; Das, A.; Higgins, R.D. Gestational age and birthweight for risk assessment of neurodevelopmental impairment or death in extremely preterm infants. *Arch. Dis. Child. Fetal Neonatal Ed.* **2016**, *101*, F494–F501. [CrossRef] [PubMed]
19. Shin, S.-H.; Kim, E.-K.; Kim, S.-H.; Kim, H.-Y.; Kim, H.-S. Head Growth and Neurodevelopment of Preterm Infants with Surgical Necrotizing Enterocolitis and Spontaneous Intestinal Perforation. *Children* **2021**, *8*, 833. [CrossRef]
20. Humberg, A.; Spiegler, J.; Fortmann, M.I.; Zemlin, M.; Marissen, J.; Swoboda, I.; Rausch, T.K.; Herting, E.; Göpel, W.; Härtel, C.; et al. Surgical necrotizing enterocolitis but not spontaneous intestinal perforation is associated with adverse neurological outcome at school age. *Sci. Rep.* **2020**, *10*, 2373. [CrossRef] [PubMed]
21. Wadhawan, R.; Oh, W.; Hintz, S.R.; Blakely, M.L.; Das, A.; Bell, E.F.; Saha, S.; Laptook, A.R.; Shankaran, S.; Stoll, B.J.; et al. Neurodevelopmental outcomes of extremely low birth weight infants with spontaneous intestinal perforation or surgical necrotizing enterocolitis. *J. Perinatol.* **2014**, *34*, 64–70. [CrossRef]
22. Keogh, M.J.; Bennet, L.; Drury, P.P.; Booth, L.C.; Mathai, S.; Naylor, A.S.; Fraser, M.; Gunn, A.J. Subclinical exposure to low-dose endotoxin impairs EEG maturation in preterm fetal sheep. *Am. J. Physiol. Regul. Integr. Comp. Physiol.* **2012**, *303*, R270–R278. [CrossRef] [PubMed]
23. Humberg, A.; Fortmann, I.; Siller, B.; Kopp, M.V.; Herting, E.; Gopel, W.; Hartel, C. German Neonatal Network; German Center for Lung Research and Priming Immunity at the beginning of life (PRIMAL) Consortium. Preterm birth and sustained inflammation: Consequences for the neonate. *Semin. Immunopathol.* **2020**, *42*, 451–468. [CrossRef] [PubMed]
24. Schlapbach, L.J.; Aebischer, M.; Adams, M.; Natalucci, G.; Bonhoeffer, J.; Latzin, P.; Nelle, M.; Bucher, H.U.; Latal, B.; the Swiss Neonatal Network and Follow-Up Group. Impact of Sepsis on Neurodevelopmental Outcome in a Swiss National Cohort of Extremely Premature Infants. *Pediatrics* **2011**, *128*, e348–e357. [CrossRef]

25. Lee, E.S.; Kim, E.-K.; Shin, S.H.; Choi, Y.-H.; Jung, Y.H.; Kim, S.Y.; Koh, J.W.; Choi, E.K.; Cheon, J.-E.; Kim, H.-S. Factors associated with neurodevelopment in preterm infants with systematic inflammation. *BMC Pediatr.* **2021**, *21*, 114. [CrossRef] [PubMed]
26. O'Shea, T.M.; Allred, E.N.; Kuban, K.; Dammann, O.; Paneth, N.; Fichorova, R.; Hirtz, D.; Leviton, A. Elevated Concentrations of Inflammation-Related Proteins in Postnatal Blood Predict Severe Developmental Delay at 2 Years of Age in Extremely Preterm Infants. *J. Pediatr.* **2012**, *160*, 395–401.e4. [CrossRef] [PubMed]
27. O'Shea, T.M.; Shah, B.; Allred, E.N.; Fichorova, R.N.; Kuban, K.C.; Dammann, O.; Leviton, A. Inflammation-initiating illnesses, inflammation-related proteins, and cognitive impairment in extremely preterm infants. *Brain Behav. Immun.* **2013**, *29*, 104–112. [CrossRef]
28. Nist, M.D.; Pickler, R.H. An Integrative Review of Cytokine/Chemokine Predictors of Neurodevelopment in Preterm Infants. *Biol. Res. Nurs.* **2019**, *21*, 366–376. [CrossRef] [PubMed]

nutrients

MDPI

Article

The Prevalence of Small for Gestational Age and Extrauterine Growth Restriction among Extremely and Very Preterm Neonates, Using Different Growth Curves, and Its Association with Clinical and Nutritional Factors

Ioanna Kakatsaki [1], Styliani Papanikolaou [1], Theano Roumeliotaki [2], Nicolina Hilda Anagnostatou [1,3], Ioanna Lygerou [1] and Eleftheria Hatzidaki [1,3,*]

[1] Neonatal Intensive Care Unit, Department of Neonatology, University General Hospital of Heraklion, 71500 Crete, Greece; joanne_k1991@hotmail.com (I.K.); stylpapa12@gmail.com (S.P.); nicolehilda@gmail.com (N.H.A.); lygerouped@gmail.com (I.L.)
[2] Clinic of Preventive Medicine and Nutrition, Division of Social Medicine, School of Medicine, University of Crete, 70013 Crete, Greece; roumeliot@uoc.gr
[3] Neonatology, School of Medicine, University of Crete, 70013 Crete, Greece
* Correspondence: el.hatzidaki@uoc.gr or elhatzidaki@gmail.com

Abstract: Monitoring the growth of neonates in the Neonatal Intensive Care Unit (NICU) using growth charts constitutes an essential part of preterm infant care. Preterm infants are at increased risk for extrauterine growth restriction (EUGR) due to increased energy needs and clinical complications. This retrospective study compares the prevalence of small for gestational age (SGA) at birth and EUGR at discharge in extremely and very preterm neonates hospitalized in the NICU of a tertiary hospital in Greece, using different growth curves, and it examines the associated nutritional and clinical factors. Fenton2013 and INTERGROWTH-21st growth curves were used to calculate z-scores of birth weight (BW) and weight, length, and head circumference at discharge. The study includes 462 newborns with a mean BW of 1341.5 g and mean GA of 29.6 weeks. At birth, 6.3% of neonates were classified as SGA based on Fenton2013 curves compared to 9.3% with INTERGROWTH-21st growth curves. At discharge, 45.9% of neonates were characterized as having EUGR based on the Fenton2013 weight curves and 29.2% were characterized based on INTERGROWTH-21st curves. Nutritional factors such as the day of initiation, attainment of full enteral feeding, and the duration of parenteral nutrition were associated with EUGR by both curves. The prevalence of SGA and EUGR neonates differs between the two growth references. This shows that further evaluation of these charts is needed to determine the most appropriate way to monitor infant growth.

Keywords: prematurity; restricted growth; EUGR; SGA; extremely preterm; very preterm; INTERGROWTH-21st; Fenton2013

1. Introduction

Assessing and monitoring the postnatal growth of prematurely born infants is fundamental to Neonatal Intensive Care Units (NICUs). However, there is no standardized approach among neonatologists regarding how the postnatal growth of preterm infants should be monitored, and the optimum pattern of growth has yet to be determined [1,2].

Growth curves serve as monitoring tools for assessing the growth of preterm infants at birth and in the postnatal period. In clinical practice, two widely utilized growth charts are the Fenton 2013 and the INTERGROWTH-21st growth charts [3]. The 2013 Fenton growth charts are one of the most commonly used reference charts and were created based on the theory that the growth of a preterm infant should follow that of a normal human fetus [4]. The use of these growth charts has been questioned in recent years since the growth of a fetus in utero and the growth of an infant ex utero are different biological processes due to environmental and nutritional factors [5]. Later developed growth monitoring tools, such as the INTERGROWTH-21st preterm postnatal growth standards, are prospectively constructed standard curves based on a subpopulation of preterm infants born from healthy mothers with no related complications in pregnancy and no evidence of fetal growth restriction [6]

Feeding practices in NICUs have exhibited significant variation, particularly in previous times [7]. Traditionally, a conservative feeding approach involved fasting shortly after birth, introducing feeds after four days, and gradually increasing feeding volume at a maximum rate of 24 mL/kg/day. This approach aimed to minimize the risks of necrotizing enterocolitis (NEC) and early onset sepsis [8,9]. Over time, a more liberal approach was followed, which involves early trophic feeding within 24–48 h after birth and gradual advancement in an effort to achieve full enteral feed in a shorter period [10].

Preterm infants are at increased risk for extrauterine growth restriction (EUGR) due to often being born small for gestational age (SGA), increased energy needs and prematurity-associated morbidities [11]. The identification of EUGR and SGA neonates is crucial as it carries significant implications to their health in the neonatal period and later in life [12–14]. Nonetheless, the prevalence of SGA and EUGR exhibits considerable variation across studies, which is closely related to the choice of a specific growth chart for assessment [15].

The aim of this study was to compare the prevalence of SGA and EUGR in infants born before the 32nd week of gestation, using the Fenton2013 and INTERGROWTH-21st growth reference curves, and determine the nutritional and clinical factors associated with restricted postnatal growth by both charts.

2. Materials and Methods

2.1. Study Setting and Population

This is a retrospective study conducted at the Department of Neonatology/Neonatal Intensive Care Unit of the University General Hospital of Heraklion (PAGNI), a tertiary referral hospital in Crete, Greece, with nearly 600 admissions annually. Preterm infants born before 32 weeks admitted to the NICU from January 2008 to December 2022, who survived until discharge to home, were considered eligible participants for the study. Exclusion criteria were major congenital malformations and genetic syndromes. The final study population consists of 462 extremely and very preterm infants. Ethical approval was obtained from the Scientific Council of the Hospital (protocol number 23000).

2.2. Indicators of Growth and Development

Birth weight, gestational age, and child's biological sex were recorded by hospital staff within 1 h after delivery. Weight, length, and head circumference (HC) were measured at discharge following standard clinical protocols. Birth and discharge weight were measured using adapted patient incubator electronic and digital infant weighing scales.

Gestational age (GA) was determined according to the last menstrual period, an early prenatal ultrasound or calculated directly in case of in vitro fertilization. Small for gestational age (SGA) was defined when birth weight was below the 10th sex-specific percentile for GA. Postmenstrual age (PMA) at discharge was calculated as gestational age plus chronological age in weeks [16]. Extrauterine growth restriction (EUGR) was defined as weight, length, or HC at discharge below the 10th sex- and postmenstrual age-specific percentile. Percentile and z-scores of weight at birth were calculated using both the Fenton growth charts and the INTERGROWTH-21st very preterm size charts [4,17]. Size at discharge was also calculated using the Fenton charts and INTERGROWTH-21st postnatal growth standards for preterm infants [4,18].

2.3. Nutritional Data

Assessed nutritional factors included in our study were the day of life that enteral and parenteral nutrition were initiated, the time to reach full feeds and the duration of parenteral nutrition. It should be noted that in the studied period of 15 years, nutrition protocols have changed, adapting to current international recommendations regarding enteral and parenteral feeding [19–26]. During the recent years, total parenteral nutrition (TPN) was initiated on the first day of life, and enteral trophic feeding started as soon as possible, either with expressed own mother's milk, when available, or with formula designed for premature infants [27]. Enteral feed volumes were gradually increased on a daily basis for each infant, provided that they tolerated the feeding, while simultaneously reducing the amount of parenteral nutrition [28].

2.4. Clinical Data

Additional information recorded for each infant included multiple gestation, duration of hospitalization (days), and morbidity data such as pneumothorax [29], bronchopulmonary dysplasia (BPD), early (<72 h) and late (≥72 h) suspected and culture-proven sepsis, anemia requiring at least one blood transfusion [30], necrotizing enterocolitis (NEC) defined according to modified Bell's criteria (stage IIIB) [31], hemodynamically significant patent ductus arteriosus (hsPDA) determined by a combination of echocardiographic and clinical criteria and requiring pharmacological treatment [32], retinopathy of prematurity (ROP) (≥Stage II) [33,34], cystic periventricular leukomalacia (PVL) and intraventricular hemorrhage (IVH) grade I–IV based on ultrasound diagnosis [35,36]. Finally, the duration in days of respiratory support, mechanical ventilation, non-invasive ventilation, and oxygen administration was recorded.

Different criteria were used to define some of the above morbidities over the years of the study. BPD until 2018 was defined as the need for supplemental oxygen for 28 consecutive days or supplemental oxygen at 36 weeks PMA; after 2019, according to Jensen et al., the definition of BPD was modified and included respiratory support plus oxygen versus oxygen only in order to classify BPD at 36 weeks PMA [37]. Sepsis is a clinical syndrome in a neonate characterized by a combination of clinical, biochemical, and microbiological data. In our study, both suspected with negative blood culture and confirmed by blood culture sepsis were assessed [38,39].

2.5. Statistical Analysis

Descriptive statistics are expressed as mean and standard deviation for continuous variables and as frequencies and percentages for binary or categorical data. The paired *t*-test was used to compare sex-specific z-scores at birth and discharge between the two growth references (Fenton2013 and INTERGROWTH-21st). Cochran's Q test was used to compare the prevalence of SGA and EUGR in the study population based on the different growth references. Bivariate comparisons of nutritional and clinical factors between the EUGR and non-EUGR groups previously defined were conducted using the parametric Student's *t*-test or non-parametric Mann–Whitney for continuous variables, and Fisher's exact test was used for categorical variables.

We used multivariate linear regression models to explore the association of sex-specific z-scores of weight, length, and HC at discharge with nutritional and clinical factors. Estimations are presented regarding β coefficients and their 95% confidence intervals (CI). For the binary outcomes of EUGR, logistic regression models were applied, and estimations are presented in terms of odds ratio (OR) and their 95% confidence interval (CI). Possible factors identified from the univariate comparisons were entered into the regression models for the multivariate models. Due to highly correlated factors, some variables were excluded according to the correlation matrix and the variance inflation factor (VIF), and only one of the highly correlated variables was included in the model. Additional sensitivity analysis was performed by stratifying admissions before and after 2018 in order to examine possible modification due to the change in nutritional feeding practices during the course of the study.

All hypothesis testing was conducted, assuming a 0.05 significance level and a 2-sided alternative hypothesis. All statistical analyses were performed using Stata Software, version 13 (Stata Corp LP, College Station, TX, USA).

3. Results

3.1. Infant Characteristics

Perinatal, clinical, and nutritional characteristics of the study population are presented in Table 1. The mean (±SD) gestational age was 29.6 (±1.7) weeks, and 17.5% of infants were born extremely preterm (<28 weeks). Newborns had a mean BW of 1341.5 (±363.3) grams, and 55.8% were male. The mean duration of hospitalization was 54 (±25.8) days. At discharge, the mean PMA was 37.3 (±2.9) weeks, and the mean weight was 2415.9 (±406.7) grams. Nutritional data indicate that parenteral feeding was introduced the first day, with a median (IQR) duration of 9 (5–18) days. Enteral feeding starting age was 4 (2–6) days, and full enteral feeding was achieved at 13 (9–22) days. The most common morbidities among preterm infants were anemia (45.7%) and late-onset sepsis (26.4%). BPD and ROP were present at 14.3% and 6.7% of cases, respectively. Mean (±SD) duration of invasive mechanical ventilation was 3.3 (±7.6) days, and non-invasive ventilation was 9.7 (±13.2) days, whereas oxygen administration was used 11.6 (±18.3) days.

Table 1. Perinatal, clinical, and nutritional characteristics of the study population (n = 462).

	Mean ± SD or *n* (%)
Perinatal characteristics	
Gestational age (weeks)	29.6 ± 1.7
Extremely preterm (<28 weeks)	81 (17.5)
Birthweight (g)	1341.5 ± 363.3
Male sex	258 (55.8)
Caesarean section	406 (88.3)
Multiple birth	194 (43.6)
At discharge	
Postmenstrual age (weeks)	37.3 ± 2.9
Weight (g)	2415.9 ± 406.7
Length (cm)	46 ± 2.8
Head circumference (cm)	33.1 ± 1.8
Nutritional information	
Parenteral feeding duration (days)	15 ± 14.5
Enteral feeding starting time (days)	4.8 ± 4.2
Full enteral feeding achieved (days)	16.4 ± 11.3
Clinical information	
Duration of hospitalization (days)	54 ± 25.8
BPD	66 (14.3)
hsPDA	43 (9.3)
Early-onset sepsis (suspected or culture proved)	49 (10.6)
Late-onset sepsis (suspected or culture proved)	122 (26.4)
NEC	8 (1.7)
IVH (≥Grade II)	53 (11.5)
ROP (≥Stage II)	31 (6.7)
Pneumothorax	21 (4.5)
Duration of respiratory support (days)	12.9 ± 17.0
Duration of mechanical ventilation (days)	3.3 ± 7.6
Duration of non-invasive ventilation (days)	9.7 ± 13.3
Duration of oxygen therapy (days)	11.6 ± 18.3
Anemia	211 (45.7)
Cystic PVL	30 (6.5)

Abbreviations: BPD, bronchopulmonary dysplasia; hsPDA, hemodynamically significant patent ductus arteriosus; NEC, necrotizing enterocolitis; IVH, intraventricular hemorrhage; ROP, retinopathy of prematurity (≥Stage II); PVL, periventricular leukomalacia.

In the course of years of the study, nutrition protocols strain to adapt to international recommendations regarding enteral and parenteral feeding, and this change is depicted in Figure 1. A significant decline is observed after year 2018 ($p < 0.001$) for the median day of enteral feeding initiation (median (IQR) before 2018: 5 (3–7) days; after 2018: 2 (2–4) days) and full enteral feeding achieved (before 2018: 14 (9–24) days; after 2018: 11 (8–17) days).

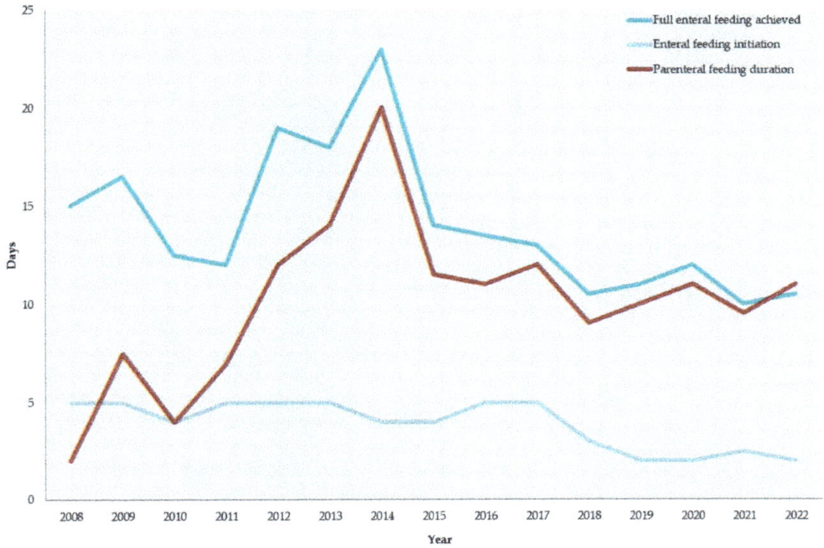

Figure 1. Median number of days of parenteral feeding duration, introduction of enteral feeding and full enteral feeding achieved by year of study.

3.2. The Fenton2013 and INTERGROWTH-21st Growth References

Infant size at birth and at discharge was examined by applying the Fenton2013 and INTERGROWTH-21st growth references, as previously described, and the results are presented in Table 2 and Figure 2. The prevalence of SGA infants at birth is 6.3% based on Fenton2013 curves and 9.3% based on INTERGROWTH-21st very preterm size at birth reference charts. Extrauterine growth, assessed by means of weight, length, and head circumference measured at discharge, was found to be significantly different between the two growth standards. The Fenton2013 growth curves produced a higher prevalence of EUGR compared to INTERGROWTH-21st for the weight (45.9% and 29.2%, respectively) and length (36% and 34.4%, respectively). Regarding HC, our study revealed a higher prevalence of EUGR when the INTERGROWTH-21st postnatal growth charts were used.

Table 2. Infant size at birth and discharge by the Fenton2013 and INTERGROWTH-21st growth references.

	Fenton2013	INTERGROWTH-21st	*p*-Value *
At birth			
Birth weight z, mean ± SD	0.1 ± 0.9	0.1 ± 1.1	0.001
SGA weight, n (%)	29 (6.3)	43 (9.3)	<0.001
At discharge			
Weight z score, mean ± SD	−1.2 ± 1.4	−0.7 ± 1.5	<0.001
Length z score, mean ± SD	−0.9 ± 1.5	−0.7 ± 2.0	<0.001
HC z score, mean ± SD	−0.1 ± 1.2	0.0 ± 1.6	<0.001
EUGR weight, n (%)	209 (45.9)	133 (29.2)	<0.001
EUGR length, n (%)	165 (36.0)	158 (34.4)	0.039
EUGR HC, n (%)	50 (10.9)	70 (15.3)	<0.001

Abbreviations: SGA, small for gestational age; HC, head circumference; EUGR, extrauterine growth restriction. * *p*-values from paired *t*-tests were used to compare sex-specific z-scores at birth and discharge, and Cochran's Q test was used to compare the prevalence of SGA and EUGR between growth references (Fenton2013 and INTERGROWTH-21st).

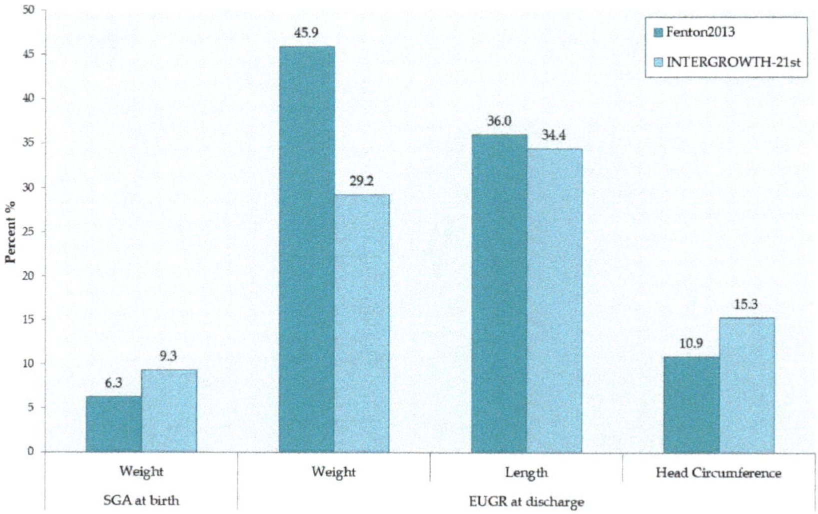

Figure 2. Prevalence of small for gestational age (SGA) and extrauterine growth restriction (EUGR) by Fenton2013 and INTERGROWTH-21st growth references.

3.3. Nutritional and Clinical Factors Associated with EUGR

Bivariate comparisons between perinatal, nutritional, and clinical information with EUGR (Table 3) showed that postnatal growth failure was more prevalent in extremely preterm infants (by Fenton, $p = 0.003$ and by INTERGROWTH-21st, $p < 0.001$) and those who had stayed longer in the NICU ($p < 0.001$, by both reference curves). Clinical conditions associated with restricted postnatal growth by both growth references were BPD, late-onset sepsis, anemia, hsPDA and ROP. In addition, EUGR infants needed more days of respiratory support, mechanical or non-invasive ventilation and oxygen supply.

Table 3. Perinatal, infant nutrition and clinical factors [1] by extrauterine restricted growth (EUGR) based on weight at discharge by the Fenton2013 and INTERGROWTH-21st growth references.

	Fenton2013			INTERGROWTH-21st		
	Restricted	Non Restricted	p-Value [2]	Restricted	Non Restricted	p-Value [2]
Perinatal factors						
Male sex	111 (53.1)	141 (57.3)	0.395	81 (60.9)	171 (53.1)	0.147
Gestational age (weeks)	29.2 ± 1.8	30.0 ± 1.5	<0.001	28.9 ± 1.9	29.9 ± 1.5	<0.001
Extremely preterm (<28 weeks)	48 (23.0)	30 (12.2)	0.003	38 (28.6)	40 (12.4)	<0.001
Birth weight (g)	1144.3 ± 288.1	1510.9 ± 334.6	<0.001	1064.2 ± 276.5	1457.5 ± 331.3	<0.001
BW z-score	−0.3 ± 0.8	0.5 ± 0.9	<0.001	−0.7 ± 1.4	0.4 ± 0.8	<0.001
SGA	26 (12.4)	3 (1.2)	<0.001	35 (26.3)	8 (2.5)	<0.001
Caesarean section	186 (89.0)	213 (87.3)	0.663	116 (87.2)	283 (88.4)	0.751
Multiple birth	114 (56.4)	131 (55.5)	0.848	78 (60.0)	167 (54.2)	0.293
Duration of hospitalization (days)	66.3 ± 27.5	43.5 ± 19.1	<0.001	75.1 ± 29.4	45.2 ± 18.2	<0.001
Nutritional factors						
Parenteral feeding duration (days)	11.5 (6–24)	8 (4–13)	<0.001	14 (8–30)	8 (4–13.5)	<0.001
Enteral feeding initiation (days)	4 (2–8)	3 (2–5)	<0.001	5 (3–9)	3 (2–5)	<0.001
Full enteral feeding achieved (days)	18 (11–27)	11 (8–16)	<0.001	19 (12–30)	11 (8–18)	<0.001

Table 3. *Cont.*

	Fenton2013			INTERGROWTH-21st		
	Restricted	**Non Restricted**	**p-Value [2]**	**Restricted**	**Non Restricted**	**p-Value [2]**
Clinical factors						
BPD	38 (18.2)	28 (11.4)	0.045	29 (21.8)	37 (11.5)	0.008
Early-onset sepsis	29 (13.9)	20 (8.1)	0.068	16 (12.0)	33 (10.3)	0.619
Late-onset sepsis	74 (35.4)	46 (18.7)	<0.001	64 (48.1)	56 (17.4)	<0.001
Anemia	117 (56.0)	92 (37.4)	<0.001	90 (67.7)	119 (37.0)	<0.001
NEC	8 (3.8)	0 (0.0)	0.002	7 (5.3)	1 (0.3)	0.001
hsPDA	31 (14.8)	11 (4.5)	<0.001	25 (18.8)	17 (5.3)	<0.001
ROP	22 (10.5)	9 (3.7)	0.005	17 (12.8)	14 (4.4)	0.002
Respiratory support (days)	17.0 ± 20.5	9.5 ± 12.5	<0.001	20.7 ± 21.1	9.7 ± 13.9	<0.001
Mechanical ventilation (days)	5.5 ± 10.4	1.5 ± 2.9	<0.001	7.0 ± 11.6	1.8 ± 4.4	<0.001
Non-invasive ventilation(days)	11.7 ± 14.8	8.0 ± 11.5	0.003	13.9 ± 15.3	8.0 ± 11.9	<0.001
Oxygen administration (days)	16.8 ± 23.0	7.2 ± 11.7	<0.001	21.0 ± 24.9	7.7 ± 13.2	<0.001
Cystic PVL	18 (8.6)	12 (4.9)	0.130	13 (9.8)	17 (5.3)	0.096
IVH (Grade ≥ II)	11 (5.3)	12 (4.9)	0.999	6 (4.5)	17 (5.3)	0.818

Abbreviations: BPD, bronchopulmonary dysplasia; BW, birth weight; hsPDA, hemodynamically significant patent ductus arteriosus; IVH, intraventricular hemorrhage (grade ≥ II); NEC, necrotizing enterocolitis; ROP, retinopathy of prematurity (≥Stage II); cystic PVL, cystic periventricular leukomalacia. [1] Numbers represent mean ± SD for parametric continuous variables, median (IQR) for non-parametric continuous variables and n (%) for categorical variables. [2] p-values obtained from independent samples t-test or Mann–Whitney non-parametric test, used to compare continuous variables between two groups, and Fisher's exact test, used to compare categorical variables.

All three nutritional factors accounted for were significantly related to postnatal growth failure with parenteral supported feeding lasting longer and full enteral feeding being achieved later by at least one week ($p < 0.001$). Further analysis revealed a significant decrease in the prevalence of EUGR after the year 2018 when nutritional practices altered toward international standards compared to previous years (36.6% compared to 51.2% by Fenton2013 ($p = 0.003$); 21.3% compared to 33.7% by INTERGROWTH-21st ($p = 0.005$)).

3.4. Multivariate Analysis

In the multivariate analysis presented in Table 4, 1 SD change of weight at discharge was increased for extreme prematurity by 0.53 (95% CI: 0.23 to 0.84) and 0.48 (95% CI: 0.17 to 0.80) based on the Fenton2013 and INTERGROWTH-21st growth references, respectively, but no effect was observed on the prevalence of EUGR. Birth weight was positively associated with weight at discharge and had a protective effect on EUGR (OR: 0.21 (95% CI: 0.14 to 0.31) by Fenton2013; OR: 0.27 (95% CI: 0.19 to 0.39) by INTERGROWTH-21st). On the contrary, long-term hospitalization was a burdensome factor for decreased weight at discharge, which was expressed in SD change by −0.04 (−95% CI: 0.04 to −0.03) and risk of EUGR (OR: 1.05 (95% CI: 1.03 to 1.07).

Weight at discharge SD score was inversely associated with the number of days needed to achieve full enteral feeding (EN), and the duration of parenteral feeding (PN) increased infant size. The day of EN initiation was a risk factor for EUGR by INTERGROWTH-21st reference (OR: 1.16 (95% CI: 1.05 to 1.25), whereas the risk of EUGR by Fenton2013 reference was higher by 7% for each day that EN was delayed (OR: 1.07 (95% CI: 1.03 to 1.12).

Lastly, the clinical conditions that retained significance in the multivariate models were anemia (β: 0.33 (95% CI: 0.10 to 0.56) and β: 0.31 (95% CI: 0.06 to 0.55)) and hsPDA (β: −0.41 (95% CI: −0.75 to −0.07) and β: −0.39 (95% CI: −0.75 to −0.04)) for Fenton2013 and INTERGROWTH-21st weight SD change, respectively. BPD was associated only with weight SD change based on INTERGROWTH-21st curves (β: 0.37 (95% CI: 0.00 to 0.73)). The risk of EUGR based on Fenton2013 curves was inversely related to anemia (OR: 0.49 (95% CI: 0.25 to 0.95)), whereas based on INTERGROWTH-21st curves, it was tripled for infants developing late-onset sepsis (OR: 3.08 (95% CI: 1.56 to 6.08)).

Table 4. Associations * of clinical and nutritional factors with extrauterine growth restriction based on the Fenton2013 and INTERGROWTH-21st weight growth references.

	Fenton2013		INTERGROWTH-21st	
	Weight z-Score	**EUGR**	**Weight z-Score**	**EUGR**
	β (95% CI)	**OR (95% CI)**	**β (95% CI)**	**OR (95% CI)**
Perinatal factors				
Extremely preterm	0.53 (0.23, 0.84)	0.49 (0.19, 1.27)	0.48 (0.17, 0.80)	0.67 (0.26, 1.76)
BW z-score	0.36 (0.26, 0.45)	0.21 (0.14, 0.31)	0.43 (0.33, 0.53)	0.27 (0.19, 0.39)
Hospitalization (days)	−0.04 (−0.04, −0.03)	1.05 (1.03, 1.07)	−0.04 (−0.04, −0.03)	1.05 (1.03, 1.08)
Nutritional factors				
PN duration (days)	0.01 (0.00, 0.02)	0.97 (0.94, 1.01)	0.01 (−0.00, 0.02)	0.99 (0.95, 1.03)
EN initiation (days)	−0.02 (−0.05, 0.00)	1.04 (0.94, 1.14)	−0.03 (−0.06, 0.00)	1.16 (1.05, 1.28)
Full EN achieved (days)	−0.02 (−0.03, −0.01)	1.07 (1.03, 1.12)	−0.02 (−0.04, −0.01)	1.03 (0.99, 1.07)
Clinical factors				
BPD	0.28 (−0.07, 0.63)	0.81 (0.27, 2.40)	0.37 (0.00, 0.73)	0.98 (0.33, 2.97)
Late-onset sepsis	−0.07 (−0.30, 0.15)	1.33 (0.70, 2.52)	−0.13 (−0.37, 0.10)	3.08 (1.56, 6.08)
Anemia	0.33 (0.10, 0.56)	0.49 (0.25, 0.95)	0.31 (0.06, 0.55)	0.55 (0.25, 1.19)
hsPDA	−0.41 (−0.75, −0.07)	2.59 (0.88, 7.61)	−0.39 (−0.75, −0.04)	1.67 (0.56, 4.95)
ROP	0.14 (−0.29, 0.57)	2.04 (0.52, 8.07)	0.08 (−0.36, 0.53)	0.99 (0.25, 3.86)
Respiratory support (days)	0.00 (−0.01, 0.01)	0.99 (0.95, 1.02)	0.00 (−0.01, 0.01)	1.00 (0.97, 1.03)
Oxygen administration (days)	0.00 (−0.00, 0.01)	1.00 (0.97, 1.03)	0.00 (−0.01, 0.01)	0.99 (0.96, 1.01)

Abbreviations: SGA, small for gestational age; PN, parenteral nutrition; EN, enteral nutrition; BPD, bronchopulmonary dysplasia; hsPDA, hemodynamically significant patent ductus arteriosus; ROP, retinopathy of prematurity (≥Stage II); cystic PVL, cystic periventricular leukomalacia. * Beta coefficients (β) and odds ratios (OR) and corresponding confidence intervals (CI) obtained using linear and logistic regression models, respectively.

Sensitivity analysis by data stratification according to the year of admission (before or after 2018) showed that the perinatal factors accounted for remained highly significant for both growth references for weight z-scores (Supplementary Table S1). Similar effects were observed for the nutritional and clinical factors, even if significance was not attained for all predictors, which was possibly due to sample size reduction. The prevalence of EUGR was lower for admissions after 2018 by both Fenton2013 (51.2% vs. 36.6%) and INTERGROWTH-21st (33.7% vs. 21.3%) weight growth references ($p = 0.003$ and $p = 0.005$, respectively). Estimates from the stratified analysis of predictors were not meaningfully changed by the year of admission (Supplementary Table S2).

4. Discussion

The present study demonstrated a difference in the proportion of infants identified as SGA at birth on the usage of INTERGROWTH-21st growth charts compared to Fenton2013, with SGA being higher on INTERGROWTH-21st. This finding is in line with the study of Tuzun et al. which revealed that one in four cases evaluated as SGA based on the INTERGROWTH-21st curves fell within the normal range according to Fenton's standards. Notably, these SGA infants did not have an increased risk of early morbidities [40]. On the contrary, in another study, Reddy et al. pointed out that neonates classified as SGA at birth by INTERGROWTH-21st and not by Fenton2013 growth charts had a higher incidence of morbidities such as sepsis and ROP [41]. In other studies, no significant difference was observed for the classification of birth weight for GA in preterm neonates born before 33 weeks between the two assessment growth charts [42,43]. It is very essential to accurately define SGA with appropriate charts, since being born SGA is associated with an increased risk of higher mortality, postnatal growth failure, and neurodevelopmental impairment at 18–22 months of corrected age [44]. Also, it has been shown that increasing SGA severity had a significant impact on neonatal outcomes among very preterm infants [45].

Our study revealed that extremely and very preterm neonates had a higher prevalence of EUGR at discharge concerning weight, according to Fenton2013 charts compared to

INTERGROWTH-21st charts. This is in accordance with other studies [46–48], and particularly, a recent study by Starc et al. reported a decreased prevalence of EUGR of weight when INTERGROWTH-21st charts were used in comparison to Fenton. The differences in outcomes between these two growth charts were expected and can be attributed to the fundamental disparities in the way they were created. The INTERGROWTH-21st charts were developed based on the growth of preterm infants developing in an extrauterine environment, while the Fenton charts were based on the growth of fetuses developing within the confines of the intrauterine setting. The extrauterine environment presents a completely different context for preterm babies, exposing them to unique metabolic responses and morbidities, which contrast significantly with the conditions experienced by fetuses in utero. A retrospective study published in 2021 presented a lower percentage of EUGR with respect to weight and length at discharge when INTERGROWTH-21st curves were used, compared to Fenton2013 curves, and this was associated with poorer language development assessed either at 12 or 24 months [43]. It is important to note that the main limitation of the INTERGROWTH-21st preterm postnatal standards is the limited number of infants born before 33 weeks' gestation who contributed to the development of the growth curves, which potentially affects the validity of the standards. Therefore, further research with large multicenter population-based data is needed to investigate the implications and effectiveness of utilizing these preterm postnatal growth curves, especially for monitoring growth in preterm infants at the earliest gestational ages [49]. In terms of HC, our study revealed a higher prevalence of EUGR when the INTERGROWTH-21st postnatal growth charts were used as the reference. However, other studies found no significant difference in the prevalence of EUGR concerning HC at discharge between the Fenton2013 and INTERGROWTH-21st growth charts [40,50].

Enteral feeding of preterm neonates has undergone significant advancements over time, and these progressions are evident in our study, which spanned fifteen years. Our study findings indicate a substantial decrease, after the year 2018, in the time it took to initiate enteral feeding and a notable reduction in the duration required to achieve full enteral feeding. According to recent meta-analyses, the prompt initiation of enteral feeding, preferably with mother's own milk, combined with a faster increment in enteral feed volumes, has been associated with a shorter duration to attain full enteral feeding, decreased length of hospitalization, and a potential decrease in the occurrence of invasive infections [51]. The previous assumption that gradually advancing milk feeds at a slow rate effectively decreases the risk of necrotizing enterocolitis in very low birth weight infants has been found to be ineffective [52].

In our study, statistically significant associations were observed between a higher decrease in weight at discharge and specific factors, including delayed initiation of enteral feeding, delayed attainment of full feedings by at least one week, and a longer duration of parenteral feeding with both Fenton and INTERGROWTH-21st charts. Furthermore, based on the Fenton 2013 reference, there was a notable 7% increase in the risk of EUGR for each day of delayed enteral nutrition initiation. Since enteral feeding is insufficient, the nutrients are delivered parenterally, and prolonged parenteral nutrition in combination with long periods of interrupted enteral feeding can lead to decreased feeding tolerance and increased risk of infection, which can negatively impact growth and development in preterm infants, as demonstrated in our research findings and other studies as well [53,54]. Indeed, an early initiation of enteral feeding is important in reducing the risk of infections, improving intestinal development and maturation, stimulating microbiome development, and simultaneously promoting growth in preterm infants [55].

Our study investigated various clinical factors that are linked to EUGR using both growth references. These factors included BPD, late-onset sepsis, anemia, hsPDA and ROP. Notably, anemia and hsPDA were identified as risk factors, as they were associated with decreased weight at discharge, according to both growth charts. Premature neonates, specifically those with hsPDA, experience reduced blood flow in the superior mesenteric artery, which raises the likelihood of developing feeding problems and consequently EUGR.

Additionally, the administration of nonsteroidal drugs for PDA treatment can potentially lead to gastrointestinal bleeding, causing these newborns to restrict their milk intake and delay the progression of enteral feeding [56]. Moreover, it is noteworthy that infants who experienced late-onset sepsis exhibited a threefold increased risk of developing EUGR when evaluated using the INTERGROWTH-21st growth curves. According to other studies, it was indicated that despite the lower prevalence of EUGR neonates based on weight according to INTERGROWTH-21st growth charts compared to Fenton, these neonates presented with a higher incidence of morbidities, and thus, these charts may be associated with adverse clinical outcomes during hospitalization [50,57].

Our research concluded that the prevalence of SGA and EUGR neonates differs between the Fenton2013 and INTERGROWTH-21st growth charts, reinforcing the importance of optimizing in-hospital and post-discharge nutritional support. Choosing an appropriate growth assessment tool for monitoring the postnatal growth of preterm infants is crucial to promote optimal neurodevelopmental outcomes and avoid excessive caloric intake that is linked to increased cardiometabolic risk later in life [58,59]. Prematurity constitutes an independent risk factor for the development of cardiovascular disease and metabolic syndrome regardless of birth weight [60]. Indeed, children born SGA, especially those who undergo rapid weight catch-up during early life, are prone to developing insulin resistance and central adiposity since early childhood. Furthermore, they may also experience cardiovascular dysfunctions in their adulthood [61]. Therefore, the best approach to address this barrier is implementing an evidenced-based enteral feeding protocol within each NICU and individualized care meeting each patient's medical needs.

Our study has several limitations. As only body sizes at birth and discharge were registered in the database, information on growth patterns such as weight loss during the first few days after delivery, body sizes at specified timing (i.e., PMA 36 weeks), or other growth indicators such as growth velocity were not provided. This restraint of available data pinpoints the importance of maintaining more comprehensive and detailed records, which could be useful for future reference to the health professionals and researchers, who can utilize this data to enhance the care and treatment offered to patients. Additionally, the present study did not investigate long-term outcomes of growth and neurodevelopment. Finally, regarding dietary data, our study did not include the advancement of enteral feed volume, the type of enteral feeding (breast milk, formula feeding) and the content of parenteral nutrition in protein, lipids, and energy.

5. Conclusions

In our study, despite the observed differences between the Fenton 2013 and INTERGROWTH-21st growth charts, it is not possible to definitively conclude that one graph is superior to the other. To evaluate the practical implications of the INTERGROWTH-21st growth charts specifically for very and extremely preterm neonates, additional validation using a large multicenter population-based dataset is necessary. It is crucial to closely monitor the growth of preterm infants using an appropriate growth curve to ensure optimal developmental and growth potential. Further research is warranted to deepen our understanding of the intricate relationship between nutrition and growth outcomes in preterm infants. By continuously refining dietary protocols and closely monitoring growth parameters, healthcare providers can enhance their ability to guide the nutritional management of them effectively. This ongoing effort is vital to improving the long-term health and overall well-being of these vulnerable individuals.

Supplementary Materials: The following supporting information can be downloaded at: https://www.mdpi.com/article/10.3390/nu15153290/s1, Supplementary Table S1: Associations of perinatal, clinical and nutritional factors with weight at discharge z scores based on the Fenton2013 and INTERGROWTH-21st weight growth references, stratified by year of hospitalization (before or after 2018); Supplementary Table S2: Associations of perinatal, clinical and nutritional factors with extrauterine growth restriction, based on the Fenton2013 and INTERGROWTH-21st weight growth references, stratified by year of hospitalization (before or after 2018).

Author Contributions: Conceptualization, I.K. and E.H.; Data curation, I.K., S.P., T.R., I.L. and E.H.; Formal analysis, T.R.; Supervision, E.H.; Writing—original draft, I.K. and T.R.; Writing—review and editing, I.K., T.R., N.H.A. and E.H. All authors have read and agreed to the published version of the manuscript.

Funding: This research received funding from the Special Account for Research Funds of University of Crete (SARF UoC), University Campus, Voutes, Heraklion P.C. 70013. (KA10773).

Institutional Review Board Statement: Ethical approval was obtained from the Scientific Council of the University General Hospital of Heraklion (PAGNI). Obtained protocol number: 23000.

Informed Consent Statement: Patient consent was waived due to the nature of the research being retrospective and anonymous. The study analyzed pre-existing data from hospital archives, and no new data was collected directly from individuals for the study. The data was already anonymized and devoid of any identifiable personal information, ensuring that the privacy and confidentiality of the individuals involved were preserved.

Data Availability Statement: The data presented in this study are available on request from the corresponding author. The data are not publicly available due to privacy or ethical restrictions.

Conflicts of Interest: All authors declare no conflict of interest.

References

1. Clark, R.H.; Olsen, I.E.; Spitzer, A.R. Assessment of neonatal growth in prematurely born infants. *Clin. Perinatol.* **2014**, *41*, 295–307. [CrossRef] [PubMed]
2. Greer, F.R.; Olsen, I.E. How Fast Should the Preterm Infant Grow? *Curr. Pediatr. Rep.* **2013**, *1*, 240–246. [CrossRef]
3. Silveira, R.C.; Procianoy, R.S. Preterm newborn's postnatal growth patterns: How to evaluate them. *J. Pediatr.* **2019**, *95*, 42–48. [CrossRef]
4. Fenton, T.R.; Kim, J.H. A systematic review and meta-analysis to revise the Fenton growth chart for preterm infants. *BMC Pediatr.* **2013**, *13*, 59. [CrossRef] [PubMed]
5. Villar, J.; Giuliani, F.; Barros, F.; Roggero, P.; Coronado Zarco, I.A.; Rego, M.A.S.; Ochieng, R.; Gianni, M.L.; Rao, S.; Lambert, A.; et al. Monitoring the Postnatal Growth of Preterm Infants: A Paradigm Change. *Pediatrics* **2018**, *141*, e20172467. [CrossRef]
6. Papageorghiou, A.T.; Kennedy, S.H.; Salomon, L.J.; Altman, D.G.; Ohuma, E.O.; Stones, W.; Gravett, M.G.; Barros, F.C.; Victora, C.; Purwar, M.; et al. The INTERGROWTH-21st fetal growth standards: Toward the global integration of pregnancy and pediatric care. *Am. J. Obstet. Gynecol.* **2018**, *218*, S630–S640. [CrossRef]
7. Klingenberg, C.; Embleton, N.D.; Jacobs, S.E.; O'Connell, L.A.F.; Kuschel, C.A. Enteral feeding practices in very preterm infants: An international survey. *Arch. Dis. Child. Fetal Neonatal Ed.* **2012**, *97*, F56–F61. [CrossRef]
8. Berman, L.; Moss, R.L. Necrotizing enterocolitis: An update. *Semin. Fetal. Neonatal Med.* **2011**, *16*, 145–150. [CrossRef]
9. Kwok, T.C.; Dorling, J.; Gale, C. Early enteral feeding in preterm infants. *Semin. Perinatol.* **2019**, *43*, 151159. [CrossRef]
10. Brune, K.D.; Donn, S.M. Enteral Feeding of the Preterm Infant. *NeoReviews* **2018**, *19*, e645–e653. [CrossRef]
11. Ruth, V.A. Extrauterine growth restriction: A review of the literature. *Neonatal Netw. NN* **2008**, *27*, 177–184. [CrossRef] [PubMed]
12. Hokken-Koelega, A.C.S.; van der Steen, M.; Boguszewski, M.C.S.; Cianfarani, S.; Dahlgren, J.; Horikawa, R.; Mericq, V.; Rapaport, R.; Alherbish, A.; Braslavsky, D.; et al. International Consensus Guideline on Small for Gestational Age: Etiology and Management From Infancy to Early Adulthood. *Endocr. Rev.* **2023**, *44*, 539–565. [CrossRef] [PubMed]
13. Lucaccioni, L.; Iughetti, L.; Berardi, A.; Predieri, B. Challenges in the growth and development of newborns with extra-uterine growth restriction. *Expert Rev. Endocrinol. Metab.* **2022**, *17*, 415–423. [CrossRef]
14. Ordóñez-Díaz, M.D.; Pérez-Navero, J.L.; Flores-Rojas, K.; Olza-Meneses, J.; Muñoz-Villanueva, M.C.; Aguilera-García, C.M.; Gil-Campos, M. Prematurity with Extrauterine Growth Restriction Increases the Risk of Higher Levels of Glucose, Low-Grade of Inflammation and Hypertension in Prepubertal Children. *Front. Pediatr.* **2020**, *8*, 180. [CrossRef]
15. Murray, Y.L.; Paul, I.M.; Miller, J.R.; Thrash, S.Z.; Kaiser, J.R. Variability in the use of growth curves between preterm and term infants in NICUs and newborn nurseries. *Pediatr. Res.* **2021**, *89*, 711–713. [CrossRef] [PubMed]
16. Engle, W.A. American Academy of Pediatrics Committee on Fetus and Newborn Age terminology during the perinatal period. *Pediatrics* **2004**, *114*, 1362–1364. [CrossRef]
17. Villar, J.; Giuliani, F.; Fenton, T.R.; Ohuma, E.O.; Ismail, L.C.; Kennedy, S.H. INTERGROWTH-21st very preterm size at birth reference charts. *Lancet* **2016**, *387*, 844–845. [CrossRef]
18. Villar, J.; Giuliani, F.; Bhutta, Z.A.; Bertino, E.; Ohuma, E.O.; Ismail, L.C.; Barros, F.C.; Altman, D.G.; Victora, C.; Noble, J.A.; et al. Postnatal growth standards for preterm infants: The Preterm Postnatal Follow-up Study of the INTERGROWTH-21(st) Project. *Lancet Glob. Health* **2015**, *3*, e681–e691. [CrossRef]
19. Agostoni, C.; Buonocore, G.; Carnielli, V.P.; De Curtis, M.; Darmaun, D.; Decsi, T.; Domellöf, M.; Embleton, N.D.; Fusch, C.; Genzel-Boroviczeny, O.; et al. Enteral nutrient supply for preterm infants: Commentary from the European Society of Paediatric Gastroenterology, Hepatology and Nutrition Committee on Nutrition. *J. Pediatr. Gastroenterol. Nutr.* **2010**, *50*, 85–91. [CrossRef]

20. Embleton, N.D.; Moltu, S.J.; Lapillonne, A.; van den Akker, C.H.P.; Carnielli, V.; Fusch, C.; Gerasimidis, K.; van Goudoever, J.B.; Haiden, N.; Iacobelli, S.; et al. Enteral Nutrition in Preterm Infants (2022): A Position Paper from the ESPGHAN Committee on Nutrition and invited experts. *J. Pediatr. Gastroenterol. Nutr.* 2022; *Ahead of Print*. [CrossRef]
21. van Goudoever, J.B.; Carnielli, V.; Darmaun, D.; de Pipaon, M.S.; Braegger, C.; Bronsky, J.; Cai, W.; Campoy, C.; Carnielli, V.; Darmaun, D.; et al. ESPGHAN/ESPEN/ESPR/CSPEN guidelines on pediatric parenteral nutrition: Amino acids. *Clin. Nutr.* **2018**, *37*, 2315–2323. [CrossRef]
22. Iacobelli, S.; Bonsante, F.; Gouyon, J.B. Fluid and electrolyte intake during the first week of life in preterm infants receiving parenteral nutrition according current guidelines. *Minerva Pediatr.* **2010**, *62*, 203–204. [PubMed]
23. Lapillonne, A.; Mis, N.F.; Goulet, O.; van den Akker, C.H.P.; Wu, J.; Koletzko, B.; Braegger, C.; Bronsky, J.; Cai, W.; Campoy, C.; et al. ESPGHAN/ESPEN/ESPR/CSPEN guidelines on pediatric parenteral nutrition: Lipids. *Clin. Nutr.* **2018**, *37*, 2324–2336. [CrossRef]
24. Mesotten, D.; Joosten, K.; van Kempen, A.; Verbruggen, S.; Braegger, C.; Bronsky, J.; Cai, W.; Campoy, C.; Carnielli, V.; Darmaun, D.; et al. ESPGHAN/ESPEN/ESPR/CSPEN guidelines on pediatric parenteral nutrition: Carbohydrates. *Clin. Nutr.* **2018**, *37*, 2337–2343. [CrossRef] [PubMed]
25. Patel, P.; Bhatia, J. Total parenteral nutrition for the very low birth weight infant. *Semin. Fetal. Neonatal Med.* **2017**, *22*, 2–7. [CrossRef]
26. Uthaya, S.; Modi, N. Practical preterm parenteral nutrition: Systematic literature review and recommendations for practice. *Early Hum. Dev.* **2014**, *90*, 747–753. [CrossRef] [PubMed]
27. De Curtis, M.; Rigo, J. The nutrition of preterm infants. *Early Hum. Dev.* **2012**, *88* (Suppl. S1), S5–S7. [CrossRef]
28. Parker, L.A.; Desorcy-Scherer, K.; Magalhães, M. Feeding Strategies in Preterm Very Low Birth-Weight Infants: State-of-the-Science Review. *Adv. Neonatal Care* **2021**, *21*, 493–502. [CrossRef]
29. Carey, B. Neonatal Air Leaks: Pneumothorax, Pneumomediastinum, Pulmonary Interstitial Emphysema, Pneumopericardium. *Neonatal Netw.* **1999**, *18*, 81–84. [CrossRef]
30. Howarth, C.; Banerjee, J.; Aladangady, N. Red Blood Cell Transfusion in Preterm Infants: Current Evidence and Controversies. *Neonatology* **2018**, *114*, 7–16. [CrossRef]
31. Müller, M.J.; Paul, T.; Seeliger, S. Necrotizing enterocolitis in premature infants and newborns. *J. Neonatal Perinat. Med.* **2016**, *9*, 233–242. [CrossRef]
32. Hamrick, S.E.G.; Sallmon, H.; Rose, A.T.; Porras, D.; Shelton, E.L.; Reese, J.; Hansmann, G. Patent Ductus Arteriosus of the Preterm Infant. *Pediatrics* **2020**, *146*, e20201209. [CrossRef] [PubMed]
33. Chiang, M.F.; Quinn, G.E.; Fielder, A.R.; Ostmo, S.R.; Paul Chan, R.V.; Berrocal, A.; Binenbaum, G.; Blair, M.; Peter Campbell, J.; Capone, A.; et al. International Classification of Retinopathy of Prematurity, Third Edition. *Ophthalmology* **2021**, *128*, e51–e68. [CrossRef]
34. Gole, G.A.; Ells, A.L.; Katz, X.; Holmstrom, G.; Fielder, A.R.; Capone Jr, A.; Flynn, J.T.; Good, W.G.; Holmes, J.M.; McNamara, J.A.; et al. The International Classification of Retinopathy of Prematurity revisited. *Arch. Ophthalmol.* **2005**, *123*, 991–999. [CrossRef]
35. Agut, T.; Alarcon, A.; Cabañas, F.; Bartocci, M.; Martinez-Biarge, M.; Horsch, S. Preterm white matter injury: Ultrasound diagnosis and classification. *Pediatr. Res.* **2020**, *87*, 37–49. [CrossRef] [PubMed]
36. Papile, L.A.; Burstein, J.; Burstein, R.; Koffler, H. Incidence and evolution of subependymal and intraventricular hemorrhage: A study of infants with birth weights less than 1500 gm. *J. Pediatr.* **1978**, *92*, 529–534. [CrossRef]
37. Thébaud, B.; Goss, K.N.; Laughon, M.; Whitsett, J.A.; Abman, S.H.; Steinhorn, R.H.; Aschner, J.L.; Davis, P.G.; McGrath-Morrow, S.A.; Soll, R.F.; et al. Bronchopulmonary dysplasia. *Nat. Rev. Dis. Primer* **2019**, *5*, 78. [CrossRef]
38. Bethou, A.; Bhat, B.V. Neonatal Sepsis—Newer Insights. *Indian J. Pediatr.* **2022**, *89*, 267–273. [CrossRef]
39. McGovern, M.; Giannoni, E.; Kuester, H.; Turner, M.A.; van den Hoogen, A.; Bliss, J.M.; Koenig, J.M.; Keij, F.M.; Mazela, J.; Finnegan, R.; et al. Challenges in developing a consensus definition of neonatal sepsis. *Pediatr. Res.* **2020**, *88*, 14–26. [CrossRef]
40. Tuzun, F.; Yucesoy, E.; Baysal, B.; Kumral, A.; Duman, N.; Ozkan, H. Comparison of INTERGROWTH-21 and Fenton growth standards to assess size at birth and extrauterine growth in very preterm infants. *J. Matern. Fetal Neonatal Med.* **2018**, *31*, 2252–2257. [CrossRef]
41. Reddy, K.V.; Sharma, D.; Vardhelli, V.; Bashir, T.; Deshbotla, S.K.; Murki, S. Comparison of Fenton 2013 growth curves and Intergrowth-21 growth standards to assess the incidence of intrauterine growth restriction and extrauterine growth restriction in preterm neonates $\leq$32 weeks. *J. Matern. Fetal Neonatal Med.* **2021**, *34*, 2634–2641. [CrossRef]
42. Lebrão, C.W.; Suano-Souza, F.I.; Sarni, R.O.S. Is the Intrauterine INTERGROWTH-21 Growth Curve Better Than Fenton's for the Classification at Birth and Prediction of Postnatal Growth in Preterm Infants? *Matern. Child Health J.* **2020**, *24*, 1446–1453. [CrossRef]
43. Yitayew, M.; Chahin, N.; Rustom, S.; Thacker, L.R.; Hendricks-Muñoz, K.D. Fenton vs. Intergrowth-21st: Postnatal Growth Assessment and Prediction of Neurodevelopment in Preterm Infants. *Nutrients* **2021**, *13*, 2841. [CrossRef]
44. De Jesus, L.C.; Pappas, A.; Shankaran, S.; Li, L.; Das, A.; Bell, E.F.; Stoll, B.J.; Laptook, A.R.; Walsh, M.C.; Hale, E.C.; et al. Outcomes of small for gestational age infants born at <27 weeks' gestation. *J. Pediatr.* **2013**, *163*, 55–60.e3. [CrossRef]
45. Minor, K.C.; Bianco, K.; Sie, L.; Druzin, M.L.; Lee, H.C.; Leonard, S.A. Severity of small-for-gestational-age and morbidity and mortality among very preterm neonates. *J. Perinatol.* **2023**, *43*, 437–444. [CrossRef]
46. Ribas, S.A.; Paravidino, V.B.; Soares, F.V.M. Comparison of growth curves in very low birth weight preterm infants after hospital discharge. *Eur. J. Pediatr.* **2022**, *181*, 149–157. [CrossRef]
47. Starc, M.; Giangreco, M.; Centomo, G.; Travan, L.; Bua, J. Extrauterine growth restriction in very low birth weight infants according to different growth charts: A retrospective 10 years observational study. *PLoS ONE* **2023**, *18*, e0283367. [CrossRef]

48. Yazici, A.; Buyuktiryaki, M.; Sari, F.N.; Akin, M.S.; Ertekin, O.; Alyamac Dizdar, E. Comparison of different growth curves in the assessment of extrauterine growth restriction in very low birth weight preterm infants. *Arch. Pediatr.* **2023**, *30*, 31–35. [CrossRef]
49. Cordova, E.G.; Belfort, M.B. Updates on Assessment and Monitoring of the Postnatal Growth of Preterm Infants. *NeoReviews* **2020**, *21*, e98–e108. [CrossRef]
50. Kim, Y.-J.; Shin, S.H.; Cho, H.; Shin, S.H.; Kim, S.H.; Song, I.G.; Kim, E.-K.; Kim, H.-S. Extrauterine growth restriction in extremely preterm infants based on the Intergrowth-21st Project Preterm Postnatal Follow-up Study growth charts and the Fenton growth charts. *Eur. J. Pediatr.* **2021**, *180*, 817–824. [CrossRef]
51. Hay, W.W. Nutritional Support Strategies for the Preterm Infant in the Neonatal Intensive Care Unit. *Pediatr. Gastroenterol. Hepatol. Nutr.* **2018**, *21*, 234–247. [CrossRef]
52. Oddie, S.J.; Young, L.; McGuire, W. Slow advancement of enteral feed volumes to prevent necrotising enterocolitis in very low birth weight infants. *Cochrane Database Syst. Rev.* **2017**, *2017*, CD001241. [CrossRef]
53. Xiang, Y.; Tang, Q.; Wang, Y.; Cai, W. Nutrition profile of very low birth weight infants with extrauterine growth restriction in NICU. *Clin. Nutr. ESPEN* **2021**, *42*, 252–257. [CrossRef] [PubMed]
54. Uthaya, S. Better preterm parenteral nutrition practice. *Early Hum. Dev.* **2021**, *162*, 105468. [CrossRef]
55. Thoene, M.; Anderson-Berry, A. Early Enteral Feeding in Preterm Infants: A Narrative Review of the Nutritional, Metabolic, and Developmental Benefits. *Nutrients* **2021**, *13*, 2289. [CrossRef] [PubMed]
56. McCurnin, D.; Clyman, R.I. Effects of a patent ductus arteriosus on postprandial mesenteric perfusion in premature baboons. *Pediatrics* **2008**, *122*, e1262–e1267. [CrossRef]
57. Anne, R.P.; Vardhelli, V.; Murki, S.; Deshabhotla, S.K.; Oleti, T.P. Comparison of Fenton, INTERGROWTH-21st, and Population-Based Growth Charts in Predicting Outcomes of Very Preterm Small-for-Gestational-Age Neonates. *Indian J. Pediatr.* **2022**, *89*, 1034–1036. [CrossRef] [PubMed]
58. Christmann, V.; Roeleveld, N.; Visser, R.; Janssen, A.J.W.M.; Reuser, J.J.C.M.; van Goudoever, J.B.; van Heijst, A.F.J. The early postnatal nutritional intake of preterm infants affected neurodevelopmental outcomes differently in boys and girls at 24 months. *Acta Paediatr.* **2017**, *106*, 242–249. [CrossRef]
59. Martínez-Jiménez, M.; Gómez-García, F.; Gil-Campos, M.; Pérez-Navero, J. Comorbidities in childhood associated with extrauterine growth restriction in preterm infants: A scoping review. *Eur. J. Pediatr.* **2020**, *179*, 1255–1265. [CrossRef]
60. García, H.; Loureiro, C.; Poggi, H.; D'Apremont, I.; Moore, R.; Ossa, J.T.; Bruera, M.J.; Peredo, S.; Carvajal, J.; Trincado, C.; et al. Insulin resistance parameters in children born very preterm and adequate for gestational age. *Endocrinol. Diabetes Metab.* **2022**, *5*, e00329. [CrossRef]
61. Cauzzo, C.; Chiavaroli, V.; Di Valerio, S.; Chiarelli, F. Birth size, growth trajectory and later cardio-metabolic risk. *Front. Endocrinol.* **2023**, *14*, 1187261. [CrossRef]

MDPI AG
Grosspeteranlage 5
4052 Basel
Switzerland
Tel.: +41 61 683 77 34

Nutrients Editorial Office
E-mail: nutrients@mdpi.com
www.mdpi.com/journal/nutrients